LAW
&
MENTAL
HEALTH
PROFESSIONALS

WASHINGTON

LAW & MENTAL HEALTH PROFESSIONALS SERIES

Bruce D. Sales and Michael Owen Miller, Series Editors

ARIZONA: Miller and Sales
CALIFORNIA: Caudill and Pope
MASSACHUSETTS: Brant
MINNESOTA: Janus, Mickelsen, and Sanders
NEW JERSEY: Wulach
NEW YORK: Wulach
TEXAS: Shuman
WASHINGTON: Benjamin, Rosenwald, Overcast, and Feldman

LAW & MENTAL HEALTH PROFESSIONALS

WASHINGTON

G. Andrew H. Benjamin
Laura A. Rosenwald
Thomas D. Overcast
Stephen R. Feldman

AMERICAN PSYCHOLOGICAL ASSOCIATION
Washington, DC

Published by
American Psychological Association
750 First Street, NE
Washington, DC 20002

Copies may be ordered from
APA Order Department
P.O. Box 2710
Hyattsville, MD 20784

In the UK and Europe, copies may be ordered from
American Psychological Association
3 Henrietta Street
Covent Garden, London
WC2E 8LU England

Typeset in Palatino by General Graphic Services, York, PA

Text and cover designer: Rubin Krassner, Silver Spring, MD
Printer: Edwards Brothers, Inc., Ann Arbor, MI
Technical/production editor: Miria Liliana Riahi

Library of Congress Cataloging-in-Publication Data
Law and mental health professionals. Washington / by G. Andrew H. Benjamin . . . [et al.].
    p. cm. — (Law & mental health professionals series)
    Includes bibliographical references and index.
    ISBN 1-55798-278-3
    1. Mental health personnel—Legal status, laws, etc.—Washington (State) 2. Mental health laws—Washington State 3. Forensic psychiatry—Washington (State) I. Benjamin, G. Andrew H. II. Series.
KFW326.5.P73L39 1995
344.797'044—dc20
[347.970444]   95-5363
                                       CIP

British Library Cataloguing-in-Publication Data
A CIP record is available from the British Library.

Printed in the United States of America
First edition

Contents

Editors' Preface

The Need to Know the Law

For years, providers of mental health services (hereinafter mental health professionals, or MHPs) have been directly affected by the law. At one end of the continuum, their practice has been controlled by laws covering such matters as licensure and certification, third-party reimbursement, and professional incorporation. At the other end, they have been courted by the legal system to aid in its administration, providing such services as evaluating the mental status of litigants, providing expert testimony in court, and engaging in therapy with court-referred juveniles and adults. Even when not directly affected, MHPs find themselves indirectly affected by the law because their clients sometimes become involved in legal entanglements that involve mental status issues (e.g., divorce proceedings or termination of parental rights hearings).

Despite this pervasive influence, most professionals do not know about, much less understand, most of the laws that affect their practice, the services they render, and the clients they serve. This state of affairs is particularly troubling for several reasons. First, not knowing about the laws that affect one's practice typically results in the MHP's not gaining the benefits that the law may provide. Consider the law relating to the incorporation of professionals. It confers significant benefit, but only if it is known about and applied. The fact that it has been enacted by the state legislature does not help the MHP, any more than an MHP will be of help to a distressed person who refuses to contact the MHP.

Second, not knowing about the laws that affect the services they render can result in incompetent performance of, and liability for, the MHP either through the civil law (e.g., malpractice law) or through criminal sanctions. A brief example may help underscore this point. When an MHP is asked to evaluate a party to a lawsuit and testify in court, the court (the law's term for the judge) is asking the professional to assess and testify about whether that litigant meets some legal standard. The court is often not concerned with the defendant's mental health per se, although this may be relevant to the MHP's evaluation of the person. Rather, the court wants to know whether the person meets the legal standard as it is set down by the law. Not knowing the legal standard means that the MHP is most likely evaluating the person for the wrong goal and providing the court with irrelevant information, at least from the court's point of view. Regretfully, there are too many cases in which this has occurred.

Third, not knowing the law that affects the clients that MHPs serve may significantly diminish their capability for handling their clients' distress. For example, a client who is undergoing a divorce and child custody dispute may have distorted beliefs about what may happen during the legal proceedings. A basic understanding of the controlling law in this area will allow the therapist to be more sensitive in rendering therapy.

The Problem in Accessing Legal Information

Given the need for this information, why have MHPs not systematically sought it out? Part of the reason lies in the concern over their ability to understand legal doctrines. Indeed, this is a legitimate worry, especially if they had to read original legal materials that were not collected, organized, and described with an MHP audience in mind. This is of particular concern because laws are written in terms and phrases of "art" that do not always share the common law definition or usage, whereas some terms and phrases are left ambiguous and undefined or are used differently for different legal topics. Another part of the reason is that the law affecting MHPs and their clients is not readily available—even to lawyers. There are no compendiums that identify the topics that these laws cover or present an analysis of each topic for easy reference.

To compound the difficulty, the law does not treat the different mental health professional disciplines uniformly or always specify the particular disciplines as being covered by it. Nor does the law emanate from a single legal forum. Each state enacts its own rules and regulations, often resulting in wide variations in the way a topic is handled across the United States. Multiply this confusion times the one hundred or so topics that relate to mental health practice. In addition, the law within a state does not come from one legal source. Rather, there are five primary ones: the state constitution; state legislative enactments (statutes); state agency administrative rules and regulations; rules of court promulgated by the state supreme court; and state and federal court cases that apply, interpret, and construe this existing state law. To know about one of these sources without knowing how its pronouncements on a given topic have been modified by these other sources can result in one's making erroneous conclusions about the operation of the law. Finally, mental health practice also comes under the purview of federal law (constitutional and statutory law, administrative rules and regulations, and case law). Federal law authorizes direct payments to MHPs for their services to some clients, sets standards for delivery of services in federal facilities (e.g., Veterans Administration hospitals), and articulates the law that guides cases that are tried in federal courts under federal law.

Purposes of This Series

What is needed, therefore, is a book for each state, the District of Columbia, and the federal jurisdictions that comprehensively and accurately reviews and integrates all of the law that affects MHPs in that jurisdiction (hereinafter state). To ensure currency, regular supplements to these books will also need to be drafted. These materials should be written so that they are completely understandable to MHPs, as well as to lawyers. To accomplish these goals, the editors have tried to identify every legal topic that affects mental health practice, making each one the subject of a chapter. Each chapter, in turn, describes the legal standards that the MHP will be operating under and the relevant legal process that the MHP will be operating within. If a state does not have relevant law on an issue, then a brief explanation of how this law works in other states will be presented while noting the lack of regulation in this area within the state under consideration.

This type of coverage facilitates other purposes of the series. Although each chapter is written in order to state exactly what is the present state of the law and not argue for or against any particular approach, it is hoped that the comprehensiveness of the coverage will encourage MHPs to question the desirability of their states' approach to each topic. Such information and concern should provide the impetus for initiating legislation and litigation on the part of state mental health associations to ensure that the law reflects the scientific knowledge and professional values to the greatest extent possible.

In some measure, states will initially be hampered in this proactivity because they will not know what legal alternatives are available and how desirable each alternative actually is. When a significant number of books in this series is available, however, it will allow for nationally oriented policy studies to identify the variety of legal approaches that are currently in use and to assess the validity of the behavioral assumptions underlying each variant, and ultimately lead to a conclusion as to the relative desirability of alternate approaches.[1] Thus, two other purposes of this book are to foster comprehensive analyses of the laws affecting

---

1. Sales, B. D. (1983). The legal regulation of psychology: Professional and scientific interactions. In C. J. Scheirer & B. L. Hammonds (Eds.), *The master lecture series: Vol. 2. Psychology and law* (pp. 5–36). Washington, DC: American Psychological Association.

MHPs across all states and of the validity of the behavioral assumptions underlying these laws, and to promote political, legislative, and legal action to change laws that are inappropriate and impede the effective delivery of services. Legal change may be required because of gaps in legal regulation, overregulation, and regulation based on invalid behavioral and social assumptions. We hope this process will increase the rationality of future laws in this area and improve the effectiveness and quality of mental health service delivery nationally.

There are three remaining purposes for this series. First, although it will not replace the need for legal counsel, this series will make the MHP an intelligent consumer of legal services. This ability is gaining importance in an era of increasing professionalization and litigiousness. Second, it will ensure that MHPs are aware of the law's mandates when providing expert services (e.g., evaluation and testimony) within the legal system. Although chapters will not address how to clinically assess for the legal standard, provider competency will increase because providers now will be sure of the goals of their service (e.g., the legal standard that they are to assess for) as well as their roles and responsibilities within the legal system as to the particular topic in issue. Third and finally, each book will make clear that the legal standards that MHPs are asked to assess for by the law have typically not been translated into behavioral correlates. Nor are there discussions of tests, scales, and procedures for MHPs to use in assessing for the behavioral correlates of the legal standards in most cases. This series will provide the impetus for such research and writing.

Content and Organization of Volumes

Each book in this series is organized into six sections. Section 1 addresses the legal credentialing of MHPs. Section 2 deals with the different business forms for conducting one's practice. Section 3 then addresses insurance reimbursement and tax deductions that clients can receive for utilizing mental health services. With the business matters covered, the book then turns to the law directly affecting service delivery. Section 4 starts by covering the law that affects the maintenance and privacy of professional information. Section 5 then considers each area of law that may require the services of MHPs. It is subdivided into five parts: families and juveniles, other civil matters, topics that apply similarly in both civil and criminal cases, criminal matters, and voluntary and involuntary receipt of state services by the clients of mental health services. The last section of the book, section 6, discusses the law that limits service delivery and that sets liability for unethical and illegal behavior as a service provider.

Collectively, the chapters in these sections represent all topics pertaining to the law as it affects MHPs in their practices. Two caveats are in order, however. First, the law changes slowly over time. Thus, a supplement service will update all chapters on a regular basis. Second, as MHPs become more involved in the legal system, new opportunities for involvement are likely to arise. To be responsive to these developments, the supplements will also contain additional chapters reflecting these new roles and responsibilities.

Some final points about the content of this book are in order. The exact terms that the law chooses are used in the book even if they are a poor choice from an MHP's point of view. And where terms are defined by the law, that information is presented. The reader will often be frustrated, however, because, as has already been noted, the law does not always define terms or provide detailed guidance. This does not mean that legal words and phrases can be taken lightly. The law sets the rules that MHPs and their clients must operate by; thus, the chapters must be read carefully. This should not be too arduous a task because chapters are relatively short. On the other hand, such brevity will leave some readers frustrated because chapters appear not to go far enough in answering their questions. Note that all of the law is covered. If there is no law, however, there is no coverage. If a question is not answered in the text, it is because Washington law has not addressed the issue. Relatedly, if an obligation or benefit is created by a professional regulation (i.e., a rule of a professional organization) but is not directly recognized by the law, it is not covered. Thus, for example, professional credentials are not addressed in these volumes.

Bruce D. Sales
Michael Owen Miller
Series Editors

Authors' Preface

The sources of the law digested in this work include the state constitution, state statutes, state administrative code, state judicial decisions, and state judicial rules. Occasionally, federal law also is reviewed when it affects the practice of mental health professionals (MHPs) within the State of Washington.

The *Washington Constitution* provides the framework for state government and establishes individual rights for the people of the state. The articles and sections of the Washington Constitution appear in the following form: Const. Art. 1, §1. This reference indicates that the citation is to the first section of the first article in the Washington Constitution.

State statutes result from legislation enacted by the state legislature. Citations of the Revised Code of Washington appear in the following form: Chapter 71.05 RCW or RCW 71.05.120. These particular citations refer to a chapter of statutes and a particular statute within the chapter.

The *Revised Code of Washington* is published by the West Publishing Company in an annotated form. The compilers often include a one-sentence summary of any reported cases that have discussed the constitutional provision or statute interpreted by the courts. Researchers use case annotations to begin research on how the constitutional provision or statute has been interpreted by the courts. The compilation also may contain references to prior statutes that have been repealed. A review of the case law and of repealed statutes can provide an understanding about how the law has changed over time and how legislative ambiguity has been clarified.

The *Washington Administrative Code* is created by state agencies operated under the authority delegated to them by the legislature to perform specific agency functions. For example, the Department of Social and Health Services has codified specific rules that regulate group homes for mentally and physically handicapped persons. These rules appear in Chapter 275-36 WAC. A rule in Title 275 would appear as WAC 275-36-010 (this rule contains all the definitions of words of art used in Chapter 275-36). Each chapter has an index that lists the subjects addressed by specific rules. After the index, a disposition of sections formerly codified in the chapter but repealed are listed. This permits a researcher to see how the code has changed over time.

Judges must apply the constitution, statutes, and code in judging the criminal and civil cases before them. When the law is ambiguous, judges will rule about what the intent of the promulgating body must have been and interpret the law in a ruling. All appellate court decisions in the State of Washington are recorded and published by West Publishing Company. A lower court decision may be appealed to the Court of Appeals, and a further appeal may go to the highest court, the state Supreme Court. Citations to these decisions appear in the following form: Bruce v. Byrne-Stevens and Associates, 113 Wash.2d 123, 774 P.2d 666 (1989). This citation refers to a decision, ruled upon in the year 1989 by the Supreme Court, that is published in volume 113, Washington Reports, Second Series, beginning on page 123 (Wash. may also appear as Wn.).The decision also appeared in a reporter of cases in the geographical region titled *Pacific Reporter*, Second Series. As with *Washington Reports*, the number preceding the reporter is the volume number and the number following is the page. A citation of a Court of Appeals decision would appear as follows: Bader v. State, 43 Wash.App. 233, 716 P.2d 925 (1986) (Wash. may also appear as Wn.). This decision that occurred in 1986 was published in the *Washington Appellate Reports* and the *Pacific Reporter, Second Series*. The volume and page number for both books is read in the same way as the above example.

State judicial rules, as contrasted with judicial decisions, are promulgated by judges of the different courts to establish procedures for general application in the particular type of court. When relevant to MHPs, rules have been cited in the digest. The rules used for the particular court can be found in your local law library. Abbreviations of the different courts that were referred to in the digest include Superior Court Administrative Rules (AR), Superior Court Civil Rules (CR), and Superior Court Criminal Rules (CrR).

Occasional reference is made to a federal court decision that interpreted or limited state law. The citations to these decisions appear from the United States District Court (F.Supp.), the United States Court of Appeals (F. or F.2nd), and the United States Supreme Court (U.S., S.Ct., or L.Ed.). Like the reports of state decisions, the number preceding the reporter is the volume number and the number following is the page. References to federal legislation appear in the form 26 U.S.C. § 213(a) (1987). This citation to the *United States Code*, the repository of federal legislation, is from title 26, section 213(a), current as of the year, 1987.

Please call or write if you have suggestions for a pocket supplement. We intend to publish one every two years or so to incorporate new statutes, rules, and judicial decisions. Although we have continually updated the manuscript, the laws are changing even as we go to press. We suggest that this text be used as a foundation from which to identify current issues and find the relevant law that sometimes may need to be updated. Before taking any action that might result in legal consequences, you are urged to consult with an attorney.

G. Andrew H. Benjamin

Acknowledgments

My professor, mentor, and friend, Bruce Sales, once gave me an empty bound book. He, of course, had in mind that I would write this book, one of 50 books in this *Law & Mental Health Professionals* series that he intends to edit. I would not have undertaken this project without his confidence in my abilities and his dolor about seeing the series completed.

My wife of 17 years, Nan Herbert, deserves the leading acknowledgment for allowing me to work on this book, at the expense of our family time. It is an enormous project that she has endured tolerantly. Her warm, loving support has made a great difference in my life.

Law student clerks Kathy Prunty, Kevin Scudder, and Sheryle Bonilla worked adeptly in gathering the materials for many of the chapters. Field reviewers and lawyers, Mark Bantz, Diane Dietrich, and Morris Rosenberg provided conscientious suggestions about how to improve our work. Mark Bantz, in particular, deserves special acknowledgment for completing so many field reviews.

G. Andrew H. Benjamin

Legal Credentialing

1.1

Licensure and Regulation of Psychiatrists

The licensure and regulation of psychiatrists is governed by the statute[1] that establishes a Board of Medical Examiners, defines terms contained within the act, establishes qualifications and procedures for licensure of physicians, defines the practice of medicine, regulates the conduct of physicians, establishes exceptions to licensure, and prescribes criminal sanctions. In general, the law regulates the practice of medicine without regard to specialty.[2] There is no separate licensure provision pertaining to the practice of psychiatry.

(A) Board of Medical Examiners[3]

The Board of Medical Examiners[4] is the administrative body that licenses and regulates psychiatrists. Examining Board members are appointed by the governor and serve five-year terms. Of the Examining Board's eight members, six must be licensed to practice medicine in the state of Washington, one must be a physician's assistant registered under RCW 18.71A, and one is a nonphysician.[5] The Examining Board meets at least four times a year

---

1. Washington Revised Code (RCW) 18.71.010 to .941; Regulation of Health Professions RCW 18.120; Uniform Disciplinary Code RCW 18.130.
2. The references to "physician" in this section therefore apply generally to psychiatrists. Note also that the law does not address the issue of the prescription of drugs, which is governed by federal law.
3. RCW 18.71.015 to .017. See also Washington Administrative Code (WAC) Chapter 308-52.
4. Hereinafter referred to as the "Examining Board."
5. RCW § 18.71.015. The physician's assistant may vote only on matters directly related to physician's assistants.

and, by majority decision, authorizes or denies applications for certification.[6]

Unlicensed practice and the issuance and denial of licenses by the Examining Board is governed by the Uniform Disciplinary Act, RCW Chapter 18.130.[7] The intent of the Act is to strengthen and consolidate disciplinary procedures for the licensed health and health-related professions and businesses and to provide both the state and the public with "awareness of accountability and confidence in the various practices of health care."[8]

The duties of the Board of Medical Examiners include

1. making rules and regulations necessary to comply with its statutory obligation;[9]
2. reviewing applications for licensing;[10]
3. approving schools of medicine for licensing purposes, and the withdrawal of approval in the event that a school ceases to comply with the requirements of the statute;[11]
4. keeping an official record of proceedings, including a register of applicants and Examining Board determinations;[12]
5. preparing, administering, or supervising the preparation and administration of qualifying examinations for applicants for certification;[13]
6. establishing continuing education requirements;[14]
7. issuing limited licenses;[15]
8. disciplining individuals defined in RCW 18.71.030(5) through (12), including students from an Examining-Board-approved school of medicine, who provide services pursuant to a regular course of study or performed under the supervision of a licensed physician,[16] and of individuals found unable to practice because of a mental or physical disability described in RCW 18.130.170.[17]

---

6. *Id.*
7. RCW 18.71.019; RCW 18.130.050(13).
8. RCW 18.130.010.
9. RCW 18.71.017. The rules are detailed in the WAC. *See* WAC 308-52-010 to -580.
10. RCW 18.71.050. The review of applications from graduates of schools of medicine outside the states, territories, and possessions of the United States is governed by RCW 18.71.051.
11. RCW 18.71.055. *See also* WAC 308-52-120.
12. RCW 18.71.060.
13. RCW 18.71.070.
14. RCW 18.71.080. *See also* WAC 308-52-405 to -425. Physicians are required to complete the equivalent of 150 hours of continuing medical education every three years.
15. RCW 18.71.095.
16. RCW 18.71.030(7).
17. RCW 18.71.230.

Physicians disciplined under this chapter have the same rights of notice, hearing, and judicial review as are provided to licensed physicians pursuant to Chapters 18.72 and 18.130 RCW.[18]

(B) Licensure

Graduates from a school of medicine located in any state, territory, or possession of the United States, the District of Columbia, or the Dominion of Canada may apply to the Examining Board for licensure. Applicants must demonstrate to the Examining Board that they[19]

1. have graduated from a school of medicine approved by the Examining Board;
2. have completed one year (two years if graduating after June, 28, 1985)[20] of postgraduate medical training in a program acceptable to the Examining Board;
3. are of good moral character;
4. are physically and mentally capable of carrying on the practice of medicine;
5. do not have a license to practice medicine that, at the time of the application, has been revoked or suspended and have not been found guilty of any conduct that would constitute grounds for refusal, revocation, or suspension of such license under the laws of the state of Washington; and
6. have passed a written examination administered by, or under the supervision of, the Examining Board.[21]

In addition to these basic requirements, graduates of foreign schools of medicine may be licensed by the Examining Board if the applicants show that they[22]

1. have completed a resident course of professional instruction equivalent to that required for applicants generally;

---

18. *Id.*
19. RCW 18.71.050.
20. RCW 18.71.050(b).
21. RCW 18.71.070. The examination also may be waived and a license granted if the applicant meets the requirements of RCW 18.71.050, has been licensed in another state or territory of the United States and Canada, and has passed satisfactorily examinations given by the national board of medical examiners. RCW 18.71.090. *See also* WAC 308-52-270.
22. RCW 18.71.051. *See also* WAC 308-52-040.

2. meet the requirements that must be met by graduates of schools of medicine, except that they need not have graduated from a school of medicine approved by the Examining Board;

3. have passed the examination given by the Education Council for Foreign Medical Graduates or have met the requirements in lieu thereof as set forth by the Examining Board; and

4. have the ability to read, write, speak, understand, and be understood in the English language.

A limited license to practice medicine may be issued, without examination, by the Examining Board to persons licensed in other states who have been hired as physicians by the Department of Social and Health Services or by a city or county health department. Such a license permits the holders to practice medicine only in connection with their duties of employment. Applicants who meet the requirements for licensing under RCW 18.71.050, except for completion of two years of postgraduate medical training, may also be issued a limited license. With this license, the resident physicians may practice medicine only in connection with their duties and not in any other form of practice.[23] All limited licenses are subject to revocation by the Medical Disciplinary Board, RCW 18.72.

Physicians invited to serve as teaching or research members of the staff of the University of Washington School of Medicine or other licensed health care facilities, or who are accepted in fellowship programs at such institutions, may also be granted limited licenses.

The practice of medicine by physicians licensed under this section is limited to the confines of the instructional or fellowship program to which they have been appointed. Limited licenses for teaching and fellowship physicians must be renewed annually.[24]

Every person licensed to practice medicine in the state of Washington must register annually with the Department of Health. Failure to renew renders a physician's license invalid, but such a license may be reinstated upon written application to the director and payment of a penalty. If a license is not renewed for three years, the license holder is required to file an original application pursuant to RCW 18.71.050. The Examining Board may permit such an applicant to be licensed without examination if it is satisfied that the applicant meets the requirements for licensure and is competent to engage in the practice of medicine.[25]

---

23. RCW 18.71.095.
24. RCW 18.71.095(4)(a) and (4)(b).
25. RCW 18.71.080. Fees for application, examination, licensing renewal, and disciplinary assessments are detailed in WAC 308-52-315. The annual license renewal date was changed to coincide with the physician's birthdate.

(B)(1) Exceptions to Licensure

The licensing law does not apply to

1. areas of medicine governed by other licensing requirements;
2. medical officers serving in the Armed Forces or public health service physicians licensed by another state so long as such physicians limit their practice to these settings;
3. students attending an Examining-Board-approved school of medicine;
4. students serving a period of postgraduate medical training sponsored by a college, university, or accredited hospital;[26]
5. persons enrolled in a physician's assistant program approved by the Examining Board; and
6. the practice of medicine in Point Roberts, Washington.[27]

Although not required to be licensed, physician's assistants[28] must be authorized by the Examining Board.[29] The practice of medicine by physician's assistants is limited to the extent permitted by the Examining Board.[30] Applications to the Examining Board may be filed by any physician licensed in the state and must detail the manner and extent to which the physician's assistant will be used and supervised, and the education, training, and experience of the physician's assistant.[31] Physician's assistants are agents for their supervising physicians,[32] and the supervising physician retains professional and personal responsibility for the practice of medicine by the assistant.[33]

26. Postgraduate medical training is defined in WAC 308-52-255.
27. RCW 18.71.030(11): "The practice of medicine, in any part of this state which shares a common border with Canada and which is surrounded on three sides by water, by a physician licensed to practice medicine and surgery in Canada or any province or territory thereof."
28. RCW 18.71A. *See also* WAC 308-52-135 to -221.
29. RCW 18.71A.020 to .030.
30. For the rules and regulations establishing qualifications and restricting the practice of physician's assistants, *see* WAC 308-52.010 *et seq.*
31. RCW 18.71A.040.
32. Washington State Nurses Association v. Board of Medical Examiners, 93 Wash.2d 117, 605 P.2d 1269 (1980) held that the Board of Examiners did not exceed its authority in authorizing physician's assistants to issue prescriptions for medication, and that nurses were not exposed to liability for administering prescriptions ordered by physician's assistants.
33. RCW 18.71A.050.

(C) Medical Disciplinary Board[34]

The Medical Disciplinary Board (Disciplinary Board) was created to administer disciplinary proceedings for licensed members of the medical profession.[35] The Disciplinary Board is composed of one elected holder of a valid license to practice medicine and surgery from each congressional district,[36] and of three members of the public, appointed by the governor, who meet the qualifications contained in RCW 70.39.020(2).[37] Each public member serves a four-year term on the Disciplinary Board, and each elected member serves two years.[38] Action taken against licensed physicians by the Medical Disciplinary Board is governed by the Uniform Disciplinary Act.[39]

(D) Disciplinary Actions Against Licensed Physicians[40]

Upon a finding that a licensed physician has committed an act of unprofessional conduct or is unable to practice with reasonable skill and safety because of a physical or mental condition, the Disciplinary Board can impose any combination of the following sanctions:[41]

1. revocation of license;
2. suspension of license;[42]
3. restriction or limitation of practice;
4. requirement to complete remedial education or treatment;

---

34. RCW 18.72. *See also* WAC 320, which details the functions of the Disciplinary Board. The Board may be contacted at Department of Health, Division of Professional Licensing, P.O. Box 9649, Olympia, WA 98504.
35. RCW 18.72.010.
36. Chapter 320-12 WAC.
37. RCW 18.72.040.
38. RCW 18.72.050.
39. RCW 18.72.154.
40. In addition to the sanctions listed here, injunctions are available to the Disciplinary Board as a means to enjoin violations of RCW 18.130.170 or RCW 18.130.180 (RCW 18.130.185). Two other violations not included here are the practice of a health profession without a license, which constitutes a gross misdemeanor (RCW 18.130.190(3)), and the use of fraudulent representation or willful misrepresentation to obtain a license, which constitutes a misdemeanor (RCW 18.130.200).
41. RCW 18.130.160.
42. Chapter 320-16 WAC allows the Disciplinary Board to suspend imposition of a suspension or revocation order or to otherwise set terms as a condition of suspending imposition of a suspension or revocation order.

5. monitoring of the practice of the physician;

6. censure or reprimand;

7. probation;

8. payment of fine;

9. denial of license;

10. corrective action;

11. refund of fees collected from the consumers.

If the Disciplinary Board believes that a physician or applicant is unable to practice with reasonable skill and safety because of a mental or physical condition, the Disciplinary Board will notify the physician or applicant of the charges and provide an opportunity for a hearing. The Disciplinary Board can require the physician or applicant to submit to a mental or physical examination.[43] If the Disciplinary Board determines that the physician or applicant is unable to practice with reasonable skill and safety, it can impose any combination of the sanctions enumerated under RCW 18.130.160.[44]

(D)(1) Unprofessional Conduct

Sanctions may also be imposed by the Disciplinary Board if any physician or applicant is found to have used unprofessional conduct, which encompasses[45]

1. the commission of any act involving moral turpitude, dishonesty, or corruption relating to the practice of the person's profession, whether the act constitutes a crime or not;

2. misrepresentation or concealment of a material fact in obtaining a license or a reinstatement thereof;

3. all advertising that is false, fraudulent, or misleading;

4. incompetence, negligence, or malpractice that results in injury to a patient or that creates an unreasonable risk such that a patient may be harmed;

5. suspension, revocation, or restriction of the individual's license to practice the profession by competent authority in any state, federal, or foreign jurisdiction;

6. the possession, use, prescription for use, or distribution of controlled substances or legend drugs in any way other than

---

43. RCW 18.130.170(2).
44. RCW 18.130.170. This section generally deals with disciplinary procedures invoked when there is reason to believe that a license holder is incapable of practicing the profession with reasonable skill and safety as a result of a mental or physical condition.
45. RCW 18.130.180.

for legitimate or therapeutic purposes, the addiction to or diversion of controlled substances or legend drugs, the violation of any drug law, or the prescription of controlled substances for oneself;

7. violation of any state or federal statute or administrative rule regulating the profession in question, including any statute or rule defining or establishing standards of patient care or of professional conduct or practice;

8. failure to cooperate with the disciplinary authority by
   a. not furnishing any papers or documents;
   b. not furnishing in writing a full and complete explanation covering the matter contained in the complaint filed with the disciplinary authority; or
   c. not responding to subpoenas issued by the disciplinary authority whether or not the recipient of the subpoena is the accused in the proceeding;

9. failure to comply with an order issued by the disciplinary authority or an assurance of discontinuance entered into with the disciplinary authority;

10. aiding or abetting an unlicensed person to practice when a license is required;

11. violations of rules established by any health agency;

12. practice beyond the scope of practice as defined by law or rule;

13. misrepresentation or fraud in any aspect of the conduct of the business or profession;

14. failure to supervise auxiliary staff adequately to the extent that the consumer's health or safety is at risk;

15. engaging in a profession involving contact with the public while suffering from a contagious or infectious disease involving serious risk to public health;

16. promotion of personal gain of any unnecessary or inefficacious drug, device, treatment, procedure, or service;

17. conviction of any gross misdemeanor or felony relating to the practice of the person's profession;

18. procuring, or aiding or abetting in procuring, a criminal abortion;

19. offering, undertaking, or agreeing to cure or treat diseases by a secret method, procedure, treatment, or medicine or the treating, operating, or prescribing for any health condition by a method, means, or procedure that the license holder refuses to divulge upon demand by the disciplinary authority;

20. willful betrayal of a practitioner–patient privilege as recognized by law;

21. violation of RCW 19.68, which makes it a misdemeanor to request, receive, or allow a rebate, refund, commission, or unearned discount from the referral of clients;

22. interference with an investigation of a disciplinary proceeding by willful misrepresentation of facts before the disciplinary authority or its authorized representative, or by the use of threats or harassment against patients or witnesses to prevent them from providing evidence in a disciplinary proceeding or in any other legal action;

23. drunkenness or habitual intemperance in the use of alcohol or addiction to alcohol; and

24. abuse of a client or patient or sexual contact with a client or patient.

A physician is also guilty of unprofessional conduct if he or she prescribes, orders, dispenses, administers, supplies, or otherwise distributes any amphetamines or other Schedule II non-narcotic stimulant drugs to any person except for therapeutic treatment of the illnesses listed in the Code, such as narcolepsy, hyperkinesis, specifically diagnosed brain dysfunctions, epilepsy, and some types of depression.[46]

Persons exempt from licensure pursuant to RCW 18.71.030(5) to (12)[47] and physician's assistants, as defined in RCW 18.71A.010,[48] are subject to discipline by the Disciplinary Board either upon a finding of an act of unprofessional conduct as defined in RCW 18.130.180 or a finding that the individual is unable to practice with reasonable skill or safety because of a mental or physical condition as described in RCW 130.170.

(D)(2) Duty to Report Unprofessional Conduct[49]

A licensed health care professional who has personal knowledge that a practicing physician has committed an act or acts constituting unprofessional conduct, or that a practicing physician may be unable to practice medicine with reasonable skill and safety to patients by reason of illness, drunkenness, excessive use of drugs, narcotics, chemicals, or any other type of material, or as a result of any mental or physical condition, must make a report to the Medical Disciplinary Board. Reporting under this statute is not required of an appointed peer review committee during the

---

46. WAC 320-18-010.
47. RCW 18.71.230.
48. RCW 18.71A.025.
49. RCW 18.72.165.

course of an investigation, or of a physician when the physician–patient is actively participating in treatment.

(D)(3) Investigation by the Disciplinary Board

The Disciplinary Board has broad powers to investigate complaints or reports of unprofessional acts and to conduct hearings as to the validity of complaints.[50] These powers include issuing subpoenas, administering oaths, implementing discovery procedures, compelling attendance of witnesses at hearings, hiring investigative staff, and imposing sanctions.[51] The Disciplinary Board initiates investigations either when it determines that a written complaint charging a license holder or applicant with unprofessional conduct merits investigation or when the Disciplinary Board is aware, without a formal complaint, that a license holder or applicant may have engaged in unprofessional conduct.[52]

If the Disciplinary Board's investigation determines that an act of unprofessional conduct has occurred, the license holder or applicant is served with a statement of charges and notice that a hearing may be requested within 20 days of being served.[53] If a hearing is requested, the license holder or applicant must be issued a notice of hearing at least 20 days prior to the hearing, specifying the time, date, and place of the hearing. The notice must also detail the procedures that will be used to conduct the hearing.[54]

Hearings conducted by the Disciplinary Board are governed by the Administrative Procedures Act, RCW 34.04.[55] If the hearing results in a finding of unprofessional conduct, the Disciplinary Board must prepare and serve findings of fact and an order as provided in RCW 34.04.120. If no unprofessional conduct is found to have been committed, the Disciplinary Board must prepare and serve findings of fact and an order of dismissal of the charges, including public exoneration of the license holder or applicant. The findings of fact and order are retained by the Disciplinary Board as a permanent record.[56] Information exempt from public disclosure under RCW 42.17 is not required to be reported.

---

50. RCW 18.130.050 to .070; RCW 18.130.100. *See also* WAC 320-108, Practice and Procedure.
51. These powers include the ability to enforce orders for the payment of fines through the Superior Court in which the hearing is held. Failure to abide by an injunction may result in a civil penalty of not more than $25,000.
52. RCW 18.130.080.
53. RCW 18.130.090(1).
54. RCW 18.130.090(2).
55. RCW 18.130.100.
56. RCW 18.130.110.

(D)(4) Impaired Physician Program

In exercising its own power to investigate complaints or reports of unprofessional acts and when there is reasonable cause to believe that the physician under investigation is impaired, the Disciplinary Board may contract with a representative group of physicians with expertise in the areas of alcoholism, drug abuse, or mental illness to evaluate the physician for the purpose of determining whether there is an impairment.[57] This group of physicians, known as the Committee, is also responsible for implementing an impaired physicians program for the detection, intervention, and monitoring of impaired physicians. The Committee has the power to

1. contract with providers of treatment programs;
2. receive and evaluate reports of suspected impairment from any source;
3. intervene in cases of verified impairment (meaning the presence of alcoholism, drug abuse, or mental illness);
4. refer impaired physicians to treatment programs;
5. monitor the treatment and rehabilitation of impaired physicians;
6. provide posttreatment monitoring and support; and
7. perform other activities as agreed upon by the Disciplinary Board and the Committee.

The Committee process is designed to complement the functions of the Disciplinary Board. The Committee is required to report statistical information and to review with the Disciplinary Board appropriate information regarding reports received, contacts or investigations made, and the disposition of each report. The identity of a physician investigated by the Committee is reported to the Disciplinary Board only when

1. the physician is found to constitute an imminent danger to the public;
2. an impaired physician refuses to cooperate with the Committee; or

---

57. RCW 18.72.301 to .321.

3. after participating in a treatment program, the physician remains unable to practice medicine with reasonable skill and safety.[58]

The records of the Committee are not subject to disclosure pursuant to RCW 42.17.

---

58. The statute emphasizes that "impairment, in and of itself, shall not give rise to a presumption of the inability to practice medicine with reasonable skill and safety."

1.2

Licensure and Regulation of Psychiatric Nurses

The licensure and regulation of psychiatric nurses[1] is governed by the statutes[2] that establish a Board of Nursing, establish qualifications and procedures for licensure of nurses, define and limit the practice of nursing, establish exceptions to licensure, prescribe sanctions for violations of laws and regulations, adopt guidelines for the issuance and denial of licenses, and provide for the discipline of license holders. The law is a generic one that regulates the practice of licensed nursing without regard to specialty.[3] There is no separate licensing procedure pertaining to the practice of psychiatric nursing.

(A) Board of Nursing[4]

The Board of Nursing is the primary administrative body that licenses and regulates nurses through the application of the Uniform Disciplinary Act, RCW 18.130.[5] It consists of seven members

---

1. RCW 71.34.020(18) defines a *psychiatric nurse* as "a registered nurse who has a bachelor's degree from an accredited college or university, and who has had, in addition, at least two years' experience in the direct treatment of mentally ill or emotionally disturbed persons, such experience gained under the supervision of a mental health professional. 'Psychiatric nurse' shall also mean any other registered nurse who has three years of such experience."
2. RCW 18.88.005 to .900; Regulation of Health Professions RCW 18.120; Uniform Disciplinary Code RCW 18.130. *See also* Chapter 308-120 WAC.
3. The law does not prohibit the practice of practical nursing (RCW 18.88.030), which is governed by RCW 18.78.
4. RCW 18.88.050.
5. RCW 18.88.086 adopts the Uniform Disciplinary Act as the governing statute for the issuance and denial of licenses and for the discipline of license holders and unlicensed practitioners under this chapter.

(six licensed registered nurses[6] and one public member[7]) appointed for five-year terms by the governor. Membership is limited to two consecutive terms.[8] The Board of Nursing has the power and/or duty to[9]

1. adopt rules and regulations;
2. approve curricula[10] and establish criteria for minimum standards for schools preparing nurses for licensure;
3. keep a record of its proceedings and report to the governor when required;
4. define what constitutes specialized and advanced levels of nursing practice;
5. adopt regulations concerning the authority of various categories of nursing practitioners to perform particular acts;
6. approve schools of nursing[11] and the establishment of basic nursing education programs;
7. establish criteria for proof of reasonable currency of knowledge and skill as a basis for safe practice after three years of nonpracticing status;
8. establish criteria for licensure by endorsement; and
9. review applications for registration and certification to the Department of Health of duly qualified license applicants.

(B) Licensure

To be licensed as a registered nurse, applicants must[12]

1. show proof of graduation from an approved school of nursing;
2. complete the Board of Nursing application requirements; and
3. pass a written examination.[13]

---

6. Nurse members of the Board of Nursing must be licensed under the statute, have at least five years' experience in the active practice of nursing, and have practiced nursing within two years of their appointment. RCW 18.88.060.
7. The public member cannot have been a member of any other licensing board or health occupation board, cannot be an employee of any health facility, and cannot derive his or her primary livelihood from the provision of health services.
8. RCW 18.88.050.
9. RCW 18.88.080.
10. See WAC 308-120-512.
11. RCW 18.88.110 and RCW 18.88.120. See also WAC 308-120-505 to -522.
12. RCW 18.88.130.
13. Subjects covered on the examination are determined by the Board of Nursing. Each written examination may be supplemented by an oral or practical examination. RCW 18.88.140. See also WAC 308-120-161 to -165.

The Board of Nursing may approve an interim permit to practice pending notification of the results of an applicant's first licensing examination. Should an applicant fail the examination, the nonrenewable permit expires upon notification.[14] Applicants are allowed to retake the examination with no fee if the examination is held within one year.

Registered nurses examined and licensed under the laws of another state may apply to the Board of Nursing for licensure without examination.[15] Applicants for licensure previously licensed in a foreign country must meet the requirements set forth in WAC 308-120-166.

Licenses issued under this statute must be renewed annually by the birthdate of the registered nurse.[16] Renewal may be conditioned upon the applicant's completion of a Board-approved continuing nursing education program.[17] Failure to renew will result in a penalty fee,[18] unless the person, by written notice to the Board of Nursing, has requested placement on the nonpracticing list.[19]

(B)(1) Exceptions to Licensure[20]

The licensing statute does not apply to

1. students enrolled in approved schools of nursing, either in their work as nurse's aides or in the practice of nursing that is incidental to their study of nursing;
2. qualified nurses from another state who accompany a patient and who reside temporarily in the state of Washington for a period of six months or less; and
3. nurses licensed in other states who are employed by the United States government.

(B)(2) Disciplinary Actions Against a Licensed Nurse

The Board of Nursing is empowered to take action against licensed nurses.[21] Investigations conducted by the Board of Nursing and the sanctions it imposes are controlled by the guidelines established in the Uniform Disciplinary Act,[22] 18.130 RCW. Upon a finding that a licensed nurse has committed an act of

---

14. RCW 18.88.140.
15. RCW 18.88.150.
16. WAC 308-120-180.
17. RCW 18.88.190. *See also* WAC 308-120-186.
18. RCW 18.88.200.
19. RCW 18.88.220.
20. RCW 18.88.280.
21. RCW 18.130.020(1)(c).
22. RCW 18.88.086.

unprofessional conduct[23] or is unable to practice with reasonable skill and safety because of a physical or mental condition,[24] the Board of Nursing may impose any combination of the following sanctions:[25]

1. revocation of license;
2. suspension of license;
3. restriction or limitation of practice;
4. completion of a program of remedial education or treatment;
5. monitoring of the license holder's practice;
6. censure or reprimand;
7. probation;
8. payment of a fine;
9. denial of license;
10. corrective action; and
11. refund of fees billed to and collected from consumers.

In addition to these sanctions, persons engaged in the following acts may be found guilty of gross misdemeanor:[26]

1. selling or fraudulently obtaining and furnishing any nursing diploma, license, record or registration, or aiding or abetting such an act;
2. practicing nursing under cover of any diploma, license, record, or registration illegally or fraudulently obtained or signed, or issued unlawfully or under fraudulent circumstances; and
3. violating any other provision of the statute governing nurses.

(B)(3) Investigations by the Board of Nursing

The Board of Nursing has broad powers to investigate complaints or reports of unprofessional acts and to conduct hearings as to the validity of such complaints.[27] These powers include issuing subpoenas, administering oaths, implementing discovery procedures, compelling attendance of witnesses at hearings, hiring investigative staff, and imposing sanctions. The Board of Nursing initiates investigations either when it determines that a written complaint charging a license holder or applicant with unprofessional conduct merits investigation, or when the Board of

---

23. Defined in RCW 18.130.180. *See* Unprofessional Conduct in chapter 1.1, Licensure and Regulation of Psychiatrists, this volume.
24. RCW 18.130.170. *See* Disciplinary Actions in chapter 1.1, Licensure and Regulation of Psychiatrists, this volume.
25. RCW 18.130.160.
26. RCW 18.88.270.
27. RCW 18.130.050 to .070.

Nursing is aware, without a formal complaint, that a license holder or applicant may have engaged in unprofessional conduct.[28]

If the investigation by the Board of Nursing determines that an act of unprofessional conduct has occurred, the license holder or applicant is served with a statement of charges and notice that a hearing may be requested within 20 days of being served.[29] If a hearing is requested, the license holder or applicant must be issued a notice of hearing at least 20 days before the hearing, specifying the time, date, and place of the hearing. The notice must also detail the procedures that will be used to conduct the hearing.[30]

Hearings conducted by the Board of Nursing are governed by the Administrative Procedures Act, RCW 34.04.[31] If the hearing results in a finding of unprofessional conduct, the Board of Nursing must prepare the findings of fact and issue an order as provided in RCW 34.04.120. Appeals from an order of the Board of Nursing are governed by the procedures detailed in RCW 34.04.[32] If no unprofessional conduct is found to have taken place, the Board of Nursing must prepare the findings of fact and issue an order of dismissal of the charges, including public exoneration of the license holder or applicant. The findings of fact and order are retained by the Board of Nursing as a permanent record [33] Information exempt from public disclosure under RCW 42.17 is not required to be reported.[34]

---

28. RCW 18.130.080.
29. RCW 18.130.090(1).
30. RCW 18.130.090(2).
31. RCW 18.130.100.
32. RCW 18.130.140.
33. RCW 18.130.110.
34. *See* chapter 4.1, Extensiveness, Ownership, Maintenance of, and Access to Records, this volume.

Licensure and Regulation of Psychologists

The licensure and regulation of psychologists is governed by statutory law and administrative regulations[1] that establish an Examining Board of Psychology, define terms contained within the act, establish qualifications and procedures for licensure of psychologists, create a Disciplinary Committee for regulating the conduct of licensed psychologists, provide for temporary permits and exemptions from licensure, establish continuing education requirements, establish a psychologist–client privilege, provide for a client's right to be informed, provide for administrative hearings, and prescribe sanctions for violations of the chapter. In addition, the Examining Board of Psychology promulgates rules necessary to execute its functions. The intent of the statute is to protect the public from the dangers of unqualified and improper practice of psychology and to provide a consistent method for regulating health care professions.[2]

(A) Examining Board of Psychology

The Examining Board of Psychology (Examining Board) is the administrative body that licenses and regulates psychologists. The Examining Board consists of nine members appointed by the governor for five-year terms. Seven of the members are psycholo-

---

1. RCW 18.83.005 to .900; RCW 18.130; Chapter 246-924 WAC.
2. RCW 18.83.005. This chapter is governed by the purposes detailed in RCW 18.120, Regulation of Health Care Professions.

gists[3] and two are public members.[4] One of the members is elected by the Examining Board to serve as chairperson.

The Examining Board has the duty to[5]

1. review applications for licensing and determine eligible applicants;
2. determine the subject matter of and administer examinations to qualified applicants;
3. keep a complete record of its proceedings;
4. adopt a code of ethics for psychologists;[6]
5. create a Disciplinary Committee within the Examining Board to investigate, hear, and rule on complaints of unethical conduct and other violations of the chapter; and
6. require licensed psychologists to obtain professional liability insurance if the Examining Board so determines.

(B) Licensure

The statutes and rules pertaining to licensure establish the qualifications that applicants must meet,[7] procedures for fees,[8] requirements for examination,[9] and exemptions to the rules.[10] The Examining Board will issue a license to an applicant who

1. is of good moral character;
2. holds a doctoral degree from a regionally accredited institution obtained from an integrated program of psychology as defined by Board rule;
3. has had at least two years of supervised experience and at least one of them subsequent to the awarding of the doctoral degree; and
4. has passed the written and oral examinations prescribed by the Examining Board.

---

3. Psychologists must be United States citizens, have actively practiced psychology in the state for at least three years immediately preceding appointment, and must be licensed under this statute. RCW 18.83.035.
4. Public members must not have trained in the field of psychology, have no connection to a commercial or professional field related to psychology, and have no substantial financial interest in a person regulated by the Examining Board in the two years prior to appointment.
5. RCW 18.83.050.
6. The code of ethics is detailed in WAC 246-924-351 to -366.
7. RCW 18.83.070. Education and experience requirements are detailed in WAC 246-924-640 to -065.
8. RCW18.83.060. Fee schedules are detailed in WAC 246-294-990.
9. RCW 18.83.070. *See* WAC 246-924-070 to -110.
10. RCW 18.83.200.

The Examining Board may waive the written examination and grant a license to an applicant who has not previously failed a Board-sanctioned examination, holds a doctoral degree with primary emphasis on psychology, is licensed or certified to practice psychology in another state having substantially equal requirements and has been licensed or certified for at least two years, or is a diplomate in good standing of the American Board of Examiners in Professional Psychology.[11]

Temporary permits to practice psychology are available (a) to applicants awaiting the results of their examinations; these permits are valid until the Examining Board completes action on the application, but not for more than one year; and (b) to persons licensed or certified in another state deemed by the Examining Board to have standards equivalent to those of the state of Washington, when such persons wish to practice in this state for not more than 90 days in a calendar year.[12]

Individuals who meet all licensing requirements, except the degree of Doctor of Philosophy or its equivalent in psychology from an accredited educational institution, may be issued certificates of qualification at the discretion of the Examining Board.[13] These certificates are granted by the Examining Board after an examination and limit the person to practicing certain functions within the practice of psychology. A licensed psychologist must periodically supervise the practice of a person who holds a certificate of qualification or, upon petition, the Examining Board may grant authority to practice without supervision.

Licenses to practice psychology must be renewed annually. Renewal coincides with the birthdate of the psychologist.[14] Upon renewal, psychologists are subject to continuing education requirements.[15] Failure to renew results in the suspension of the license,[16] which may be reinstated by paying a renewal fee for each year for which the psychologist fails to renew. However, no renewal license will be issued unless the Examining Board finds that the psychologist has not violated any of the provisions of this chapter since suspension of the license.

---

11. RCW 18.83.170. Diplomate status is an alternative to licensure in another state.
12. RCW 18.83.082.
13. RCW 18.83.105.
14. WAC 246-924-120.
15. RCW 18.83.090. The law requires the equivalent of 60 credit hours of continuing psychological education every three years. See WAC 246-924-180 to -340.
16. RCW 18.83.100.

(B)(1) Exceptions to the Regulations

Any person who claims to be a psychologist without possession of a valid license, temporary permit, or certificate of qualification is subject to an injunction, criminal prosecution, and suspension or revocation of his or her license.[17] Exempt from these provisions are persons who[18]

1. teach, lecture, consult, or engage in research in psychology in furtherance of a position in a college or university in this state;
2. hold valid school psychologist credentials from the Washington State Board of Education, but only when practicing psychology during the course of employment;
3. are employed by a local, state, or federal government agency for which psychologists must qualify under federal or state certification or civil service regulations, but only when executing the functions of employment;
4. are employed by a business or industry not engaged in offering psychological services to the public, but only when executing the functions of employment, provided that a person exempt under these regulations shall not engage in the clinical practice of psychology;
5. are students of psychology, psychology interns, or residents in psychology preparing for the profession of psychology in a training institution or facility, and who are designated as psychology trainees or psychology students; or
6. have received a doctoral degree from an accredited school with an adequate major in sociology or social psychology and have passed comprehensive examinations in the field of social psychology. These persons may use the title of "social psychologist."

In addition, these regulations should not be construed as prohibiting individuals from offering counseling or guidance, provided that they do not represent themselves as psychologists.[19]

---

17. RCW 18.83.190.
18. RCW 18.83.200.
19. RCW 18.83.210.

(C) Regulation by the Disciplinary Committee

Within the structure of the Examining Board, the Disciplinary Committee hears and rules on complaints of unethical conduct and other violations discussed in this chapter.[20] Investigations by the Disciplinary Committee and the sanctions that it can impose are governed by the guidelines of the Uniform Disciplinary Act,[21] Chapter 18.130 RCW. Sanctions can be imposed on a licensed psychologist who has committed an act of unprofessional conduct[22] or is unable to practice with reasonable skill and safety because of a physical or mental condition.[23] In addition, sanctions can be imposed under RCW 18.130.160[24] for the following reasons:[25]

1. failing to maintain the confidentiality of client information under RCW 18.83.110;[26]

2. violating the ethical code developed by the Examining Board under RCW 18.83.050;

3. failing to inform prospective research subjects or their authorized representatives of the possible serious effects of participation in research and failing to undertake reasonable efforts to remove the possible harmful effects of participation;

4. practicing in an area of psychology in which the person is clearly untrained or incompetent;

5. failing to exercise appropriate supervision over persons who must practice under the supervision of a psychologist;

6. using fraud or deceit in the procurement of a psychology license or knowingly assisting another in the procurement of such a license through fraud or deceit;

7. failing to maintain professional liability insurance when required by the Examining Board;

---

20. RCW 18.83.050(6).
21. RCW 18.83.054.
22. Defined in RCW 18.130.180. *See* Unprofessional Conduct in chapter 1.1, Licensure and Regulation of Psychiatrists, this volume.
23. RCW 18.130.170. *See* Disciplinary Actions in chapter 1.1, Licensure and Regulation of Psychiatrists, this volume.
24. *See* Disciplinary Actions in chapter 1.1, Licensure and Regulation of Psychiatrists, this volume.
25. RCW 18.83.121.
26. Confidential communications between a client and a psychologist are privileged from compulsory disclosure in the same manner in which attorney-client communications are privileged.

8. violating any state statute or administrative rule specifically governing the practice of psychology; and

9. gross, willful, or continued overcharging for professional services.

In addition to the violations referenced above, unlicensed persons who improperly use a designation implying that they are licensed psychologists or licensed psychologists who practice while holding a suspended or revoked license are guilty of a gross misdemeanor.[27]

(C)(1) Investigations By the Examining Board

The Examining Board conducts investigations through the Disciplinary Committee. In addition to the broad powers under the Uniform Disciplinary Act, the Disciplinary Committee is authorized to[28]

1. maintain records of all activities and to publish and distribute, to all psychologists, abstracts of significant Committee activities; and

2. obtain the written consent of the complaining client or patient, or of their legal representative, or of any person who may be affected by the complaint in order to gain access to confidential or privileged information.

Action taken by the Disciplinary Committee pursuant to an investigation or hearing that finds a licensee guilty of unprofessional conduct is reported to the appropriate national and state organizations that represent the profession of psychology.[29]

(D) Duty To Disclose Information to Client

Washington law explicitly protects, as confidential and privileged, the communications between psychologists and their patients,[30] subject to the limitations under RCW 71.05.250.[31] However, there are four exceptions to this general rule:

---

27. RCW 18.83.180.
28. RCW 18.83.135.
29. RCW 18.83.155.
30. RCW 18.83.110. *See also* chapter 4.2, Confidential Relations and Communications and chapter 4.3, Privileged Communications, this volume.
31. When a petition is filed seeking 14-day involuntary treatment or 90 days of less restrictive alternative treatment, the court may determine that, to protect the detained person or the public, waiver is necessary for obtaining a sufficient psychiatric or psychological evaluation.

1. when reasonable cause exists to believe that a child, adult dependent person, or an elder has suffered abuse or neglect, then the psychologist has a duty to report the matter to the authorities;[32]

2. at a probable cause hearing for either a 14-day or a 90-day involuntary commitment;[33]

3. if the client actually threatens to inflict physical violence on reasonably identifiable victims;[34] and

4. in a criminal, civil, or administrative agency action when a client who is a criminal defendant raises a mental disability defense;[35] or when, as a criminal defendant, the client is being evaluated to determine competency to stand trial;[36] or when a client, having agreed to be evaluated at the request of a state agency, manifests his or her intention not to keep the communication confidential;[37] or when a client brings charges against the psychologist in a civil action, such as for malpractice or personal injury.[38]

One result of this intrusion into the arena of protected conversation is that a client may make self-incriminating statements without knowing the probable consequences thereof.

To offset this possible result, the statute imposes, upon a psychologist, the duty to disclose certain information to the clients.[39] At the commencement of psychological services, a psychologist must inform the clients of the following:

1. the clients' right to refuse treatment,

2. the clients' responsibility for choosing the provider and treatment modality that best suit their needs, and

---

32. RCW 26.44.030 and .040. State v. Fagalde, 85 Wash.2d 730, 539 P.2d 86 (1975). *See* chapter 5A.6, Reporting of Adult Abuse and chapter 5A.8, Reporting of Child Abuse, this volume.
33. Peterson v. State, 100 Wash.2d 421, 671 P.2d 230 (1983). *See* chapter 4.3, Privileged Communications and chapter 5E.4, Involuntary Civil Admission of Mentally Ill Adults, this volume.
34. RCW 71.05.120; *see* chapter 6.5, Malpractice Liability, this volume.
35. *See* chapter 5D.9, Criminal Responsibility, this volume.
36. *See* chapter 5D.5, Competency to Stand Trial, this volume.
37. Matter of Welfare of Henderson, 29 Wash. App. 748, 630 P.2d 944 (1981). This determination requires a balancing of the benefits of the privilege against the public interest in full revelation of all the facts. *See* chapter 4.3, Privileged Communications, this volume.
38. *See* chapter 6.5, Malpractice Liability, this volume.
39. RCW 18.83.115. *See* chapter 6.1, Informed Consent for Services, this volume.

3. the extent of confidentiality and privilege to which they are entitled, as described in this chapter.[40]

Psychologists must also disclose their relevant education and training, the therapeutic orientation of their practice, the proposed course of treatment when known, the rights of clients regarding treatment, financial requirements, and other information that the Examining Board may require.[41] The receipt of these disclosures must be acknowledged in writing both by the psychologists and their clients.

---

40. The statute does not indicate whether exceptions to the confidentiality standard must be disclosed, but responsible practice would include informing the client of any relevant exceptions. *See* chapter 4.3, Privileged Communications, this volume.
41. RCW 18.83.115(1). The Examining Board of Psychology updated these standards in June 1993.

1.4

Unlicensed Psychologists

The laws in some states allow subdoctoral psychologists to maintain independent psychology practices. While recognizing the value of these practitioners, other states limit the independent practice of subdoctoral psychologists in various ways. Washington law follows the latter approach.

(A) Psychologists Exempted from Licensure

As noted in chapter 1.3, the law provides that a person must obtain a license to use the title of psychologist. Exceptions to this rule are granted for persons who[1]

1. teach, lecture, consult, or engage in research in psychology in furtherance of a position in a college or university;

2. hold valid credentials as school psychologists from the Washington State Board of Education;[2]

3. are employed by a local, state, or federal government agency, and are qualified for employment under federal or state certification or civil service regulations (the title of psychologist may be used only when conducting employment-related activities);

---

1. RCW 18.83.200.
2. Certification and academic requirements for school psychologists are governed by WAC 180-84-015, -020, and -025. *See* chapter 1.6, Certification and Regulation of School Psychologists, this volume.

4. are employed by a business or industry engaged in offering psychological services to the public (the title of psychologist may be used only when conducting employment-related activities, provided that the individual does not engage in the clinical practice of psychology);

5. are students of psychology, psychological interns, or residents in psychology preparing for the profession of psychology in a training institution or facility (such individuals may use the title of psychology trainee or psychology student);

6. have received a doctoral degree from an accredited school with an adequate major in sociology or social psychology, and have passed comprehensive examinations in the field of social psychology (these persons may use the title of social psychologist); or

7. are issued temporary permits, granted to applicants awaiting examination results and to out-of-state psychologists who wish to practice in this state, for not more than 90 days in a calendar year.[3]

Individuals not licensed or not falling under one of these exemptions cannot represent themselves as psychologists.

---

3. RCW 18.83.082.

1.5

Registration and Certification of Social Workers, Mental Health Counselors, and Marriage and Family Therapists

Beyond the practices of psychiatry and psychology, there is a variety of disciplines, theories, and techniques used by counselors who practice under a variety of titles. While recognizing the right of these individuals to practice their skills freely, the state of Washington has chosen to regulate them as a means of protecting the health and safety of the public and of ensuring that citizens can choose the practitioner who best suits their needs and purposes.[1] The statute governing the registration and certification of these counselors requires that the public be educated about the responsibilities of such practitioners and about the rights and responsibilities of their clients.[2]

(A) Certification

To charge a fee or to practice as certified social workers, mental health counselors, or marriage and family therapists, all counselors must be registered with the Department of Licensing.[3] A counselor may be any individual, practitioner, therapist, or analyst who counsels members of the public for a fee.[4] The term

---

1. RCW 18.19.010.
2. RCW 18.19.050(3).
3. RCW 18.19.030.
4. RCW 18.19.020(6).

counseling includes the use, for a fee, of therapeutic techniques that "offer, assist or attempt to assist an individual or individuals in the amelioration or adjustment of mental, emotional or behavioral problems, and include therapeutic techniques to achieve sensitivity and awareness of self and others and the development of human potential."[5]

In addition to social workers, mental health counselors, marriage and family therapists, and hypnotherapists, the law applies also to counseling professions that are not yet defined or identified. One of the powers delegated to the Director of Licensing is to "develop a dictionary of recognized professions and occupations providing counseling services to the public."[6] Thus, the identification of counseling professions will be a continuing process, and subsequently persons may be subject to registration even though their profession is not currently listed in the statute.

(B) Authority of the Director of Licensing

The Director of Licensing has to power to[7]

1. set fees for registration, certification, and renewal;
2. issue registrations to qualified applicants;
3. set educational ethical and professional standards of practice for certification;
4. prepare and administer an examination to all qualified applicants for certification;
5. establish criteria for evaluating the ability and qualifications of persons applying for certification, including standards for passing the examination and standards of qualifications for certification to practice;
6. evaluate and designate schools for accreditation and establish standards and procedures for accepting alternative training in lieu of such education;
7. issue certificates to any applicant who has met the education, training, and conduct requirements established for certification; and
8. set competence requirements for maintaining certification.

---

5. RCW 18.19.020(5). The statute makes it clear that the practice of hypnotherapy is not limited to counseling.
6. RCW 18.19.050(1)(l).
7. RCW 18.19.050.

Issuance and denial of certification and registration is governed by the Uniform Disciplinary Act.[8] The governing body for the registration process is the Department of Licensing. Five-member advisory committees are established for each category of counseling designated by the Director of Licensing.[9] Members of the committees are appointed by the Director to provide advice on certification issues. Four must be currently registered or certified in the category designated by that committee. The fifth member is a representative of the public.[10] Members of the committees may be appointed for one-, two-, or three-year terms, but no member may serve for more than two consecutive terms.

Applicants for registration must register as counselors with the Director of Licensing and include a description of their therapeutic orientation, discipline, theory, or technique. An applicant may register as a hypnotherapist if he or she uses hypnosis as a treatment modality.[11]

(C) Requirements for Social Worker Certification[12]

A certified social worker certificate will be issued to any applicant who meets the following requirements:

1. a minimum of a master's degree from an accredited graduate school of social work approved by the Director of Licensing;

2. a minimum of two years of postmaster's degree social work conducted under the supervision of a social worker certified under this chapter or of a person deemed acceptable to the Director of Licensing. This practice must consist of at least 30 hours per week for two years or at least 20 hours per week for three years; and

3. the successful completion of an examination.[13]

---

8. RCW 18.19.050(2). *See* chapter 1.1, this volume.
9. RCW 18.19.070.
10. RCW 18.19.070(3).
11. RCW 18.19.090.
12. RCW 18.19.110.
13. An applicant may retake the examination if he or she receives a failing score. Upon failure of four examinations, the Director of Licensing may invalidate the original application and require remedial education prior to admission to future examinations. RCW 18.19.140(4). An applicant is exempt from examination upon a showing of qualification and proof that he or she is currently credentialed under the laws of another jurisdiction. RCW 18.19.160(1).

Successful applicants for certification in social work are deemed competent in the professional application of social work values, principles, and methods. The social work profession "requires knowledge of human development and behavior, knowledge of social systems and social resources, adherence to the social work code of ethics, and knowledge of and sensitivity to ethnic minority populations."[14] The methods used by social workers include, but are not limited to, evaluation, assessment, treatment of psychopathology, consultation, psychotherapy and counseling, prevention and educational services, administration, policy making, research, and education directed toward client services.[15]

(D) Requirements for Mental Health Counselor Certification[16]

A certified mental health counselor certificate will be issued to any applicant who meets the following requirements:[17]

1. a master's or doctoral degree in mental health counseling or a related field from an approved school, or completion of at least 30 graduate semester hours or 45 graduate quarter hours in the field of mental health counseling, or the substantial equivalent in both subject content and extent of training;

2. postgraduate, supervised mental health counseling practice;

3. successful completion of an examination,[18] submission of necessary documents, and payment of required fees; and

4. 24 months of postgraduate professional experience working in a mental health counseling setting that meets the requirements established by the Department of Health.

The purpose of certification of mental health counselors is to ensure that the counselor can "assist the client in achieving effective personal, organizational, institutional, social, educational, and vocational development and adjustment and to assist the client in achieving independence and autonomy in the helping relationship."[19] Mental health counselors certified under this chapter engage in the aspect of counseling that emphasizes "well-

---

14. RCW 18.19.110(3).
15. RCW 18.19.110(3).
16. RCW 18.19.120.
17. RCW 18.19.120(1).
18. RCW 18.19.120(2).
19. RCW 18.19.120(4).

ness" rather than illness in their application of therapeutic principles, methods, and procedures.

(E) Requirements for Marriage and Family Therapist Certification[20]

A certified marriage and family therapist certificate will be issued to any applicant who meets the following requirements:[21]

1. a master's or doctoral degree in marriage and family therapy, or its equivalent, from an approved school that shows evidence of the following coursework:
   a. marriage and family systems;
   b. marriage and family therapy;
   c. individual development;
   d. assessment of psychopathology;
   e. human sexuality;
   f. research methods;
   g. professional ethics and law; and
   h. a minimum of one year in the practice of marriage and family therapy under the supervision of a qualified marriage and family therapist;

2. two years of postgraduate practice of marriage and family therapy under the supervision of a qualified marriage and family therapist; and

3. passing scores on both written and oral examinations.[22]

As defined by the statute, the practice of marriage and family therapy "involves the assessment and treatment of impaired marriage or family relationships including, but not limited to, premarital and postdivorce relationships and the enhancement of marital and family relationships via use of educational, sociological, and psychotherapeutic theories and techniques."[23]

---

20. RCW 18.19.130.
21. RCW 18.19.130(1).
22. RCW 18.19.130(1)(b).
23. RCW 18.19.130(3).

(F) Renewal of Registration and Certification

Certified social workers, mental health counselors, and marriage and family therapists must be registered with the Department of Licensing.[24] The requirements for registration are defined in RCW 18.19.090. Applicants must complete the required application and not have engaged in unprofessional conduct as defined in the Uniform Disciplinary Act.

(G) Exemptions to Certification[25]

The certification requirements listed in this chapter do not apply to the following practices:

1. the practice of a profession by a person who is registered, certified, licensed, or similarly regulated under the laws of this state and who is performing services within the person's authorized scope of practice, including an attorney admitted to practice in this state when providing counseling incidental to and in the course of providing legal counsel;

2. the practice of counseling by an employee or trainee of any federal agency or the practice of counseling by a student of a college or university, if the employee, trainee, or student is practicing solely under the supervision of and accountable to the agency, college, or university through which he or she performs such functions as part of his or her position for no additional fee other than ordinary compensation;

3. the practice of counseling by a person who does not charge a fee;

4. the practice of counseling by a person offering services for public and private nonprofit organizations or charities not primarily engaged in counseling for a fee;

5. evaluation, consultation, planning, policymaking, research, or related services conducted by social scientists for private corporations or public agencies;

6. the practice of counseling by a person under the auspices of a religious denomination, church, or organization or the practice of religion itself; and

---

24. RCW 18.19.030.
25. RCW 18.19.040.

7. counselors whose official residency is not the state of Washington and who provide up to 10 days per quarter of training or workshops in the state so long as they do not hold themselves out to be registered or certified in Washington State.

(H) Regulation

The discipline of certified practitioners and registrants under this chapter is governed by the Uniform Disciplinary Act, RCW 18.130.[26]

(I) Disclosure[27] and Confidentiality[28]

At the commencement of any program of treatment, each person registered or certified under RCW 18.19 must inform clients of

1. the right of clients to refuse treatment,
2. the responsibility of clients to choose the provider and treatment modality that best suits their needs,
3. the extent of confidentiality provided under the statute,
4. relevant education and training,
5. the therapeutic orientation of the practice,
6. the proposed course of treatment when known,
7. financial requirements, and
8. other information that the Director of Licensing may require.

The disclosure of this information must be acknowledged in writing both by the counselor and the client, but disclosure should not be taken as a guarantee of effectiveness.

The written acknowledgement of the disclosure statement and the information acquired from a client during the rendering of the professional services are confidential. The counselor has a duty to maintain this confidentiality at all times, except:

1. with the written consent of the client or, in the case of death or disability, the client's personal representative, other person authorized to sue, or the beneficiary of an insurance policy on the client's life, health, or physical condition;

---

26. RCW 18.19.050(2). *See* chapter 1.1, this volume.
27. RCW 18.19.060.
28. RCW 18.19.180.

2. that a counselor is not required to treat as confidential a communication that reveals the contemplation or commission of a crime or harmful act;

3. if the client is a minor, and the information acquired by the counselor indicates that the minor was a victim or subject of a crime, the counselor may testify fully upon any examination, trial, or other proceeding in which the commission of the crime is the subject of the inquiry;

4. if the client waives the privilege by bringing charges against the counselor;

5. in response to a subpoena from a court of law or the Director of Licensing; or

6. as required under RCW 26.44 when there is suspicion of child abuse.

1.6

Certification and Regulation of School Psychologists

The Washington State Board of Education certifies school psychologists under the category of Specialized Personnel.[1] This certification is independent of the Examining Board of Psychology, which specifically exempts school psychologists from regular licensure (see chapter 1.3).[2]

(A) Certification

The requirements for certification are set out to ensure that the school psychologist is competent in psychological techniques and skilled in applying them to the education setting. In the course of his or her work, a school psychologist may perform the following functions:[3]

1. measuring the intellectual, social, and emotional development of children and interpreting the results of psychological studies;

2. diagnosing educational and personal disabilities and collaborating in the planning of reeducational and therapeutic studies;

3. identifying exceptional children and collaborating in the planning of appropriate educational and social placements and programs;

---

1. Chapter 180-84 WAC.
2. RCW 18.83.200(2).
3. WAC 180-84-015. The authority to promulgate these rules is set out in RCW 28A.04.120 and RCW 28A.70.005.

4. developing ways to facilitate the learning and adjustment of children;

5. helping teachers and administrators to understand child behavior and intellectual and personality differences as they apply to the individual pupil and the class;

6. serving in a consultative capacity in curriculum planning; and

7. encouraging and initiating research and helping to use research findings for the solution of school problems.

The rules governing the certification of school psychologists establish three levels of certification:[4]

1. Provisional Certificate, which requires

   a. a master's degree with a major in psychology or completion of the course work toward a master's degree but not of the thesis requirement, and

   b. 15 credit hours of professional education courses, including practice teaching or directed laboratory experiences in a school situation.

2. Standard Certificate, which requires

   a. fulfillment of all the requirements for the Provisional Certificate,

   b. a master's degree with a major in psychology, and

   c. successful completion of two years of experience as a school psychologist, one of which must be under supervision.

3. School Psychologist in a Supervisory Capacity, which requires

   a. a doctorate in psychology,

   b. defined experience as a school psychologist, and

   c. fulfillment of the requirements for the Provisional and Standard Certificates.

(B) Education

The rules governing the educational requirements for school psychologists list three areas of required study:[5]

1. Basic Education Areas, which require a minimum of 15 quarter hours of credit in

   a. directed laboratory experience in a school setting,

   b. education of the exceptional child, and

---

4. WAC 180-84-020.
5. WAC 180-84-025.

c. philosophy, organization, and administration of the American school system;

2. Basic Psychology Areas, which include studies in
   a. introductory psychology,
   b. statistics,
   c. child growth and development,
   d. psychology of adjustment or mental hygiene,
   e. psychology of learning, and
   f. social psychology or sociology; and

3. Clinical Psychology and Personality Areas, which include study in
   a. abnormal psychology,
   b. personality theory,
   c. tests and measurements,
   d. individual intelligence testing—children,
   e. individual intelligence testing—adults,
   f. introduction to personality testing,
   g. interviewing and counseling,
   h. diagnosis of the exceptional child, and
   i. practicum in diagnosis and report writing.

(C) Regulation

As an employee of the Washington State Board of Education, the conduct of a school psychologist is subject to the provisions contained in Washington law[6] relating to the regulation of school employees. Under these provisions, a certified employee may be discharged only upon a showing of "sufficient cause."[7] Examples of sufficient cause include:

1. use of habit-forming drugs without a prescription from a licensed practitioner of medicine or of dentistry;[8]

2. unauthorized use of alcoholic beverages on school premises or at a school-sponsored activity off the school premises;[9]

3. failure to maintain good order and discipline in the classroom;[10]

---

6. WAC 180-44; WAC 180-75; RCW 28A.58.099(1).
7. RCW 28A.58.099(1).
8. WAC 180-44-060.
9. Id.
10. WAC 180-44-020.

4. commission of or being found guilty of (a) immorality, (b) violation of a written contract, (c) intemperance, (d) a crime against the law of the state, or (e) an act of unprofessional conduct, the nature of which justifies the revocation of the individual's certificate;[11] or

5. conviction of any crime involving the physical neglect of children, injury to children (except from motor vehicle violations), or the abuse of children.[12]

Upon receipt of a written complaint, the Office of the Superintendent for Certification investigates the allegations. If sufficient cause for revocation is found, the holder of the certificate is notified by certified mail and informed of the appeal procedures available under the law.[13] If the proposed action is not appealed within 30 days from the date of mailing, the order of revocation will be signed by the Superintendent of Public Instruction. An individual who has had his or her certification revoked may reapply for certification one year from the date of revocation.[14]

---

11. WAC 180-75-035(1).
12. WAC 180-75-035(2).
13. *See* WAC 180-75-020, -030, and -033.
14. WAC 180-75-035. *See also* RCW 28A.70.180.

1.7

Certification and Regulation of School Social Workers

The Washington State Board of Education certifies school social workers under the category of Specialized Personnel.[1] This certification is issued independently of the Advisory Committee for Social Workers, which exempts from regular certification persons who are certified under the laws of Washington and who are performing services within the person's authorized scope of practice (see chapter 1.5).[2]

(A) Certification

The requirements for certification are set out to ensure that the school social worker is competent both to help the school identify children who present social and emotional difficulties and to enable these children to make satisfactory progress in the classroom. To achieve this goal, school social workers participate in

1. consultation service to teachers, principals, and other school personnel;
2. individual or group help to parents and children; and
3. liaison services in using community resources for the benefit of children.

The rules governing school social workers establish two levels of certification:[3]

---

1. Chapter 180-84 WAC. The authority to promulgate these rules is set out in RCW 28A.04.120 and RCW 28A.70.005.
2. RCW 18.19.040(1).
3. WAC 180-84-060.

1. Provisional Certificate, which requires

   a. a master's degree from a school of social work accredited by the Council on Social Work Education or the following combinations:

       (1) a bachelor's degree from an approved institution;

       (2) one full year of postgraduate study in a school of social work accredited by the Council on Social Work Education and one full year of directed field placement in an agency approved by the school of social work; and

       (3) two years of successful experience under the supervision of a qualified supervisor in an approved family or children's agency, or two years of successful teaching experience;

   b. completion of a minimum of 15 quarter hours of professional education courses, including practice teaching or directed laboratory experiences in a school situation and orientation to the school philosophy, methods, organization, and group activity; and

2. Standard Certificate, which requires

   a. fulfillment of all requirements for the Provisional Certificate;

   b. a master's degree from a school of social work accredited by the Council on Social Work Education; and

   c. completion of two years of successful experience as a school social worker.

(B) Education

The rules governing the educational requirements for school social workers[4] emphasize a specialized social work skill through knowledge of behavior causation, human growth and community resources, and the ability to work with professional personnel in the school and the community. For undergraduate preparation, a broad liberal arts education with a concentration in social work is recommended.

A master's degree in social work requires

1. completion of the prescribed curricula in a school of social work for a two-year postgraduate study accredited by the Council on Social Work Education;

---

4. WAC 180-84-055.

2. six quarters of directed laboratory experience in an approved social agency, clinic, or institution for two to three days a week; and

3. completion of either an individual or a group research project.

(C) Regulation

As an employee of the Washington State Board of Education, the conduct of a school social worker is subject to the provisions contained in Washington law[5] relating to the regulation of school employees. Under these provisions, a certified employee can be discharged only upon a showing of "sufficient cause."[6] Examples of sufficient cause include

1. use of habit-forming drugs without a prescription from a licensed practitioner of medicine or of dentistry;[7]

2. unauthorized use of alcoholic beverages on school premises or at a school-sponsored activity off the school premises;[8]

3. failure to maintain good order and discipline in the classroom;[9]

4. commission of or being found guilty of (a) immorality, (b) a violation of written contract, (c) intemperance, (d) a crime against the law of the state, or (e) an act of unprofessional conduct, the nature of which justifies the revocation of the individual's certificate;[10] or

5. conviction of any crime involving the physical neglect of children, injury to children (except from motor vehicle violations), or the abuse of children.[11]

Upon receipt of a written complaint, the Office of the Superintendent for Certification investigates the allegations. If sufficient cause for revocation is found, the holder of the certificate is notified by certified mail and informed of the appeal procedures available under the law.[12] If the proposed action is not appealed within 30 days from the date of mailing, the order of revocation will be signed by the Superintendent of Public Instruction. An individual who has had his or her certification revoked may reapply for certification one year from the date of revocation.[13]

---

5. WAC 180-44; WAC 180-75; RCW 28A.58.099(1).
6. RCW 28A.58.099(1).
7. WAC 180-44-060.
8. *Id.*
9. WAC 180-44-020.
10. WAC 180-75-035(1).
11. WAC 180-75-035(2).
12. *See* WAC 180-75-020, -030, and -033.
13. WAC 180-75-035. *See also* RCW 28A.70.180.

1.8

Certification and Regulation of Hypnotists

In some states, the law regulates hypnosis and the professional title of hypnotist by prescribing education, experience, and skills. In those states, mental health professionals would have to obtain certification to use the title of hypnotist. In the state of Washington, hypnotherapists, for the purposes of the state's Omnibus Credentialing Act for Counselors, Chapter 18.19 RCW, are considered counselors regulated under that Act (see chapter 1.5). However, RCW 18.19.020(5) clarifies that nothing limits hypnotherapy to counseling settings, that is, hypnotherapy may be used in a variety of medical and dental settings.

1.9

Certification and Regulation of Polygraph Examiners

The use of polygraph testing and the licensing of polygraph examiners is widely divergent among states. The state of Washington does not regulate or certify polygraphy, license polygraph operators, or provide standards for training polygraph operators (see chapter 5C.3, Polygraph Examinations and Polygraph Evidence). The use of polygraph testing is limited in this jurisdiction.[1]

---

1. *See* RCW 49.44.120. Lie detector examinations may be used as a condition of employment or of continued employment only in law enforcement, drug-dispensing, or national security agencies. Case law also has restricted polygraph use: State v. Grisby, 97 Wash.2d 493, 647 P.2d 6 (1982), *cert. denied*, 459 U.S. 1211 (1982); State v. Young, 89 Wash.2d 613, 574 P.2d 1171, *cert. denied*, 439 U.S. 870 (1978).

1.10

Sunset of Credentialing Agencies

The *sunset law*[1] is the means by which the legislature reviews and revises most facets of state government, from entire departments to small commissions. The law works by automatically terminating the authority of a state agency[2] to continue to operate. The sunset law ensures that the past work, efficiency, and effectiveness of each agency is reviewed periodically by the legislature.[3] After these mandatory reviews, the legislature either extends the termination date or terminates the agency.

(A) Operation of the Law

Under the sunset law, each agency is reviewed by three different entities: the Legislative Budget Committee, the Office of Financial Management, and the appropriate committee of reference.

(A)(1) Legislative Budget Committee

The initial review is conducted by the Legislative Budget Committee. A report on the agency must be completed on or before June 30 of the year before the date established for termination.[4] In

---

1. Chapter 43.131 RCW.
2. State agencies include state offices, departments, boards, commissions, regulatory entities and, where provided by law, other programs and activities involving less than the full responsibility of a state agency. RCW 43.131.030(4).
3. RCW 43.131.020.
4. RCW 43.131.050. In Washington, June 30 is used as the standard termination date for state agencies. By reviewing groups of agencies at the same time, the legislature is able to modify and consolidate agency conduct better as a means of preventing duplicative activity. RCW 43.131.120(1)(b).

reviewing a regulatory agency, the Legislative Budget Committee considers the following factors:[5]

1. the extent to which the regulatory entity has permitted qualified applicants to serve the public;

2. the extent to which the regulatory entity has restricted or inhibited competition or otherwise adversely affected the state's economic climate;

3. the extent to which the system of regulation has contributed directly or indirectly to increasing or decreasing the costs of any goods or services involved;

4. the duties of the regulatory entity and the costs incurred in carrying out such duties;

5. whether the regulatory entity has operated in the public interest, including the extent to which the regulatory entity has

   a. sought and achieved public participation in making the rules and decisions, including consideration of recommending appointment of one or more "public" members to the entity;

   b. processed to completion in a timely and equitable manner the formal complaints filed with it;

   c. implemented an effective system of evaluating the impact on the public of its rules and decisions regarding economy, availability, and improvement of the services rendered to the persons it regulates;

   d. initiated administrative procedures or recommended statutory changes to the legislature that would benefit the public as opposed to the persons it regulates; and

   e. identified the needs and problems of the recipients of goods and services provided by those regulated;

6. the extent to which persons regulated by the regulatory entity have been encouraged to participate in assessing problems in their profession, occupation, or industry that affect the public;

7. the impact and effectiveness of the regulatory entity with regard to the problems or needs that the entity is intended to address;

8. the consequences of eliminating or modifying the program of the regulatory entity;

---

5. RCW 43.131.060.

9. the extent to which the regulatory entity has duplicated the activities of other regulatory entities or of the private sector; and

10. the extent to which the absence or modification of regulation would adversely affect the public health, safety, or welfare.

If the agency being reviewed by the Legislative Budget Committee is a state agency other than a regulatory agency, the Committee will consider the extent to which[6]

1. the state agency has complied with legislative intent;

2. the state agency has operated in an efficient and economical means that have resulted in optimal performance;

3. the state agency has operated in the public interest by effectively providing a needed service that should be continued rather than modified, consolidated, or eliminated;

4. the state agency has duplicated the activities of other state agencies or of the private sector; and

5. the termination or modification of the state agency would adversely affect the public health, safety, or welfare.

(A)(2) Office of Financial Management

Upon completion of its report, the Legislative Budget Committee transmits the report to the Office of Financial Management for a fiscal review. The fiscal report must be completed on or before September 30 of the year prior to the date established for agency termination.[7] The completed fiscal report is then transmitted back to the Legislative Budget Committee, which prepares a final report. The final agency report is transmitted to all members of the legislature, the state agency concerned, the governor, and the state library.[8]

(A)(3) Committees of Reference

The final review of the agency is conducted by the appropriate committees of reference.[9] Committees of reference are standing legislative committees designated by the Senate and House of Representatives to consider termination, modification, or reestablishment of state agencies. In considering the report received from the Legislative Budget Committee, the committees of reference are empowered[10] to hold public hearings, to hear testimony from

---

6. RCW 43.131.070.
7. RCW 43.131.050.
8. *Id.*
9. RCW 43.131.030(1).
10. RCW 43.131.080.

interested parties, and to conduct additional meetings to determine whether a state agency has demonstrated a public need for its continued existence. A determination by a committee of reference that a state agency should be reestablished or modified must take the form of a bill and is subject to passage by the Senate and House of Representatives.

(B) Scheduling for Sunset Review

The Select Joint Committee is responsible for monitoring the schedule of agencies to be reviewed under the sunset law. [11] It consists of five senators and five representatives nominated by the senate president and speaker of the house, respectively.[12] In scheduling a sunset review, the Committee must take into consideration:[13]

1. identifying state agencies that may be subject to termination;
2. scheduling agencies with similar functions for termination on the same date so duplicative activities are easier to recognize; and
3. scheduling agencies so as not to overburden any one committee of reference during a legislative session.

---

11. RCW 43.131.120(1).
12. RCW 43.131.115.
13. RCW 43.131.120(1).

Forms of Business Practice

2.1

Sole Proprietorships

Mental health professionals (MHPs) who do not work for an employer typically organize their practices in one of three forms: sole proprietorship, professional corporation (see chapter 2.2), or partnership (see chapter 2.3). MHPs who practice alone and without any formal business organization are termed *sole proprietors*. Unlike partnerships and professional corporations (see chapters 2.2 and 2.3), there is no law regulating this type of business entity directly. Thus, sole proprietors need to abide only by the laws regulating businesses in general.

2.2

Professional Corporations[1]

MHPs who do not work for an employer may organize their practices into professional corporations. The value of offering professional services[2] through a professional corporation is that it offers many of the tax and practice benefits of regular business incorporation.

(A) Benefits of Incorporation

There are three main benefits that MHPs can derive from professional incorporation. First, certain tax deductions are available only to a professional corporation (e.g., for the purchase of health insurance, death benefits, and retirement plans). Second, when there is more than one MHP shareholder in the corporation, the professional liability (e.g., for malpractice) of each shareholder engaged in conduct on behalf of the corporation is shared by the corporation, thereby reducing the financial burden to any one person.[3] Finally, meeting the requirements of corporation law, such as holding shareholder meetings and issuing regular re-

---

1. The material in this chapter is only an introduction to the law and is not a comprehensive analysis of the benefits and drawbacks of professional incorporation as opposed to other forms of doing business.
2. Chapter 18.100 RCW, Professional Service Corporations, covers practitioners who must hold proof of a license including, but not limited to, the following licensed professionals: certified public accountants, chiropractors, dentists, osteopaths, physicians, podiatrists, chiropodists, architects, veterinarians, and attorneys at law.
3. RCW 18.100.070.

ports, may cause professionals to be more sensitive to the business aspects of their practices.[4]

(B) Incorporation and Operational Procedures

MHPs who wish to incorporate must meet two basic requirements:

1. Each professional must be licensed or otherwise legally authorized to provide a professional service;[5] and
2. All professional shareholders must be engaged in providing the same professional service (e.g., licensed psychologists providing psychological services).[6]

A professional corporation may engage only in the business of rendering the professional service for which it was incorporated, though the professional corporation is free to invest in real estate, personal property, mortgages, stocks, bonds, insurance, or other types of investments.[7] Stock of the professional corporation may be held only by individuals duly licensed or otherwise legally authorized to render the same specific professional services as those for which the professional corporation was incorporated.[8]

To the extent that the provisions for incorporating as a professional corporation conflict with the regular incorporation procedures listed under the Washington Business Corporation Act,[9] the rules governing incorporation of the professional corporation prevail. Where there is no conflict, such as with the articles of

---

4. For more information on incorporation and the particular benefits available, MHPs should seek the advice of a tax consultant and a business planning attorney.
5. RCW 18.100.050.
6. RCW 18.100.065. Thus, a nonphysician health care professional, such as a psychologist or midwife licensed under the applicable provisions of the RCW, cannot be admitted as a shareholder (i.e., incorporating professional) in a professional corporation organized to provide medical services. Likewise, a professional corporation organized to provide a broad range of health care services may not admit a nonphysician health care professional as a shareholder. Op. Atty. Gen. 1980, L.O. No. 18.
7. RCW 18.100.080.
8. RCW 18.100.090. Shares that pass to ineligible shareholders because of a death or of a transfer by operation of law or court decree must be transferred to an eligible shareholder within 12 months or the shares will be canceled and the ineligible person will have a right to payment of the shares. *See* RCW 18.100.110.
9. Chapter 23A RCW.

incorporation, bylaws, and shareholder's meetings, MHPs should follow the procedures set out in the Business Corporation Act.

The support staff employed by a professional corporation do not have to be licensed professionals. The clerks, secretaries, bookkeepers, technicians, and other assistants employed by a professional corporation are considered, by custom and practice, to be support staff.[10]

(C) Liability and Accountability

Unlike regular business corporations that can indemnify individuals from liability, shareholders in a professional corporation remain personally and fully liable and accountable for any negligent or wrongful acts committed by them or by anyone under their direct supervision and control.[11] In addition, if there is more than one shareholder, each is potentially responsible for the professional acts of the other shareholders of the corporation. If questionable conduct has taken place as an extension of the rendering of services on behalf of the corporation, the corporation is liable for any negligent or wrongful acts of misconduct committed by its directors, officers, shareholders, agents, or employees.[12]

The professional corporation, by implication, is accountable to the board that grants professional licenses or certificates to its shareholders as well as to the secretary of state. A professional corporation is required to follow the guidelines established by Chapter 18.100 RCW, including providing services only in the area for which the professional corporation was organized. In addition, if any director, officer, shareholder, agent, or employee of a professional corporation becomes legally disqualified to render professional services, such person must sever all employment with, and financial interests in, the corporation. Failure to comply constitutes a ground for dissolution of the corporation.[13]

---

10. RCW 18.100.060.
11. RCW 18.100.070.
12. *Id.*
13. RCW 18.100.100.

(D) Termination of the Professional Corporation

The professional corporation continues until the last surviving shareholder dies, or until a voluntary or involuntary dissolution occurs pursuant to the laws governing dissolution of regular business corporations.[14]

---

14. RCW 23B.14.

Partnerships[1]

MHPs who do not work for an employer may organize their practices into a partnership.

A *partnership* is a form of doing business in which two or more persons agree to carry on as coowners of a business for profit. This business arrangement allows the partners to pool their resources to undertake projects that would be financially or technically difficult for either partner alone. The law may find a joint endeavor to be a legal partnership, even though the individuals engaged in it may not consider it so and may not call it a partnership. Such a finding could result in a forced sharing of profits and debts as well as in shared liability for a wrongful act or breach of trust committed by a partner. MHPs should be aware of this form of business organization whether they form a legal partnership or whether they merely work in a close business relationship with other persons, which could be construed to be a partnership.

(A) Formation of a Partnership[2]

A partnership is formed when two or more persons agree to carry on as coowners of a business for profit.[3] The existence of a

---

1. The material in this chapter is only an introduction to the law and is not a comprehensive analysis of the benefits and drawbacks of partnership as opposed to other forms of doing business.
2. The law governing general partnerships is the Uniform Partnership Act, adopted in every state except in Louisiana. In Washington, the Act was adopted in RCW 25.04.
3. RCW 25.04.060(1).

partnership depends on the intention of the parties and may be implied from the facts and circumstances surrounding the business relationship.[4] Receipt of a share of profits of a business is *prima facie* evidence that a partnership exists.[5] For instance, two psychiatrists who work out of a building owned jointly under a common name will not have partnership status forced upon them unless they also had the intent to share the profits of their services.

Intent is also a factor in determining which persons make up the partnership. This determination is important for reasons of liability. Persons, who by means of writing, speech, or conduct represent themselves or consent to being represented by someone else as members of an existing partnership, or group of persons not actually in a partnership, will be considered to be partners and may be held liable to a person to whom such a representation was made if the person relied on such a representation.[6]

Partners are not required to share equally in profits and losses. Generally, profits and losses are assigned to the partners according to their respective share in the partnership. For example, if a partnership consists of two persons, one of whom initially contributed $50,000 to the partnership and the other $100,000, the latter may legitimately take 66% of the profits. However, partners may agree to allocate partnership income and losses in different proportions although the Internal Revenue Service will not recognize losses in excess of a partner's investment in a partnership.[7]

Partnership status is not invoked by mere part ownership, that is, by the sharing of gross receipts.[8] Similarly, the presence of a profit-sharing plan is not determinative of the existence of a partnership, nor does the partnership require a formal declaration or filing of a business purpose. Rather, any agreement between parties, even an oral one, that meets the definition outlined above suffices to initiate a partnership.

(B) Rights and Duties Between Partners

A partnership is more than a business relationship. The law imposes, on the partners, duties to govern their interactions and

---

4. Thornton Estate, 18 Wash.2d 72, 499 P.2d 864 (1972).
5. RCW 25.04.070(4).
6. RCW 25.04.160.
7. For information regarding the tax consequences of partnerships, MHPs should seek the advice of a tax consultant or business planning attorney.
8. RCW 25.04.070.

grants rights to protect their interest in the partnership. Subject to specific agreement between partners, these include the right to

1. be repaid for contributions to the partnership and to share equally in profits of the partnership;[9]
2. indemnity from liability reasonably incurred from ordinary conduct taken on behalf of the partnership;[10]
3. equal say in the management and conduct of partnership business;[11]
4. consent to the addition of new members into the partnership;[12]
5. inspect and copy the partnership books;[13] and
6. a formal accounting of the partnership affairs under certain circumstances.[14]

Correspondingly, partners have a duty to

1. share in the losses of the partnership;[15]
2. share with partners any information affecting the partnership;[16] and
3. account for all benefits to the partnership.[17]

In general, the law views each partner as an agent of the partnership. The acts of each partner bind the partnership so long as the partner acts in the natural course of the partnership's business and within his or her authority.[18] It is outside a partner's authority, individually or in a number less than the total of the partners, to

1. assign the partnership property in trust for creditors;
2. dispose of the goodwill of the business;[19]
3. perform any other act that would make it impossible to carry on the ordinary business of the partnership;
4. acknowledge responsibility in any suit against the partnership; or

---

9. RCW 25.04.180(1).
10. RCW 25.04.180(2).
11. RCW 25.04.180(5).
12. RCW 25.04.180(7).
13. RCW 25.04.190.
14. RCW 25.04.220.
15. RCW 25.04.180(1).
16. RCW 25.04.200.
17. RCW 25.04.210.
18. RCW 25.04.090
19. *Goodwill* refers to the reputation of the business. As it pertains to the sale of a business, it is equal to the difference between the purchase price and the value of the net assets of the business.

5. submit a partnership claim or liability to arbitration or reference.[20]

Perhaps most important, any wrongful act or omission of any partner acting in the ordinary course of business of the partnership that results in a loss, injury, or penalty accrues to all the partners.[21] Therefore, if any partner breaches the trust of a client by misapplying money or property received, the partnership is bound to make good the loss.[22] Partners are jointly and severally liable for such losses, which means that a wronged person may sue one, several, or all of the partners to recover what has been lost.[23]

(C) Dissolution of a Partnership

The dissolution of a partnership involves the dissociation of the partners from their partnership agreement. Upon dissolution, the authority of any partner to act for the partnership is terminated.[24] The partnership itself is not terminated until the winding up of partnership affairs is completed.[25] The dissolution of the partnership, however, does not discharge the partners or partnership from liability that may have accrued prior to dissolution.

A partnership is dissolved by[26]

1. the term or undertaking specified in the partnership agreement;
2. the express will of any partner when no definite term or particular undertaking is specified; in other words, when the partners have not agreed to conduct a particular business activity for a specified length of time and one of the partners wishes to dissolve the partnership, that person may do so;
3. the expulsion of any partner from the business in accordance with the agreement among the partners;
4. a violation of the agreement among partners when one of the partners expressly intends for the partnership to be dissolved;
5. any event that makes it unlawful for the business of the partnership to be conducted or for the members of the partnership to conduct it;

---

20. RCW 25.04.090(3).
21. RCW 25.04.130.
22. RCW 25.04.140.
23. RCW 25.04.150.
24. RCW 25.04.330.
25. RCW 25.04.300.
26. RCW 25.04.310 and .320.

6. the death of any partner;

7. the bankruptcy of any partners; or

8. the decree of a court when

    a. a partner has been found to be mentally ill in a judicial proceeding or has been shown to be of unsound mind;

    b. a partner becomes in some way incapable of fulfilling his or her part of the partnership contract;

    c. a partner has been guilty of conduct that tends to affect prejudicially the carrying on of the partnership business;

    d. a partner willfully or persistently breaches the partnership agreement or otherwise conducts himself or herself, in matters relating to the partnership, in such a way that it is not reasonably practicable to carry on the business in partnership with that person;

    e. the business of the partnership can only be carried on at a loss; or

    f. other circumstances render dissolution equitable.

2.4

Health Maintenance Organizations[1]

A *health maintenance organization* (HMO) offers health care services to individuals or a group for a single fee, usually paid annually, with little or no additional cost. The services are provided by health care practitioners who are HMO employees or by other practitioners who contract with the HMO on a fee-for-service basis. The overall costs of care through an HMO are kept low primarily by limiting the organization's expenses to the prepaid amount and by efficient use of centralized administration.

(A) Benefits for Mental Health Services

HMOs are encouraged by the state of Washington as a means of providing persons with competitively priced, alternative health care delivery systems.[2] The law requires that HMOs offer comprehensive health care services, including, at a minimum, basic consultative, diagnostic, and therapeutic services; emergency and preventive care; and inpatient and outpatient hospital and physician care.[3]

In addition, HMOs must offer optional supplemental coverage for mental health treatment. Services can be provided by the HMO itself or through referral to a[4]

---

1. Chapter 48.46 RCW.
2. RCW 48.46.010.
3. RCW 48.46.020(2).
4. RCW 48.46.290(1).

1. physician,
2. licensed psychologist,
3. licensed community health agency, or
4. state hospital.

The costs of treatment must be covered at the usual and customary rates, but different rates can be set for each of the three groups of providers above. Because these outside referrals are more expensive to the HMO, they are monitored carefully and not made often unless the treatment expertise is not available through the HMO staff.

(B) Benefits for Chemical Dependency Treatment[5]

HMOs must provide benefits for the treatment of chemical dependency in covered persons by an approved alcoholism or drug treatment facility.[6] As is the case of mental health treatment, the costs of treatment must be covered at the usual and customary rates for any referrals to professionals outside the HMO.

---

5. *Chemical dependency* is defined as an "illness characterized by a physiological of (sic) psychological dependency, or both, on a controlled substance regulated under chapter 69.50 RCW and/or alcoholic beverages. It is further characterized by a frequent or intense pattern of pathological use to the extent the user exhibits loss of self-control over the amount and circumstances of use; develops symptoms of tolerance or physiological and/or psychological withdrawal if use of the controlled substance or alcoholic beverage is reduced or discontinued; and the user's health is substantially impaired or endangered or his or her social or economic function is substantially disrupted." RCW 48.46.355.
6. RCW 48.46.350. Criteria for approval of treatment facilities are contained in RCW 70.96A.020(3).

2.5

Preferred Provider
Organizations

A *preferred provider organization* (PPO) is a group of health care providers and hospitals that contracts with employer, union, or third-party payors (such as Blue Cross/Blue Shield) to provide services to the employees, members, or insureds for a discounted fee in return for an exclusive service arrangement. Members of the PPO see patients in their own offices. There is no specific Washington law that regulates the formation or operation of PPOs.

2.6

Individual Practice Associations

An *individual practice association* (IPA) is a group of health care providers that contracts to provide services for an organization that provides a prepaid health plan, frequently an HMO.[1] The members of the IPA practice in their own offices but are compensated by the organization on a fee-for-service or fee-per-patient basis. There is no Washington law regulating the formation or operation of IPAs.

---

1. An IPA is a new form of health care organization, and an exact definition has not yet been adopted.

2.7

Hospital, Administrative, and Staff Privileges

The law in many states governs which classes of mental health practitioners are eligible for agency and hospital staff and administrative privileges. In the state of Washington, hospitals are licensed under two statutes that distinguish hospitals[1] from state mental institutions and private psychiatric hospitals.[2] The governing body of each institution is required to set standards and procedures to be applied by the hospital and its medical staff in considering and acting on applications for staff membership or professional privileges.[3] Staff membership and privileges at state mental institutions and private psychiatric hospitals are governed by the rules and regulations of the Department of Social and Health Services.[4]

(A) Hospital-Staff Privileges: Medical

The State Board of Health is responsible for establishing rules and procedures for the licensing and regulation of hospitals. Each hospital is required to have a governing body responsible for adoption of policies concerning the purposes, operation, and maintenance of the facility. With the approval of the governing body, the medical staff (appointed by the governing body) implement bylaws, rules, and regulations, including qualifications for

---

1. Licensed under RCW 70.41.090.
2. Licensed under RCW 71.12.460.
3. RCW 70.43.010.
4. For the Washington Administrative Code provisions pertaining to hospitals, *see* WAC 248-18 *et seq.*; for private psychiatric hospitals and alcoholism treatment hospitals, *see* WAC 248-22, *et seq.* to 248-26 *et seq.*

medical staff membership,[5] procedures for delineation of hospital-specific clinical privileges, and organization of the medical staff.[6] State law prohibits discrimination in extension of staff membership and professional privileges, but extends that protection only to physicians, osteopaths, and podiatrists.[7]

(A)(1) Psychiatric Unit Staff Privileges

If a hospital operates a psychiatric unit, the regulations require that qualified personnel, in the form of a multidisciplinary treatment team,[8] be available to operate it properly. Clinical responsibility for services is assigned to an MHP.[9] The following personnel are required:

1. a psychiatrist with medical staff privileges who will be available for consultation;

2. a full-time psychiatric nurse responsible for the nursing care;

3. social work, occupational therapy, and recreational services provided with the ongoing input of professionals (social worker, occupational therapist, and recreational therapist) experienced in working with mentally ill patients; and

4. a psychologist to direct psychological evaluations.

The work of all professionals is identified in an individualized treatment plan prepared for each patient.

(A)(2) Private Psychiatric and Alcohol Unit Staff Privileges

The regulations governing administrative and staff privileges in private psychiatric and alcoholism hospitals differ from those applicable to hospitals in general. Although the relationship between the governing body and the medical staff is much the same, the regulations specifically define medical staff to mean physicians and other medical practitioners.[10] Also, the requirements

---

5. The governing body is responsible for ensuring that each individual granted clinical privileges has the appropriate and current qualifications. RCW 43.70.040; WAC 246-318-030.
6. WAC 246-318-033.
7. RCW 70.43.020. "The governing body ... shall not discriminate against a qualified person solely on the basis of whether such person is licensed under chapters 18.71 [physicians], 18.57 [osteopaths], or 18.22 [podiatrists]."
8. WAC 246-318-280(1)(j). This team consists of individuals from the various treatment disciplines and clinical services who assess, plan, implement, and evaluate treatment for patients under care.
9. WAC 246-318-280(2).
10. WAC 248-22-001(28).

for staff differ between private psychiatric hospitals and private alcoholism hospitals.[11] Private psychiatric hospitals must provide

1. medical services (and each patient must be admitted by a member of the medical staff);
2. a staff psychiatrist available for consultation daily;
3. nursing, social work, occupational therapy, and recreational therapy services provided by professionals experienced in working with psychiatric patients; and
4. psychological services under the auspices of medical services.

A psychologist, who must provide documented evidence of skill and experience in working with psychiatric patients, is responsible for supervision and coordination of psychological services. However, private alcoholism hospitals need to provide only medical, nursing, and alcoholism counseling services.

---

11. WAC 246-322-070(6). Private psychiatric and alcoholism hospitals may provide special services, either by contract or by direct employment and at the direction of a staff physician or other appropriate clinical staff, to meet the needs of patients. Such services must be provided by qualified individuals.

2.8

Zoning for Community Homes

Zoning regulations are the laws by which state and local governments control the residential and commercial growth of communities and areas. These laws can be and have been used to exclude certain classes of people thought to be undesirable from particular communities or areas within communities. For example, some zoning boards have prohibited community homes for the mentally disordered from locating in single-family residential neighborhoods even though such a placement would have been in the best interests of the community home residents. The laws of some states specifically prohibit this form of discrimination by designating certain community group homes as family residences.[1] However, Washington law does not provide any specific protection to community or group homes. Rather, they are subject to the planning, zoning, sanitary and building laws, and ordinances and regulations that are applicable to the locality in which they are situated.[2]

Washington law provides that housing authorities of first class counties may establish and operate group homes or halfway houses to serve juveniles released from state juvenile or correctional institutions or to serve the developmentally disabled.[3]

---

1. For example, *see* Arizona Revised Statutes Section 36-582.
2. RCW 35.82.120. *See also* RCW 35.82.285. For a general description of the law regarding zoning enforcement, *see* Rorick, M. H. Zoning—Judicial Enforcement of the Duty to Serve the Regional Welfare in Zoning Decisions, 55 Wash. L. Rev. 485 (1980). SAVE v. City of Bothell, 89 Wash.2d 862, 576 P.2d 401 (1978).
3. RCW 35.82.285.

However, such facilities can be established only after an appropriate public hearing.[4] The only specific statutory limitation is that the housing authority cannot acquire property for group homes or halfway houses through the exercise of eminent domain.[5]

---

4. Chapter 42.30 RCW.
5. RCW 35.82.285.

Insurance Reimbursement and Deductions for Services

3.1

Insurance Reimbursement for Services

As a general rule, health insurance carriers (insurers) have considerable discretion in defining the coverage of mental health services under the health insurance policies that they issue. In many states, health insurance policies limit the scope of covered mental health services and restrict reimbursement to specified MHPs. In response, many states require the inclusion of some specified minimum level of mental health coverage into all health insurance policies offered in the state.[1] Although not specifically defining the mental health services that must be offered, Washington law requires each carrier to offer supplemental benefits for mental health treatment and specifies that reimbursement must be made for such services when provided by psychiatrists, psychologists, and community mental health agencies.[2]

(A) Types of Insurance Affected

The law specifies that providers of three types of health insurance must offer supplemental coverage for mental health treatment: (a) group and blanket disability insurance,[3] (b) health care service contractors,[4] and (c) health maintenance organizations.[5]

---

1. Note that the U.S. Supreme Court has held that such mandatory minimum mental health benefit statutes are not preempted by federal law (e.g., Employee Retirement Income Security Act or the National Labor Relations Act. Metropolitan Life Insurance Co. v. Commonwealth of Massachusetts, 471 U.S. 724 (1985).
2. The law does not refer to other types of registered or certified MHPs in private settings.
3. RCW 48.21.240.
4. RCW 48.44.340.
5. RCW 48.46.290.

(B) Authorized Providers

The law requires that benefits be provided under the authorized coverage regardless of whether treatment is rendered by a licensed physician, a licensed psychologist, a community mental health agency licensed by the Department of Social and Health Services,[6] or a state hospital.[7]

Payment for such treatment is to be at the usual and customary rate, but separate rates may be established for the providers authorized under the law. In addition, the treatment may be subject to insurance provisions regarding reasonable deductible amounts and copayments (*see* chapter 6.6, i.e., fraud).

---

6. To qualify under these provisions, community mental health agencies must have in effect a plan for quality assurance and peer review, and the treatment must be supervised by a licensed physician or licensed psychologist.
7. RCW 48.21.240(2); RCW 48.44.340(2); RCW 48.46.290(2).

3.1A

Impact Assessment for Mandated Health Coverage

The Washington legislature recognized that mandated health coverage under insurance policies improved access to health care services, and that such access could provide social and health benefits that may be in the public interest. However, the Legislature also recognized that the cost implications of mandated health benefit coverage should be of concern, and that the merits of mandated health coverage must be weighed against a variety of consequences, including the cost of such coverage. As a result of these concerns, Washington requires that all legislative proposals for mandated health benefits be accompanied by a systematic impact assessment report.[1] The Department of Health must review such reports and make recommendations as requested by the relevant legislative committees.[2]

(A) Guidelines for Assessing Impact

The law provides guidelines for the assessment report on any proposed mandated health coverage.[3] These guidelines include, but are not limited to,

1. the social impact, including answers to the following questions:

   a. to what extent is the treatment or service generally used by a significant portion of the population;

---

1. RCW 48.42.060.
2. RCW 48.42.070.
3. RCW 48.42.080.

b. to what extent is the insurance coverage already generally available;

c. if coverage is not generally available, to what extent does the lack of coverage result in persons avoiding necessary health care treatments;

d. if coverage is not generally available, to what extent does the lack of coverage result in unreasonable financial hardship;

e. what is the level of public demand for the treatment or service;

f. what is the level of public demand for insurance coverage of the treatment or service; and

g. what is the interest level of collective bargaining agents in negotiating privately for inclusion of this coverage in group contracts.

2. the financial impact, including answers to the following questions:

a. to what extent will the coverage increase or decrease the cost of the treatment or service;

b. to what extent will the coverage increase the appropriate use of the treatment or service;

c. to what extent will the mandated treatment or service be a substitute for more expensive treatment or service;

d. to what extent will the coverage increase or decrease the administrative expenses of insurance companies and the premium and administrative expenses of policyholders; and

e. what will be the impact of this coverage on the total cost of health care.

3.2

Mental Health Benefits in State Insurance Plans

In some states, the law mandates that any health insurance plan provided for state government employees include certain mental health benefits. Washington law, however, does not specify which mental health benefits must be offered to state employees.[1]

---

1. It is not a violation of law for the State Employees' Insurance Board to provide state employees with the option of coverage by an HMO that restricts the availability of the services of licensed health practitioners, including psychologists, to those provided either directly through the HMO or, upon referral, by a primary care physician employed by the HMO. Op. Atty. Gen. 1986, L. O. No. 11.

3.2A

Washington State Health Insurance Pool

The Washington State Health Insurance Pool (hereinafter referred to as the Pool) was created to ensure access to health insurance coverage to all residents of the state who were denied health insurance for any reason. It is intended to make available an adequate level of health insurance coverage, defined to include specified mental health benefits.

(A) Administration of the Pool

The Pool is governed by a nine-member Board of Directors made up of representatives of the general public, health care providers, and insurance carriers,[1] and administered by an insurance carrier selected by competitive bidding.[2] Membership in the Pool consists of all commercial insurers that provide disability insurance, health care service contractors, and health maintenance organizations doing business in the state.[3] Members are subject to an annual assessment to help pay claims under the Pool and to cover its administrative expenses.[4]

---

1. RCW 48.41.040(2).
2. RCW 48.41.080.
3. RCW 48.41.030(12).
4. RCW 48.41.050(5).

(B) Eligibility for Coverage

The Pool covers any state resident, and his or her dependents[5] , who provides evidence of

1. rejection of coverage for medical reasons,
2. imposition of restrictive insurance riders,
3. an up-rated premium, or
4. a preexisting condition limitation.[6]

In addition, any person whose health insurance coverage is involuntarily terminated for any reason other than nonpayment of premium may apply for coverage under the Pool.[7]

The following are not eligible for coverage under the Pool:[8]

1. persons eligible for medical assistance;
2. persons who have terminated their coverage under the Pool, unless (a) 12 months have elapsed since termination, or (b) the person can show continuous insurance coverage (other than the Pool) that has been involuntarily terminated for any reason other than nonpayment of premiums;
3. any person on whose behalf the Pool has paid out $500,000 in benefits; and
4. inmates of public institutions and persons whose benefits are duplicated under public programs.

(C) Services Covered

The Pool pays the usual, customary, and reasonable charges for medically necessary health care services rendered or furnished for the diagnosis or treatment of illnesses, injuries, and conditions. The minimum covered mental health benefits include, but are not limited to,[9]

1. hospital services, but limited to a total of 180 inpatient days in a calendar year and limited to 30 days inpatient care for mental and nervous conditions, or alcohol, drug, or chemical dependency or abuse per calendar year;

---

5. RCW 48.41.140.
6. RCW 48.41.100(1).
7. RCW 48.41.100(3).
8. RCW 48.41.100(2).
9. RCW 48.41.110.

2. professional services, other than dental; or[10]

3. the first 20 outpatient professional visits for the diagnosis or treatment of one or more mental or nervous conditions or alcohol, drug, or chemical dependency or abuse rendered during a calendar year by one or more physician, psychologist, or community mental health professionals, or, at the direction of a physician, by other qualified licensed, health care practitioners.

The law also permits the Pool to employ cost containment measures that may allow the Pool to operate in a cost-effective manner.[11]

(D) Deductibles and Coinsurance

The Pool offers coverage at two levels of annual deductible payment, $500 and $1,000,[12] and imposes a coinsurance requirement of 20% of the eligible expenses in excess of the annual deductible payment.[13] However, the combined out-of-pocket expense for an insured client for one year cannot exceed[14]

1. $1,500 per individual or $3,000 per family per year for the $500 deductible coverage, or

2. $2,500 per individual or $5,000 per family per year for the $1,000 deductible coverage.

---

10. *Professional services* are those "rendered by a health care provider or, at the direction of a health care provider, by a staff of registered or licensed practical nurses or other health care providers." RCW 48.41.110(1)(b).
11. RCW 48.41.110(2).
12. RCW 48.41.120(1).
13. RCW 48.41.120(2). The coinsurance requirement means that, after the individual has incurred and paid eligible expenses up to the deductible amount, the Pool will pay only for 80% of the subsequent eligible expenses.
14. RCW 48.41.120(3).

3.3

Tax Deductions for Services

Payments for mental health services may be deductible either as an individual medical deduction or as a business expense, depending on the nature of the service and the use by the recipient–taxpayer.

(A) Mental Health Services as a Medical Deduction

Professional services relating to the diagnosis and treatment of mental or emotional disorders are allowable as medical deductions under federal tax law.[1] In addition to a deduction for the services of a psychiatrist, federal law also provides that[2]

> Amounts paid to psychologists, qualified and authorized under state law to practice psychology, for services rendered by them in connection with the diagnosis, cure, mitigation, treatment, or prevention of disease or for the purpose of affecting any structure or function of the body, constitute expenses paid for medical care within the meaning of section 23(x) of the Internal Revenue Code and may be deducted in computing net income for federal income tax purposes to the extent provided therein.

However, such deductions are not unlimited.[3]

---

1. In many states, such expenses are allowable deductions from income for state income tax purposes as well. However, Washington does not have a state income tax.
2. Rev. Rul. 143, 1953-2 C.B. 129.
3. Rev. Rul. 75-187, 1975-1 C.B. 92. Amounts paid by a husband and wife for meals and lodging at a hotel, at which they stayed on the advice of their psychiatrists while they received psychiatric treatment for sexual inadequacy and incompatibility, are not deductible as medical expenses; however, the amounts paid for the therapy are deductible.

The Internal Revenue Service also allows deductions for payments made to other types of health care providers:[4]

> Accordingly, it is held that amounts paid for medical services rendered by practitioners, such as chiropractors, psychotherapists, and others rendering similar type services, constitute expenses for "medical care" within the provisions of section 213 of the Code, even though the practitioners who perform the services are not required by law to be, or are not (even though required by law) licensed, certified, or otherwise qualified to perform such services.

(B) Mental Health Services as a Business Deduction

The use of mental health services by a taxpayer who operates a business is deductible as a trade or business expense. Federal law provides that "there shall be allowed as a deduction all the ordinary and necessary expenses paid or incurred during the taxable year in carrying on any trade or business."[5] The key words in interpreting the rule are *ordinary*, defined to mean common and accepted, and *necessary*, defined to mean appropriate and helpful.[6]

---

4. Rev. Rul. 63-91, 1963-1 C.B. 54.
5. 26 U.S.C. § 162(a).
6. Welch v. Helvering, 290 U.S. 111 (1933).

Privacy of Professional Information

Extensiveness, Ownership, Maintenance, and Access to Records

The requirements governing the extensiveness and maintenance of and access to records differ across settings and among types of MHP. The following subsections discuss differences among practitioners in public or private institutional settings as well as among psychiatrists, psychologists, and certified practitioners in noninstitutional settings.

The statutes and regulations are silent as to ownership of the clinical records of a client in either a public or private institutional or noninstitutional setting. Yet, the absence of guidelines about ownership of records within the statutes or regulations suggests that a common-law, property right of client ownership of records may exist.[1] Under this theory, the practitioner is regarded only as a preparer and custodian of the records. Other jurisdictions that have ruled on this issue have held that either the client owns the records[2] or the practitioner owns the records.[3]

(A) Public or Private Institutional Settings

The requirements regarding the extensiveness and maintenance of and access to records are established for all mental health practitioners through statutory or administrative code require-

---

1. Oliver v. Harborview Medical Center, 94 Wash.2d 559, 618 P.2d 76 (1980). WAC 248-22-041; WAC 275-19-170; WAC 275-55-263; WAC 275-56-330.
2. Wallace v. University Hospitals of Cleveland, 164 N.E.2d 917 (1959).
3. Estate of Finkle, 305 N.Y.S. 2d 343 (1977); People v. Cohen, 414 N.Y.S. 2d 642 (1979).

ments that apply to various settings. In addition, each setting may create standards for its own records. During a civil or criminal action against a practitioner for breaching some duty or breaking a law, unless records meet the statutory and setting standards, the practitioner's defense will appear weak to the factfinder(s) at trial; proper record-keeping adds to the credibility of the practitioner.[4]

(B) State Mental Health Institutions[5]

(B)(1) Extensiveness of Records

The law mandates that the records of voluntary patients in state facilities include the following:

1. a consent signed by the patient indicating voluntary admission to the institution and the receipt of information about patients' rights (see chapter 5E.3 for the delineation of the due process and custodial rights of patients);[6]

2. documentation showing a periodic review of the patient's treatment program, progress, goals for future treatment, and the consideration of a less restrictive treatment;[7] and

3. notation about disclosures of information, including the date of the disclosure, the circumstances of the disclosure, the names and relationships to the patient of the persons or agencies to whom the disclosures were made, and the content of the information disclosed.[8]

Records of involuntary patients are required to be more extensive. They must include the following information:

1. sufficient factual data to complete a petition and testify before a superior court that the patient "as a result of a mental disorder presents a likelihood of serious harm to others or himself or herself or is gravely disabled and that there are no

---

4. Peck J. A., & Campion, T. F. *Ingredients of a psychiatric malpractce lawsuit*, 51 Psychiatric Q. 236–241 (1979); Pope, K. S., Simpson, N. H., & Weiner, M. F. *Malpractice in outpatient psychotherapy*, 32 Am. J. of Psychotherapy 593–601 (1978).

5. Legislated requirements for client records exist for group homes for the mentally and physically handicapped (Chapter 275-36 WAC), child care agencies (Chapter 388-73 WAC), and adult family homes (Chapter 388-76 WAC). The staffing at these settings generally does not include licensed or certified MHPs. Therefore, the particular standards for these settings are not discussed here.

6. WAC 275-55-040.

7. WAC 275-55-081.

8. RCW 71.05.420.

less restrictive alternatives in the best interest of such person or others" (see chapter 5E.4 on involuntary commitment);[9]

2. a consent signed by the patient that indicates agreement to continue treatment during the 24-hr period before any commitment hearing—all treatment can be refused except emergency lifesaving treatment and physical restraints or seclusion, if necessary to protect the patient or others from injury;[10]

3. a notation that the patient, orally or in writing, and when possible, a responsible member of the patient's family or another person designated by the patient, has received in writing notice as to the patient's confinement rights;[11]

4. a treatment and medication history with other diagnostic and prognostic information that indicates why involuntary inpatient treatment is in the best interest of the committed person or of others;[12] and

5. notations about any disclosures of information concerning the patient.[13]

The regulations do not mention documenting progress notes, reevaluating the treatment plan, or goals for future treatment and less restrictive treatment. However, many institutional practitioners regularly include this type of information.

(B)(2) Maintenance of Records

No requirements exist as to the length of time for which records are to be stored. However, because no law exists addressing this issue under Chapter 71.05 RCW, the Health Care Information Act (Chapter 70.02 RCW) may apply.[14] Under that law, a record must be maintained for at least one year[15] following receipt of authorization to disclose information from the record,[16] during the pendency of a request for examination and for copying,[17] or a request for disclosure, or a request for a record correction.[18]

(B)(3) Client Access

Under the Public Disclosure Act,[19] clients of any public institution or health agency may inspect or copy their records. If the clients

9. RCW 71.05.230.
10. WAC 275-55-161.
11. WAC 275-55-211.
12. RCW 71.05.390(g).
13. RCW 71.05.420.
14. RCW 70.02.900.
15. RCW 70.02.160.
16. RCW 70.02.40.
17. RCW 70.02.80.
18. RCW 70.02.100.
19. Chapter 42.17 RCW.

request access to the records, the burden of proof falls on the agency to justify why the records should not be disclosed, and the clients will be awarded all costs, including reasonable attorney's fees, if they win the case.[20] Unless disclosure of the information in the clients' records would violate personal privacy or vital state government interests, the court will rule in favor of the clients' right to access.[21] An agency may remove any material confidential to another person or compiled and released to the agency by an outside practitioner, but the remainder of the record must be made available.

(C) County Mental Health Settings

The Community Mental Health Services Act applies to all county mental health programs. One of the underlying purposes of the Act was to provide "accountability of services through state-wide standards for management, monitoring, and reporting of information."[22] It also is possible that the standards at various settings exceed the promulgated standards. Each setting must establish written policies and procedures about client rights, records, record entry, service planning, operations, and services.[23]

(C)(1) Extensiveness of Records

A screening interview may precede an intake evaluation. If the person is acutely or chronically mentally ill or seriously disturbed, and the setting can provide the service, the first available intake will be assigned otherwise an appropriate referral will be made.[24] Screening dispositions must be recorded, although the setting's standards will determine how much detail is necessary.[25]

At the intake evaluation, the following is assessed and must be documented:[26]

1. a clear statement of the presenting problems in the client's or guardian's own words;

2. a psychosocial, substance abuse, and medical history;

---

20. RCW 42.17.340(1); Oliver v. Harborview Medical Center, 94 Wash.2d 559, 618 P.2d 76 (1980).
21. *Id.*
22. Chapter 71.24 RCW; RCW 71.24.025(5); WAC 275-56-015(8).
23. WAC 275-56-110; WAC 275-56-310 for general outline of required policies and procedures related to client records.
24. WAC 275-56-255(2).
25. WAC 275-56-255(3).
26. WAC 275-56-260.

3. a history of mental health treatment covering at least the last two years;[27]

4. if the client is younger than 18 years of age, a developmental, academic, and learning problem history;

5. a mental status examination;

6. direct observations about the client's behavior;

7. a summation of the client's current level of functioning, strengths, needs, and problems, with a determination of whether the person is acutely or chronically mentally ill or seriously disturbed, and a provisional *Diagnostic and Statistical Manual–III (DSM-III)* diagnosis;[28]

8. the name and telephone number of the client's most recent physician and the date of the last examination or treatment;

9. the need and justification for special psychiatric, psychological, neuropsychological, or medical examinations, tests, or procedures;[29]

10. a drug-use profile to include the names, dosages, prescribing person's name, dates of use, reasons for changes or discontinuance, and any significant side effects of all prescribed and nonprescribed drugs used during the previous six months;[30] and

11. cross references to the records of any immediate family members who may be clients at the setting.[31]

If the county setting is an institutional setting, the records also must include the promulgated requirements that apply to a voluntary or involuntary admission.[32]

From the onset, a client may be served by both a primary therapist and by a case manager who should confer regularly and document the conferences.[33] An individualized treatment plan

---

27. If inpatient or residential treatment has occurred during this period, either the records or summaries of them must be included within the client's record (WAC 275-56-315(5)).

28. American Psychiatric Association, Committee on Nomenclature and Statistics. (1980). *Diagnostic and Statistical Manual of Mental Disorders* (3rd ed.). Washington, D.C.: Author.

29. Before diagnosis of primary degenerative dementia with senile or presenile onset is made, all other forms of treatable medical or mental disorders must be ruled out, WAC 275-56-260(5).

30. WAC 275-56-265.

31. WAC 275-56-315(9).

32. *See* State Mental Health Institutions in text above. In addition, the certification standards for a county facility regulate record keeping as well as other staff responsibilities. However, the regulations of the Community Mental Health Services Act exceed in scope the certification standards previously promulgated by the legislature. *See* WAC 275-55-263.

33. WAC 275-56-270.

must be developed for each client and contain the following elements:[34]

1. the problems to be addressed by the treatment;

2. the goals of the treatment and anticipated changes in client behavior, skills, attitudes, or circumstances, and a time frame for attainment of the goals and termination of services;

3. the services and specific treatment modalities that the client will use, the expected referrals for those services that the practitioner is not able to provide,[35] and the identification of the primary therapist and/or case manager;

4. a justification of how the services, modalities, and referrals will address the needs and treatment goals of the client;

5. a review updating the plan each 90 days for outpatient, day-treatment, or community support services;

6. a signed consent from the client or guardian as to the initial plan and any significant subsequent changes to the plan (see chapter 6.1, Informed Consent for Services).

The requirements for group treatment plans are much less thorough. Practitioners are required to record the goals of the group, the modalities and approaches intended to produce these goals, and the common needs and characteristics of the clients within the group.[36] Outpatient group records must contain cross references to individual client records[37] as well as documentation about the fees to be charged for services.[38]

For both individual and group records, the practitioners should make brief progress notes. Frequency varies with the type of service: outpatient services, after each client contact; day treatment, at least weekly; and emergency services, after each instance.[39] Progress notes must document the date, nature of service, progress toward established goals, changes in treatment

---

34. WAC 275-56-275.
35. WAC 275-56-315, the record shall contain a report of each collateral contact.
36. WAC 275-56-280. Also, group records are to include the name of the staff responsible for leading the group, a current roster of all clients, brief notes documenting group activities and events, and modifications in the group plan, WAC 275-56-320.
37. WAC 275-56-315(4).
38. WAC 275-56-315(1)(b).
39. WAC 275-56-285(1). If practitioners use a problem-oriented record system, regardless of the type(s) of service, they need enter only the date, type of each contact, and a narrative summary of the client's progress at least every 30 days.

plan, referrals, and extraordinary events,[40] and be signed by the treating practitioner.[41] Changes in the treatment plan must include a periodic assessment of the need for continued treatment and the projected length of time that the additional treatment would take.[42] Whenever possible, the clinical supervisor must participate in the formal progress assessment, reviewing, approving, and signing summaries prepared by the primary therapist or by the case manager.[43]

If medications are used, the treatment must be reviewed by a physician every three months.[44] A registered nurse or a licensed practical nurse may administer them under the supervision of a physician.[45] The client record must indicate the following:[46]

1. name of the medication;

2. dosage and method of administration;

3. purpose of medication;

4. dates prescribed, reviewed, or renewed;

5. observed effects and side effects, including laboratory findings and corrective actions taken for side effects;

6. reasons for change or termination of medication; and

7. the name and signature of the prescribing person. (A signed consent for use of any medication also is required.)[47]

If the client transfers to another setting or formally terminates treatment, a summary of the treatment is to be entered in the client's record within 14 days.[48] The case need not be closed when a documented, planned leave does not exceed 90 days.[49] Unexplained interruptions in client contact must be followed up and

---

40. WAC 275-56-305 defines and establishes procedures for extraordinary events. These events include (a) injury to the client or staff, (b) suicide or homicide by the client, (c) client behaviors so bizarre or disruptive as to threaten the program, and (d) disaster or threatened disaster of a natural or human origin. Each of these events shall be reported to an appropriate supervisory staff, administrator, or governing body. Although reporting is curbed by the confidentiality provisions (see chapter 4.2, Confidential Relations and Communications), all disclosures outside the setting must be documented as described above (RCW 71.05.420; WAC 275-56-315(1)(c)). A review of each occurrence is required by one or more MHPs not participating in the treatment. A review, corrective action plan, and its implementation shall be documented within the client's record when appropriate.
41. WAC 275-56-285(2).
42. WAC 275-56-285(4).
43. WAC 275-56-285(5).
44. WAC 275-56-295(2).
45. Id.
46. WAC 275-56-295(3).
47. WAC 275-56-315(1)(d).
48. WAC 275-56-290(1) and (2).
49. WAC 275-56-290(3).

documented by the primary therapist or case manager, and the case must be closed within 90 days of the last attempt to reach the client.[50]

In telephone and outreach emergency services, the extensiveness of documented records is reduced. After each contact, the practitioner must document the following, when possible:[51] client name (name of person and agency if other than client), address (note location), telephone number, and time of initial contact or outreach; responsible staff involved and names of persons and agencies cooperating in the emergency response; nature of the emergency; summary of services provided; referrals or other disposition; follow-up summary; and condition of the client at termination of contact. Any departures from the written protocol of the setting are to be documented.[52] Decisions not to respond with outreach services require recording as well.[53]

(C)(2) Maintenance of Records

All client records must be maintained in locked cabinets or in a fully enclosed room with a locked door; they may be checked out during the day, but must be returned to the record storage area at the end of the day.[54] Records must be retained for a least five years after the last contact with the client. However, a termination summary and reports of special assessment or examination procedures are to be retained at least ten years.[55] Emergency records, such as for telephone or outreach services, must be maintained for at least two years.[56]

(C)(3) Client Access

When a client asks to review the case record, the practitioner must grant this request within seven days, after removing any material confidential to another person[57] or records received from other practitioners. Although the records should be reviewed in the

---

50. WAC 275-56-290(3).
51. WAC 275-56-325.
52. WAC 275-56-350(c); WAC 275-56-355(a).
53. WAC 275-56-355(2).
54. WAC 275-56-330.
55. WAC 275-56-335(3). If the client is a minor, the records must be retained for the longer of either three years beyond the 18th birthday or five years beyond the last contact, WAC 275-56-335(2).
56. Id.
57. WAC 275-56-235(2). A parent or guardian of a child 13 years of age or younger may request a review of the record, but a practitioner may refuse the request if there is reason to believe that the parent or parent surrogate has harmed the child. Unless a minor older than 13 years requests to review the records and consents to having the parent or guardian present, records cannot be accessed by anyone other than the minor. See also RCW 13.50.100(4)(a).

presence of a staff member of the setting (in part, to answer questions), the client should be provided with sufficient time and privacy to review the record.[58] The fact and content of the review session should be documented in the client's record.[59]

(D) Department of Corrections

(D)(1) Extensiveness of Records

All client records are referred to as *medical records* because allied health professionals may treat clients only under the supervision of a licensed physician.[60] Internal written policies and procedures exist for the screening, referral, and care of mentally ill, developmentally disabled, or alcohol- or other substance-addicted prisoners.[61] The legislature has mandated that the following health care records be maintained for all findings, diagnoses, treatments, dispositions, prescriptions, and administration of medications; notes concerning patient education; notations of place, date, and time of medical encounters and of terminations of treatment.[62] The legislature also requires that records include detailed reports of admission evaluations and recommendations, progress notes regarding continuing health status, results of consultations, reports of tests done, and reports made by outside consultants.[63]

(D)(2) Maintenance of Records

The law does not specify how long records should be kept. So long as the prisoner is within state institutions, the records must be transferred with the inmate.[64]

(D)(3) Client Access

Treatment records are not exempted from disclosure.[65] A client may gain access to these records under the Public Disclosure Act.[66]

---

58. WAC 275-56-235(2)(c).
59. *Id.*
60. WAC 137-91-050.
61. WAC 289-20-105.
62. WAC 289-20-150.
63. WAC 137-91-060.
64. *Id.*
65. WAC 137-08-150(1)
66. *See* chapter 4.5.

(E) Private Psychiatric Hospitals

(E)(1) Extensiveness of Records

Each hospital must have written policies and procedures about admission criteria, treatment methods, and retention of patients.[67] Unless a comprehensive health assessment and medical history about a client are completed within 14 days before admission and the information is recorded in the clinical record, the regulations require that a new assessment and history be recorded within 48 hours of admission.[68] Within 72 hours of admission, a psychiatric evaluation (including a provisional *DSM-III* diagnosis) must be documented[69] and a comprehensive, individualized treatment plan developed.[70] The psychiatric condition of the patient must be described clearly, including a history of findings and treatment rendered.[71] The plan should be implemented, reviewed, and modified as indicated.[72] Any orders for drug prescriptions, medical treatment, and discharge must be signed by the physician.[73] Finally, an adequate clinical record must be maintained for every patient, with each entry being dated and authenticated.[74] Although there is no specific definition of *adequate*, presumably, the record must be sufficient to provide clinical services.

(E)(2) Maintenance of Records

Records must be retained for 10 years after the last contact with the patient.[75] However, if the patient is younger than 18 years of age, the records must be retained until the patient obtains the age of 21 years or for at least 10 years, whichever is longer.[76]

The records are to remain at the hospital in event of transfer of ownership.[77] But if the hospital ceases operation, arrangements for preservation of the records must be approved by the Washington Department of Social and Health Services.[78]

---

67. WAC 248-22-021(1).
68. WAC 248-22-021(4)(a)(ii).
69. WAC 248-22-021(4)(a)(iii).
70. WAC 248-22-021(2)(a)(ii).
71. WAC 248-22-041(7).
72. WAC 248-22-021(2)(a)(ii).
73. WAC 248-22-021 (4)(a)(iv).
74. WAC 248-22-041(3).
75. WAC 248-22-041(9)(a).
76. *Id.*
77. WAC 248-22-041(9)(c).
78. WAC 248-22-041(9)(d).

(E)(3) Client Access

Access to clinical records is regulated, in part, by the policies of the setting.[79] Statutory language states that records at public or private agencies may be disclosed only when those receiving services (or their guardians) designate persons to whom records may be released.[80]

Patients may not be denied access to their records,[81] However, access to records of juveniles is treated differently. If it is determined by the agency that release of the records is likely to cause severe psychological or physical harm to the juvenile or to his or her parents, the agency may withhold the information.[82]

(F) Alcohol and Drug Treatment Facilities

(F)(1) Extensiveness of Records

Residential and outpatient facilities must maintain client records that include the following information:[83]

1. an intake form with the client's full name, gender, birth date, date of admission, address, and telephone number or of the client's next of kin or other responsible person, and name and city of the client's physician, if any;

2. an evaluation of the client's involvement with alcohol or drugs supported by a list of signs and symptoms;

3. a treatment plan that establishes objectives for addressing specific problems, time-linked means to be used in reaching the objectives, and anticipated length of treatment or physicians' standing orders if the client is in an inpatient detoxication facility;

4. progress notes relating the client's response to treatment and noting all significant events;

5. formal reviews of the treatment plan to assess the adequacy of the plan in light of the client's status and progress as required by WAC 275-19-165(5);

6. authentication of each entry by the practitioners;

7. a copy of any program rules signed and dated by the client;

---

79. Oliver v. Harborview Medical Center, 94 Wash.2d 559, 618 P.2d.76 (1980).
80. RCW 71.05.390(3).
81. RCW 70.02.090.
82. RCW 13.50.100(4). A court may determine that a limited release is appropriate. *See also* WAC 275-56-235(2), *supra* Footnote 57.
83. WAC 275-19-170(3).

8. a consent to treatment, signed and dated by the client;

9. any authorizations for release of information;

10. a copy of the client's aftercare plan;

11. date of discharge, a summary of the client's progress in meeting the objectives outlined in the treatment plan or, if a detoxication facility, a summary of the client's physical condition after detoxication or drug withdrawal; and

12. any medical records, including findings from the physical examination, orders for any drug or medical treatment, and medical progress notes.[84]

Often, alcohol and drug treatment involve the continuation of treatment in other settings. If the client provides a release of information, the following documentation must be sent to the new setting before the arrival of the client:[85] a copy of the intake form, the evaluation, the treatment history, the reason for the referral, the court mandated or agency recommended follow-up treatment, and a copy of the discharge summary.

(F)(2) Maintenance of Records

Client files must be kept for at least five years after the last contact or discharge of the client.[86] With the client's consent, records may be sent to any other approved treatment center if the original treatment facility closes. When consent is not obtained, the record must be sealed and labeled as follows:[87] Records of (insert name of approved treatment facility) required to be maintained, pursuant to WAC 275-19-170, until a date not later than December 31, (insert year). The sealed records must be forwarded to the Washington Department of Social and Health Services.[88]

(F)(3) Client Access

If clients wish to review their own treatment records, the treatment facilities must provide a review in the presence of a staff person.[89]

(F)(4) Access by Department of Social and Health Services

The clinical records at any approved facility may be open for inspection to verify the provision of services and compliance with

---

84. WAC 248-26-050(3).
85. WAC 275-19-165(10).
86. WAC 275-19-170(2).
87. Id.
88. Id.
89. WAC 275-19-075(1)(f). However, see supra Footnote 82. Access to records may be treated differently.

Chapter 275-18 WAC.[90] Presumably, the intention of this regulation is to prevent fraud. There is no indication of the extent to which the department may review records.[91]

(G) Private Practitioners in Noninstitutional Settings

The Uniform Health Care Information Act enacted in 1991 greatly affected access to client records.[92] The law applies to all health care providers who are licensed, certified, or registered to practice within the state of Washington.[93] However, this chapter does not apply to MHPs in some instances or to those within state-approved alcohol and drug treatment programs even when they are private.[94]

(G)(1) Extensiveness

The Uniform Health Care Information Act specifies that the following written notice of information practices be entered into the record:[95]

NOTICE

We keep a record of the health care services that we provide to you.

You may request to see and to make a copy of that record. You may also ask us to correct that record. We will not disclose your record to others unless you direct us to do so or unless the law authorizes or compels us to do so. You may see your record or get more information about it at. . . .

In addition, all disclosures of health care information must be documented, except disclosures to third-party health care payors.[96] To be valid, a disclosure authorization to the health care provider must[97]

1. be in writing, dated, and signed by the patient or client;

2. identify the nature of the information to be disclosed;

---

90. WAC 275-19-060(1).
91. *See* chapter 4.2 for discussion about restricting review by state agency of confidential, clinical records.
92. Chapter 70.02 RCW.
93. RCW 71.02.010(7).
94. RCW 71.02.900(2). Statutory construction would lead a court to apply the law of the Health Care Information Act unless it provided less procedural protection than Chapters 70.41, 71.05, 71.12, 71.24, 71.34, 10.77 RCW.
95. RCW 71.02.120.
96. RCW 71.02.020.
97. RCW 71.02.030(3).

3. identify the name, address, and institutional affiliation of the person to whom the information is to be disclosed;

4. identify the provider who is to make the disclosure; and

5. identify the patient or client.

(G)(2) Maintenance

Under the Act, health care providers must create reasonable safeguards to secure the health care information that they maintain.[98] The providers must maintain a record of existing health care information for at least one year following:[99] a receipt of authority to disclose the information, a request for correction or amendment of the record, or a request for examination and copying of the record. No other holding period for records is specified.

(G)(3) Client Access

An MHP may not deny access to cient records.[100] If the client is a juvenile, access to the records may be limited.[101] Information may be withheld if its release is likely to cause severe psychological or physical harm. If such circumstances exist, the court must determine what limited release is appropriate.[102] The providers may charge a fee not to exceed the usual charge of a basic office visit for searching, duplicating, and editing the record and do not have to honor an authorization until the fee is paid.[103]

If patients or clients send a written request to examine or copy all or part of their record, the providers must, as soon as possible but no later than 15 working days:[104]

1. make the information available for examination during regular business hours;

2. inform the patient if the information does not exist or cannot be found;

3. inform the patient if the record is maintained by another health care provider and provide its name and address, if known;

4. specify in writing the unusual circumstances delaying the fulfillment of the request and state when the information will be

---

98. RCW 71.02.150.
99. RCW 71.02.160. A juvenile's record is controlled by RCW 13.50. *See supra* Footnote 82.
100. *See supra* Footnote 57.
101. RCW 13.50.100(4).
102. RCW 13.50.100(4)(a).
103. RCW 71.02.030.
104. RCW 71.02.080.

available but, in no case, should the delay be longer than 21 working days from receipt of the request; or

5. deny the request, in whole or part, as specified above.

The provider must provide an explanation of any code or abbreviation used in the record, but need not rewrite the record.[105] Examination and copying of the record may be denied until the actual cost for providing the health care information is paid.[106]

(H) Psychiatrists

There are few laws pertaining to the extensiveness and maintenance of or to client access to psychiatric records specifically.

(H)(1) Maintenance of Records

The principles of medical ethics suggest that client records be held in perpetuity.[107] When a physician retires or dies, clients should be notified and urged to find a treating practitioner who would receive the records upon authorization of the client.

(H)(2) Client Access

Upon request of the client, physicians should provide a summary of the record.[108] (See footnote 100.) Client access to information cannot be denied except to juveniles, as specified earlier.

(H)(3) Access by the Board of Medical Examiners

Physicians engage in unprofessional conduct if they refuse to cooperate with the disciplinary authority by not furnishing client records or not submitting a response to the matter contained in a complaint.[109] Violation of the above law may result in restriction, suspension, or revocation of the psychiatrist's license.[110] Failure to abide by the ethical principles may also result in civil liability.

---

105. RCW 71.02.070(2).
106. *Id.* Corrections or amendments to the record and to the process by which a statement of disagreement is created are specified by RCW 71.02.100 and .110.
107. Washington State Medical Association Principles of Medical Ethics, § 7.03.
108. *Id.* at § 7.02.
109. RCW 18.130.180(8).
110. RCW 18.130.110.

(I) Psychologists

There are few laws pertaining specifically to the psychologists' record-keeping duties. A general rule states that "in those areas in which recognized standards do not yet exist, psychologists (may) take whatever precautions are necessary to protect the welfare of their clients."[111]

(I)(1) Extensiveness of records

At the start of any professional relationship (see chapter 6.1), psychologists are required to disclose and to document client receipt of information relating to the right of the client to refuse treatment; the responsibility of clients for choosing the provider and treatment modality that best suits their needs; the extent to which confidences can be protected; the relevant education and training of the psychologist; the therapeutic orientation of the practice; the proposed course of treatment when known; and any requirements for payment of services.[112]

(I)(2) Maintenance of Records

Psychologists must make provisions for maintaining confidentiality in the storage and disposal of records.[113]

(I)(3) Client Access

Client access to information cannot be denied except to juveniles, as specified earlier (see footnote 100).

(I)(4) Access by the Examining Board of Psychology

Psychologists are guilty of unethical practice if they fail to cooperate with the Disciplinary Committee of the licensing board, to furnish documents, or to respond to the matter contained in a complaint,[114] which may encompass material within client records. However, to obtain information that otherwise might be confidential or privileged, the Committee must first obtain the written consent of the complaining client(s), or of the legal representative, or of any person affected by the complaint.[115] Violation of this law may result in restriction, suspension, or revocation of the psychologist's license. Failure to abide by the laws may result also in civil liability.

---

111. WAC 308-122-620.
112. RCW 18.83.115(1).
113. WAC 308-122-650.
114. RCW 18.83.120(7).
115. RCW 18.83.135(14).

(J) Practitioners Certified by the Omnibus Credentialing Act for Counselors[116]

(J)(1) Extensiveness of Records

Practitioners certified under this Act are required to disclose and to document, at the start of any professional relationship, that the client received information regarding the right of clients to refuse treatment; the responsibility of the clients for choosing the provider and treatment modality that best suits their needs; the extent to which confidences can be protected; the relevant education and training of the counselor; the therapeutic orientation of the practice; the proposed course of treatment when known; any requirements for payment of services; and a statement indicating that *registration* of the practitioner does not include recognition of any practice standards nor does it necessarily imply the effectiveness of any treatment.[117]

(J)(2) Maintenance of Records

The Health Care Information Act appears to be the only law establishing any requirements for maintenance of records.

(J)(3) Client Access

Client access to information cannot be denied except to juveniles, as specified earlier (see footnote 100).

(J)(4) Access by Board Regulating MHPs Registered or Certified Under Chapter 18.19 RCW

Counselors are guilty of unethical practice if they fail to cooperate with the Disciplinary Committee, to respond to matter contained in a complaint,[118] or to furnish documents, including material within client records that may be subpoenaed because of the complaint.[119] Violation of the above laws may result in restriction, suspension, or revocation of the counselor's registration or certification and also in civil liability.

---

116. *See* chapter 1.5.
117. RCW 18.19.060.
118. RCW 18.130.180(8).
119. RCW 18.19.180(5).

(K) General Recommendations for All Types of Practitioners

(K)(1) Extensiveness of Records

It is likely that the courts in the state of Washington will apply a high standard of care to the practice of mental health.[120] The absence of records may be construed, by a fact finder, as an indication that the practitioner has evaded reasonable case-management duties, at best, or destroyed documentation about the case, at worst.[121] At a minimum, practitioners should document the following:

1. informed consent of the client to treatment (see chapter 6.1);
2. a listing of the symptoms and the therapeutic needs of the client;
3. whether any symptoms may be due to physiological causes, a note about referring the client to a physician for a physical examination if a recent examination cannot be documented, or documentation that the client refused such a referral;
4. previous records of any recent counseling that the client may have obtained or a notation that the client would not provide consent to obtain earlier records;
5. treatment decisions and progress toward treatment goals;
6. evaluation results and treatment decisions about extraordinary client events (e.g., actual threats of danger to self or others); and
7. notation about the release of any information to others.

(K)(2) Maintenance of Records

Although there is no specific requirement, the accepted period of time for maintaining records appears to be five years after the termination of treatment. This is the standard that applies in most public and private institutional settings. Practitioners are urged to make provisions for the maintenance of their records should the practice end (e.g., death of the practitioner).

(K)(3) Client Access

Client access to information cannot be denied except to juveniles, as specified earlier, see footnote 100.

---

120. Peterson v. State of Washington, 100 Wash.2d 421, 671 P.2d 230 (1983).
121. Pope, K. S., Simpson, N. H., & Weiner, M. F. *Malpractice in outpatient psychotherapy*, 32 Am. J. of Psychotherapy, 593–601 (1978); Rheingold, P. D. *How to know a good medical malpractice case*, 70 Am. Bar Assoc. J., The Lawyers Magz. 70–74 (1984).

Confidential Relations and Communications

A *confidential communication* is written or verbal information conveyed by the client to a practitioner in the course of a professional relationship. Confidentiality requirements for some health care providers may be found in the professional ethics codes[1] and, for other providers, in the law.[2] It is commonly accepted that effective evaluation and treatment require the revelation of the deepest thoughts and secrets of the client while protecting the client from the embarrassment, scandal, or incrimination that might result if the information were to be released. Central to providing the full benefit of professional treatment to the client is the encouragement of candor.[3] Thus, client communications are kept confidential, unless the client provides written consent to release confidential information or to waive the privilege of confidentiality (see chapter 4.3).

(A) Laws or Rules that Apply to All Health Care Professionals

The principle of confidentiality was reconfirmed recently by the Uniform Health Care Information Act (UHCIA), which states that

---

1. American Medical Association. (1980). *Principles of Medical Ethics*. Washington, DC: Author. American Psychological Association. (1981). Ethical principles of psychologists. *American Psychologist*, 36, 633–38.
2. For instance, for social workers, mental health counselors, and marriage and family therapists, the duty to protect client confidences is established by RCW 18.19.180.
3. RCW 71.05.390; Taylor v. U.S., 222 F.2d. 398, 401 (D.C. Cir. 1955); State v. Sullivan, 60 Wash.2d. 214, 225, 373 P.2d 474, 480 (1962).

any licensed, certified, or registered health care provider may not disclose health care information about a patient to any other person without the patient's written authorization.[4] The UHCIA does not modify the terms or conditions of disclosure and of rules adopted about disclosure that apply to MHPs.[5] Nevertheless, the following UHCIA changes will affect how MHPs respond to protecting confidences.

(B) Mental Health Care Providers

Disclosure of information may be made only with the written, dated, and signed authorization of the patient. The authorization must specify[6]

1. the nature of the information to be disclosed;

2. the name, address, and institutional affiliation of the person to whom the disclosure is to be made;

3. the identity of the provider making the disclosure; and

4. the identity of the patient.

The provider must retain the written authorization in the patient's records and must chart each disclosure, except to third party payors. No statement limiting redisclosure must accompany the released information. An authorization lapses automatically in 90 days from the date signed,[7] unless a patient revokes it in writing.[8]

Disclosure of client records without authorization are significantly limited by specific laws.[9] As a result, the UHCIA section does not apply to MHPs.[10] Mental health client confidences may be disclosed only[11] among professional persons providing ser-

---

4. The UHCIA went into effect on July 28, 1991 and is codified in RCW 70.02 *et seq.*
5. RCW 70.02.900(2).
6. RCW 70.02.030.
7. *Id.*
8. RCW 70.02.040.
9. RCW 71.05.390 specifies several possible disclosures without client authorization for purposes of continuity of care, quality assurance, claim reimbursements, and various notifications because of duties to report. *But see* chapter 5A.7, Reporting of Adult Abuse and Neglect, and chapter 5A.8, Reporting of Maltreatment of Minors.
10. RCW 70.02.050 would not apply because RCW 70.02.900(2) states that the laws established under Chapters 71.05 and 71.34 RCW and rules adopted under these provisions are not modified by the UHCIA. The principle of statutory construction would not be applied because the UHCIA is less specific then the other laws that exist.
11. RCW 71.05.390. Also *see* RCW 71.05.630(2); it is discussed fully at footnote 92, chapter 5E.4, Involuntary Civil Admission of Mentally Ill Adults.

vices or referrals to the client; during guardianship proceedings; to the extent necessary for a recipient to make a claim for aid, insurance, or medical assistance; for program evaluation and/or research so long as specific protections are followed; to the courts as necessary during involuntary commitment proceedings; to law enforcement and public health officers or to personnel of the Department of Corrections;[12] to the attorney of the detained person; to the prosecuting attorney for purposes of committing the person to involuntary treatment; to appropriate law enforcement agencies and to reasonably identifiable victims whose health and safety have been threatened or who have been repeatedly harassed; to persons designated by statute when the person detained is a sex offender;[13] to the patient's next of kin or guardian in the event of his or her death; and to persons designated by a court who has ordered the release of records, only upon good cause shown, if the court finds that appropriate safeguards for strict confidentiality will be maintained.

If an MHP violates any provision of the UHCIA, the violation may result in a civil law suit by the patient for actual damages caused as well as for attorney's fees.[14] However, there are other laws still in force that, in some instances, provide liquidated or treble damages for violating confidences obtained from a recipient of voluntary or involuntary services at either public or private agencies.[15] Furthermore, practitioners may be the object of civil suits by clients who have been harmed by breaches of confidentiality (see chapter 6.5).

(C) Alcohol and Drug Treatment Providers

The confidentiality of alcohol and drug treatment records for health care providers who work within state-approved alcohol and drug treatment settings are regulated by both state and federal laws, with federal law superseding state law, unless the state law is more restrictive.[16] Disclosure of information must be

---

12. RCW 71.05.390(7) specifies many restrictions.
13. RCW 71.05.280(3); RCW 71.05.320(2)(c); RCW 71.05.425.
14. RCW 70.02.170.
15. RCW 71.05.390 and .440.
16. RCW 70.96A.150; WAC 275-19-074, -075; WAC 248-18-235; WAC 248-22-041; WAC 248-18-235. The Public Health Service of the Department of Health and Human Services of the United States, pursuant to § 408 of the Drug Abuse Prevention, Treatment and Rehabilitation Act (42 U.S.C. § 290dd-3); see 42 C.F.R. § 2.1 et seq. (1991).

made in accordance with the written, dated, and signed authorization of the patient.

The authorization must address[17]

1. the nature and extent of the information to be disclosed;
2. the name, address, and institutional affiliation of the person to whom the disclosure is to be made;
3. the identity of the provider making the disclosure;
4. the identity of the patient;
5. the need for the disclosure; and
6. the revocation of the authorization, including the expiration date of said authorization.

The provider must retain the written authorization in the patient's records and must chart each disclosure.[18] A statement limiting redisclosure must accompany the information released.[19] A patient may revoke an authorization at any time, even orally; the authorization will lapse automatically 90 days from the date on which it was signed.[20]

Alcohol and drug treatment client confidences are subject to disclosure only when the patient provides a release;[21] for good cause upon court approval to issue a subpoena compelling production of records or testimony;[22] to comply with state laws mandating the reporting of suspected child abuse or neglect;[23] when a patient commits a crime on the program premises or against program personnel, or threatens to do so;[24] to the extent necessary to meet a medical emergency;[25] and for research and audit purposes so long as specific protective measures are followed.[26] It is unclear whether a health care provider must report an actual threat of physical violence against a reasonably identifiable victim[27] and disclose to the public health officer the identities of partners of a client who is HIV infected.[28] Health care providers who face this conflict in law should seek legal counsel and obtain a written opinion as to how to meet the conflicting requirements of confidentiality and those of protecting third parties.

---

17. 42 CFR § 2.31.
18. WAC 275-19-170.
19. *See* 42 CFR § 2.32 for specific language to use in the prohibition.
20. RCW 70.02.040 is more specific than the federal law, so it would be applied.
21. RCW 70.96A.150(1)(a).
22. RCW 70.96A.150(1)(b); 42 C.F.R. § 2.61(a).
23. RCW 70.96A.150(1)(c).
24. RCW 70.96A.150(1)(d).
25. 42 CFR § 2.51.
26. 42 CFR § 2.53.
27. RCW 71.05.120.
28. RCW 70.24.105(2)(g); WAC 248-100-072.

(D) Liability for Violation

Violations of confidentiality may result in suspension or revocation of license or in censure or probation (see chapter 1.1). Failure to abide by a law that prescribes a minimum standard of conduct may result in civil liability for negligence (see chapter 6.5). Clients also may bring suit on the basis of other legal theories. Chapter 6.6 describes other actions that have been used with varying degrees of success.

4.3

Privileged
Communications

The confidentiality standards (see chapter 4.2) may not protect client disclosures from being revealed at a court hearing. However, most written or verbal information conveyed by the client to a practitioner in the course of a professional relationship is protected from disclosure in the courtroom by privileged communications statutes. The privileged communications statutes are designed solely to protect the client and will not protect all communications. The law views the willful betrayal of a health care practitioner–patient privilege as unprofessional conduct.[1] During the informed consent process, practitioners should advise their clients of the extent to which their communications can be protected.

(A) Privilege for Psychiatrists

The physician–client privilege is codified in two separate statutes that cover both civil and criminal actions. The statute that applies to civil actions appears broader as it covers all communications in physician–client relationships, not only the communications with the client's physician:

> A physician. . .shall not, without the consent of his patient, be examined in a civil action as to any information acquired in attending such patient, which was necessary to enable him to prescribe or act for the patient.[2]

---

1. RCW 18.130.180.
2. RCW 5.60.060(4).

In contrast, the statute that applies to criminal actions is narrowed to only "regular" physicians:

> In criminal prosecutions. . . regular physicians. . .shall be protected from testifying as to confessions, or information received from any defendant.[3]

Although undefined, presumably, a *regular* physician is one who has treated the defendant before the alleged crime occurred.

(B) Privilege for Psychologists

The psychologist–client privilege assures that

> Confidential communications between a client and a psychologist shall be privileged against compulsory disclosure to the same extent and subject to the same conditions as confidential communications between attorney and client.[4]

The law remains unclear as to whether such language protects psychologist–client confidences to a greater extent than physician–client confidences.[5] In a case involving attorney–client privilege, an attorney refused to reveal information based on a good-faith claim of privilege at the lower court level, and could not be held in contempt of court pending appellate review of the issue.[6]

(C) Privilege for Health Care Providers Certified by the Omnibus Credentialing Act[7]

Unlike physicians and psychologists, other health care providers may testify and reveal communications about the contemplation or commission of a crime or harmful act regardless of the client's wishes.[8]

---

3. RCW 10.52.020.
4. RCW 18.83.110.
5. Petersen v. State of Washington, 100 Wash.2d 421, 429 (1983).
6. Seventh Elect Church v. Rogers, 102 Wash.2d 527, 688 P.2d 506 (1984).
7. Chapter 18.19 RCW.
8. RCW 18.19.180(2) and (3). Information communicated to practitioners during the treatment of alcohol abusers or of users of narcotic or dangerous drugs is considered to be privileged in criminal proceedings, RCW 69.54.070.

(D) Assertion and Waiver of the Privilege

The court will not assume that a privilege exists merely on the assertion that the practitioner has seen the client in a professional capacity. Usually, a lawyer representing the client and a lawyer seeking to limit the protection of privilege will base their arguments on the following facts before the judge arrives at a determination:

1. did the client see the mental health practitioner in a professional capacity;
2. is the communication confidential;
3. has the client waived the privilege.

The first question is answered easily if the practitioner is licensed or certified, and the client believes that the consultation with the practitioner is for evaluation or treatment; who employed the practitioner is unimportant.[9] Even if the practitioner is unlicensed or uncertified and no fee has been paid, it is the client's belief in the status of the relationship with the practitioner that would give rise to the privilege.[10]

As to the second question, the privilege extends only to information acquired when the practitioner is professionally attending to the client. This would include communications or information obtained by observation or during the interaction between the practitioner and the client.[11]

The privilege may be waived expressly or by implication (i.e., the client acts in a way that indicates an intent to waive). Common examples of waiver occur when the[12]

---

9. State v. Gibson, 3 Wash. App. 496, 476 P.2d 727(1970).
10. *Id.*, a case applying to a psychiatrist–client relationship. *See* State v. Fagalde, 85 Wash.2d 730, 539 P.2d 865 (1975), a case involving a psychologist–client relationship, with other precedents being established by the attorney–client cases of McGlothlen, 99 Wash.2d 515, 663 P.2d 1330 (1983); and Heidebrink v. Moriwaki, 38 Wash. App. 388, 685 P.2d 1109 (1984), *reversed on other grounds*, 104 Wash. 2d 392, 706 P.2d 212 (1985).
11. For psychiatrist–client relationships, *see* State v. Gibson, 3 Wash. App. 496, 476 P.2d 727 (1970), and State v. Broussard, 12 Wash. App. 355, 529 P.2d 1128 (1974). For psychologist–client relationships, *see* State v. Dorman, 30 Wash. App. 351, 633 P.2d 1340 (1981), information privileged only if attorney is consulted in the capacity of legal advisor; Somers v. Olwell, 64 Wash. 2d 828, 394 P.2d 681 (1964), information privileged only if communicated or delivered by client to attorney while attorney was acting as legal advisor.
12. In general, *see* Aronson, Robert H. (1994). *The Law of Evidence in Washington*. Salem, NH: Butterworth Legal Publishers. Note that the death of the client does not serve as a waiver, Martin v. Shaen, 22 Wash.2d 505, 156 P.2d 640 (1945).

1. client fails to assert privilege at first opportunity in a judicial setting (e.g., at trial, in a deposition, or in response to interrogations);[13]

2. client discloses the communication to a third person who is not in a protected relationship (e.g., client agrees to an evaluation at the request of a state agency with the results of the evaluation to be used in an agency action,[14] or the client makes an admission to a police officer);[15]

3. client files a legal action against the practitioner;[16]

4. client/defendant raises a mental disability defense in a criminal trial or asserts that he or she is incompetent to stand trial (see chapters 5D.5 and 5D.9);[17] or

5. client's lawyer introduces testimony describing the evaluation and treatment of an illness at trial.[18]

The practitioner cannot refuse to release information to the court once the privilege is waived, even if the disclosures might be injurious to the client. Yet under the rules of evidence the information still may be ruled inadmissible if the probative value is outweighed by the prejudicial effect.[19]

In the absence of the client waiver, the privilege should be asserted by the practitioner.[20]

---

13. *Id.*

14. In re Henderson, 29 Wash. App. 748, 630 P.2d 944 (1981).

15. State v. Clark, 26 Wash.2d 160, 173 P.2d 189 (1946); however, if the third person is an agent of the physician or psychologist, including a police officer present for the protection of the practitioner, so long as the communication was intended to be confidential, it remains privileged. State v. Gibson, 3 Wash. App. 496, 476 P.2d 727 (1970).

16. Randa v. Bear 50 Wash.2d 415, 312 P.2d 640 (1957); however, if the personal inquiry of the client does not involve the treating MHP, unless the practitioner is included on the list of the client's witnesses, waiver will not be found. Phipps v Sasser, 74 Wash.2d 439, 445 P.2d 624 (1968).

17. State v. Tradewell, 9 Wash. App. 821, 515 P.2d 172 (1973), *reh. den.* 83 Wash.2d 1005 (1974), *cert. denied,* 416 U.S. 985 (1975).

18. Randa v. Bear 50 Wash.2d 415, 312 P.2d 640 (1957).

19. *See* Wash. R. Evid., 403.

20. Psychologists may depend upon attorney–client privilege law that provides great protection to an attorney who refuses to reveal information based on a good-faith claim of privilege at the lower court level. The practitioner cannot be held in contempt of court pending appellate review of the issue. Seventh Elect Church v. Rogers, 102 Wash.2d 527, 683 P.2d 506 (1984).

(E) Statutory Exceptions on the Scope of the Privilege

There are three general exceptions to the scope of the privilege. First, the different Boards of Examiners may subpoena attendance and production of documents or other information pertaining to investigations of their rules, regulations, or orders (see chapters 1.1 to .4). However, the specific Board must obtain the written consent of any client(s) who may be affected by the release of information that would otherwise be confidential or privileged.

A second limitation involves child, adult dependent, or elder abuse or neglect (see chapters 5A.7 to .10). Not only do practitioners have a duty to report abuse or neglect, but they must also testify as to communications by a perpetrator client or a victim client. As Aronson noted,[21] "under the spirit of this exception courts have found the privilege inapplicable in child dependency hearings[22] and in parental termination proceedings."[23] Repeatedly, Washington courts have found a broad legislative intent to permit as much information as possible to be considered in making a decision about the best interests of a child. For instance, in divorce actions in which a permanent parenting plan remains in dispute, circumstances indicating child neglect, a chronic physical or mental impairment, or alcohol or drug addiction may limit the privilege that protects mental health records from disclosure and the provider from having to testify at a deposition or a trial.[24]

The third limitation arises when a court, hearing a petition for involuntary commitment, finds that it is unreasonable to obtain an evaluation from any practitioner other than the one doing the treating.[25] In this instance, the treating-practitioner–client privilege will be construed as waived, and the practitioner must testify at either a 14-day or a 90-day probable cause hearing for detaining the client (see chapter 5E.4).[26]

(F) Liability for Violations

The law and responsible practice suggest that practitioners must inform their clients as to the statutory limitations of protecting confidentiality in legal proceedings (see chapter 6.1). Practitioners

---

21. *Supra*, Footnote 12.
22. In re Welfare of Coverdell, 39 Wash. App. 887, 696 P.2d 1241 (1975).
23. In re Welfare of Dodge, 29 Wash. App. 486, 628 P.2d 1343 (1974).
24. Marriage of Nordby, 41 Wash. App. 531, 705 P.2d 277 (1985).
25. RCW 71.05.250.
26. In re R., 97 Wash.2d 182, 641 P.2d 704 (1982).

who testify improperly may face civil liability for violating the duty to maintain confidences,[27] and disciplinary action by their Board for willful betrayal of a practitioner–patient privilege.[28]

---

27. State v. Mark, 23 Wash. App. 392, 597 P.2d 406 (1979). In dicta, the Washington Supreme Court stated that a physician would not be held liable for divulging privileged communications if the physician is ordered to testify.
28. RCW 18.130.180(20).

Search, Seizure, and Subpoena of Records

Search of an MHP's office and seizure of any property (including records) may occur only during a criminal investigation of the practitioner or of the client. If a court demands, from the practitioner, information that was obtained in a professional relationship with a client, the demand usually will be in the form of a subpoena. Both types of requests, search, or subpoena may affect confidential (see chapter 4.2) and privileged communications (see chapter 4.3). However, the seizure or subpoena of records does not necessarily mean that they ultimately will be admissible in court. That determination will be made at trial.

(A) Search and Seizure

The law in this area concerns a governmental official's search or seizure of things or places in which an individual has a reasonable expectation of privacy. Although warrantless searches are sometime permitted, they are restricted to exigent circumstances such as "real danger to the police or the public or a real danger that evidence. . . might be lost."[1] Search and seizure typically is authorized by a written order from a court upon request of a peace officer or of a prosecuting attorney.[2] A warrant may be issued to seize any[3]

1. evidence of a crime;

---

1. State v. Counts, 99 Wash.2d 54, 659 P.2d 1087 (1983) *citing* U.S. v. Bulman, 667 F.2d 1374, 1384 (11th Cir. 1982).
2. Superior Court Criminal Rules, 2.3(a).
3. Superior Court Criminal Rules, 2.3(b).

2. contraband, fruits of crime, or things otherwise criminally possessed;

3. weapons or other things by means of which a crime has been committed or reasonably appears about to be committed;

4. person for whose arrest there is probable cause or who is unlawfully restrained.

There must be an affidavit or sworn testimony establishing grounds (probable cause) for issuing the warrant; the warrant must describe the specific property or person to be seized and be used within 10 days of being issued.[4] Lawful entry into private premises requires that the police officers have a search warrant, announce their identity and purpose, and then ask for admittance. The officer may break into the building if exigent circumstances arise to justify forced entry.[5] Furthermore, the officer may search any person as a protection against concealed weapons[6] or when it appears that the sought after property is concealed on the person.[7] Additional property not listed on the warrant may be seized if it is in plain view while a valid search warrant is being executed.[8]

Police officers must seize property in the following manner:[9] a copy of the warrant and a receipt for the property taken must be given to the person present when the property is taken. If no person is present, a copy of the warrant and receipt may be posted, and an inventory of the property must be made in the presence of at least one other person. Persons objecting to any aspect of a search should contact their attorney rather than interfere with the peace officers.[10] The attorney may return to the court that issued the warrant to argue, in a written motion, whether the property is the same as that specified within the warrant or whether probable cause existed to seize the item. If the court is convinced, the items will be restored to the person from whom they were taken.[11] Also, a cause of action can be filed against the peace officers if they did unnecessary damage while conducting a search.[12]

---

4. Superior Court Criminal Rules, 2.3(c).
5. RCW 10.31.040; State v. Edwards, 20 Wash. App. 648, 581 P.2d 154 (1978).
6. State v. Hobart, 94 Wash.2d 437, 617 P.2d 429 (1980). A search may not go beyond what is necessary to detect the presence of weapons.
7. State v. Ryan, 163 Wash. 496, 1 P.2d 893 (1931); State v. Ringer, 100 Wash.2d 686, 674 P.2d 1240 (1983).
8. State v. Helmka, 86 Wash.2d 91, 542 P.2d 115 (1975).
9. Superior Court Criminal Rules, 2.3.
10. It may be requested that items that are seized or given up because of a subpoena remain in a sealed envelope until a Judge has ruled on a motion to overturn the original warrant or subpoena.
11. Superior Court Criminal Rules, 2.3(e).
12. Goldsby v. Stewart, 158 Wash. 39, 290 P. 422 (1930).

(B) Subpoena

A *subpoena* is a written order of the court compelling a witness to appear and give testimony. Although the law, in most cases, does not require that the subpoena be in a particular format, it should contain the name of the court, title of the action, and the time and place where the testimony is expected to be given.[13] It also may extend to documentary evidence and other tangible things in possession or control of the witness (referred to as a *subpoena duces tecum*).

Service of a subpoena is made by delivering a copy directly to the witness and tendering the fees for one day's attendance, meals, and mileage allowed by law.[14] Witnesses subpoenaed in a criminal case may be compelled to attend and testify without their fees and mileage being first paid or tendered.[15] Failure, by the practitioner, to obey a subpoena may result in a contempt of court proceedings. If the subpoena commands production of documentary evidence that would be unreasonable and oppressive to produce in court, the practitioner (usually through the practitioner's or client's attorney) may make a timely motion to quash entirely or modify in part the subpoena or condition compliance upon payment of the reasonable cost of producing the evidence.[16]

The mere issuance of a subpoena does not override the practitioner–client privilege (see chapter 4.3). The practitioner must assert the privilege until the client expressly waives it (e.g., when the client discloses the information in such a way as to extinguish the privilege, see chapter 4.3) or the court orders the privilege waived as a matter of law. Failure, by a practitioner, to assert the privilege in court may result in civil liability (see chapter 6.5).

(B)(1) Alcohol and Drug Treatment Records

The confidentiality of alcohol and drug treatment records for health care providers, who work within state-approved, alcohol and drug treatment settings, are regulated by both state and

---

13. Superior Court Civil Rules, 45(a).
14. RCW 5.56.010. The practitioner must demand the fee when the subpoena is served, otherwise payment will not be required if practitioner lives in the same county or within 20 miles of the trial location.
15. Ferguson, R. D. (1985). Wash. Practice. *Crim. Prac. and Proc.*, § 3305 at 156-7.
16. Superior Court Civil Rules, 45(b). For a deposition (Superior Court Civil Rule 45(d)(i)), a *subpoena duces tecum* may be served on the practitioner. The sought-after written records must be produced for inspection or copying within the time specified by the subpoena, or a written objection must be served on the opposing attorney. After an objection is served, only a court order may force disclosure.

federal laws.[17] Alcohol and drug treatment client confidences are subject to disclosure for good cause upon the court approving the issuance of a subpoena to compel production of records or testimony.[18] The procedures and criteria for obtaining orders authorizing disclosures for noncriminal purposes are specified by federal law:[19]

1. The application may be filed by any person with a legally recognized interest in using the patient records as evidence. The application must use a fictitious name to refer to the patient and may not disclose any identifying information about the patient unless the patient has waived confidentiality or given consent to disclosure or the court has ordered the record sealed from public scrutiny.

2. Adequate notice must be given to the patient whose records are being sought in a manner that will not disclose patient identifying information to other persons. An opportunity to file a written response to the application must be provided.

3. Any oral argument, review of the evidence, or hearing on the application must be held in the judge's chambers to avoid disclosure of confidential information to anyone other than a party to the proceeding, the patient, or the person holding the record unless the patient requests an open hearing.

4. An order authorizing disclosure may be entered only if the court determines that good cause exists because other ways to obtain the information are not available or are ineffective and the public interest in the disclosure outweighs the potential injury to the patient, to the treatment provider–patient relationship, and to the treatment services.

5. An order must limit disclosure of those parts of the patient's record that are essential to fulfill the objective of the order and to those persons whose need for information is the basis of the order, and include other methods to protect patient confidences, such as ordering the information sealed from public scrutiny.

---

17. RCW 70.96A.150; WAC 275-19-074 to -075; WAC 248-18-235; WAC 248-22-041; WAC 248-18-235. The Public Health Service of the Department of Health and Human Services of the United States, pursuant to § 408 of the Drug Abuse Prevention, Treatment, and Rehabilitation Act (42 U.S.C. § 290dd-3), *see* 42 C.F.R. § 2.1 *et seq.* (1991).
18. RCW 70.96A.150(1)(b); 42 C.F.R. § 2.61(a).
19. 42 C.F.R. § 2.64 (1991).

4.5

Public Disclosure Act

Washington's Public Disclosure Act[1] is modeled on the federal Freedom of Information Act.[2] Public agencies have a duty to make their records available to the public for inspection and for copying.[3] A request for records may be made of a mental health provider in public practice.

(A) Who May Request Public Records

Personal records maintained on clients at public institutions or public health agencies are exempted from third party inspection.[4] On the other hand, clients of a public institution or health agency can gain access to inspect or copy their records under the Act.[5]

(B) Legal Test Applied

The burden of proof falls on the agency to prevent disclosure. Unless the disclosure of a client's record would violate personal

---

1. Chapter 42.17 RCW.
2. 5 U.S.C. § 552-552a.
3. RCW 42.17.250.
4. RCW 42.17.310(1)(a).
5. Oliver v. Harborview Medical Center, 94 Wash.2d 559, 618 P.2d 76 (1980). An agency may remove any material confidential to another person or records released to the agency by other agencies or professionals before allowing the client to inspect or copy his or her record, RCW 42.17.310(3).

privacy or a vital governmental interest, Washington courts will rule in favor of the client's right to access.[6]

(C) Probable Outcome of a Lawsuit

If the public agency denies the patient access to his or her records and fails to prevail in an action challenging the client's right to access to the records, the client's costs of the law suit, including reasonable attorney's fees, will be assessed by the court to the agency.[7]

---

6. *Id*. RCW 42.17.340(1).
7. After the Oliver decision, *id.*, the Community Mental Health Act established standards for client access to records in county mental health settings: WAC 275-56-235. *See* chapter 4.1, County Mental Health Settings: Client Access.

Practice Related to the Law

Families and Juveniles

5A.1

Competency to Marry

In the state of Washington, persons 18 years of age or older may marry. However, a minimum mental status must exist at the time of the marriage. MHPs may be called upon to evaluate and to testify about the mental status of a party at the time of the marriage if competency to marry becomes an issue.

(A) Who May Challenge the Marriage

A marriage is voidable[1] by the party laboring under a disability.[2] An example of such a disability occurs when consent to marry is obtained through force or fraud.

If either party is 17 years of age or younger, the marriage is void.[3] Any interested party, for instance a parent or legal guardian, may challenge the validity of the marriage. However, a superior court judge can approve the necessity of the marriage.[4]

---

1. *Voidable* designates a marriage that is subject to an impediment but is considered valid unless set aside by court decree. In re Romano's Estate, 40 Wash.2d 796, 246 P.2d 501 (1952).
2. RCW 26.04.010 and .130.
3. *Void* is used to designate any marriage that is an absolute nullity, incapable of satisfaction. In re Romano's Estate, 40 Wash.2d 796, 246 P.2d 843 (1952). If either party is 17 years of age or younger, the marriage is void because of a want of legal age. RCW 26.04.010 and .130.
4. RCW 26.04.010.

(B) Test for Determining Challenge

A marriage is voidable if either person lacks the mental capacity to consent to marry. To invalidate a marriage because of mental incapacity, it must be shown clearly and convincingly that, at the time of the marriage, the disabled party was unable to understand the nature of the marriage contract and of the duties and responsibilities that it entails, or that the disabled party did not give "free and intelligent consent."[5] Examples of mental incapacity include intoxication at the time of the marriage or the use of force to obtain the consent to marry.

If either party is less than 17 years of age, the marriage is void. To approve the necessity of the marriage, a judge considers the statutory goals of marriage, in particular, whether the minor could promote the welfare of any children that may be produced by the marriage.[6]

(C) Legal Procedure Related to a Challenge

The hearing challenging the validity of a marriage must occur while both parties to an alleged marriage are living; at least one party is a resident of the state; and either party, both parties, or the guardian (see chapter 5A.11, Guardianship for Minors) of the alleged incapacitated spouse files a petition to declare the marriage invalid.[7] MHPs can provide expert testimony as to whether a disability existed at the time of the marriage and caused mental incapacity. They also might be called upon to evaluate whether a minor had developed sufficient capacity to parent and promote the welfare of any children.

---

5. In re Gallagher's Estate, 35 Wash.2d 512, 213 P.2d 621 (1950).
6. Singer v. Hara, 11 Wash. App. 247, 522 P.2d 1187 (1974).
7. RCW 26.09.040. In re Romano's Estate, 40 Wash.2d 796, 246 P.2d 501 (1952).

5A.2

Guardianship for Adults

The legislature has recognized that certain persons who are emotionally or cognitively disabled must be protected legally. Appointment of a guardian arises for some incapacitated individuals who cannot exercise their rights or provide for their basic needs, without assistance, in conducting their day-to-day affairs.

(A) Definition of Incapacity

Two types of adults may be deemed incapacitated by the Superior Court:[1]

1. A person may be deemed incapacitated if the court determines that a significant risk of personal harm exists based upon a demonstrated inability of the person to provide adequately for nutrition, health, housing, or physical safety.

2. A person may be deemed incapacitated if the court determines that the individual presents a significant risk of causing financial harm based upon a demonstrated inability to manage property or financial affairs.

A determination of incapacity exists as a legal, not as a medical decision, on the basis of a determination of management insufficiencies over time.[2] Age, eccentricity, poverty, or medical

---

1. RCW 11.88.010.
2. *Id.*

diagnosis[3] alone are not sufficient to justify a finding of incapacity.[4] The court may appoint limited guardians for persons capable of managing some of their personal or financial affairs.[5]

In all proceedings to appoint a guardian or a limited guardian, the court must be presented with a written report from a physician or a psychologist selected by the guardian *ad litem*,[6] who has expertise in the type of incapacity that the person is believed to have developed and who has examined the person within 30 days of the report to the court. The report must contain[7] a summary of all known and relevant medical, functional, neurological, psychological, or psychiatric evidence about the person's incapacity; the findings of the examining physician or psychologist as to the condition of the allegedly incapacitated person; current medications and their effects upon the person's ability to understand or participate in guardianship proceedings; opinions on the specific assistance that the person needs, and the identity of persons with whom the physician or psychologist has met or spoken regarding the person.[8]

(B) Guardianship

The guardian or limited guardian acts as a fiduciary on behalf of the incapacitated person.[9] The court determines the extent to which the incapacitated person is unable to care for himself or

---

3. In fact, if the person is committed involuntarily to a mental health or alcohol institution for care, this action does not determine whether the person is legally incompetent to handle his or her financial interests. A separate proceeding to appoint a guardian must be pursued to declare someone incompetent or disabled and in need of a guardian. In re Pfeiffer, 10 Wash.2d 703, 118 P.2d 158 (1941).
4. RCW 11.88.010(1)(c).
5. RCW 11.88.010(2).
6. RCW 11.88.045(4). A guardian *ad litem* is appointed by the court to represent the allegedly incapacitated person. Such representation involves a full investigation into the allegations; meaningful consultation with the client; examination of records and witnesses; and zealous, affirmative advocacy to protect rights, offer relevant defenses, or make legal claims on behalf of the client. A guardian *ad litem* may not waive the fundamental rights of the client without evidence of the client's specific, knowing consent. In re Quesnell, 83 Wash.2d 224, 517 P.2d 568 (1973).
7. *Id.*
8. This chapter creates an exception to the physician–patient and psychologist–client privilege for purposes of filing the report with the court. Matter of Guardianship of Atkins, 57 Wash. App. 771, 790 P.2d 210 (1990).
9. As a fiduciary, the guardian has a duty of loyalty in managing the ward's property. A guardian is personally liable for any losses sustained by the ward from self-dealing. Appropriate equitable relief is supposed to deter future breaches of fiduciary duties. This would leave the ward in the same position that he or she would have occupied if the breach had not occurred. In re Eisenbery, 43 Wash. App. 761, 719 P.2d 187 (1986).

herself or to manage his or her financial interests. It will restrict legal rights only to the extent necessary to protect and to assist the person.[10] Under a limited guardianship, the person is not presumed to be completely incapacitated and will not lose any legal rights, except those specifically restricted by the court order; in addition, the limited guardianship lapses after a specific period of time.[11] Presumably, if the court finds that the person is unable to function more globally, a full guardianship will be created and the legal rights will be restricted more broadly. The discussion in the rest of this chapter applies to either form of guardianship, except in a few areas where the differences are noted.

(B)(1) Application and Preparation for the Guardianship Hearing

Any person or entity may petition the Superior Court for a finding of incapacity and the appointment of a guardian.[12] Upon receipt of the petition, the court must appoint a guardian *ad litem*[13] who will represent the best interests of the allegedly incapacitated person.[14] This representative must be known by the court to be free of influence from anyone interested in the result of the proceeding and have acquired the requisite knowledge, training, or experience to perform the duties.[15]

As soon as practicable following appointment, the guardian *ad litem* must meet with the allegedly incapacitated person and explain in plain language the substance of the petition, the nature of the proceedings, the person's right to contest the petition, the identification of the proposed guardian, the right to a jury trial for determining whether the person is incompetent, the right to independent legal counsel, and the right to be present in court at the hearing on the petition.[16]

---

10. A person against whom guardianship proceedings are being conducted is presumed to have capacity until entry of an order to the contrary. In re Quesnell, 83 Wash.2d 224, 517 P.2d 568 (1973).
11. RCW 11.88.010.
12. RCW 11.88.030.
13. Such a person must meet specific requirements before being appointed guardian *ad litem*. RCW 11.88.090(3). The fee for the services shall be determined by the court and may be charged to the incapacitated person; the county, if such payment would result in substantial hardship; or the petitioner of the guardianship, if the petition is found to be frivolous or not made in good faith. RCW 11.88.090(8).
14. RCW 11.88.090(2). Upon application of a relative or friend, a guardian *ad litem* may be appointed also for an insane person who is a party in a lawsuit. RCW 4.08.060. If the insane person objects to the appointment, an adjudication for guardianship must be pursued and, in either case, the guardian *ad litem* has no authority to waive any substantive right of the ward. In re Houts, 7 Wash. App. 476, 499 P.2d 1276 (1972).
15. *Id.*
16. RCW 11.88.090(5).

The guardian *ad litem* also must meet with the proposed guardian and ascertain knowledge of a guardian's duties and steps to take to meet the needs of the allegedly incapacitated person.[17] Friends and relatives of the person and others with a significant interest in the allegedly incapacitated person must be consulted.[18] A written evaluation from a psychiatrist or psychologist also shall be obtained and submitted to the court along with other written or oral reports from qualified professionals, as necessary.[19]

The guardian *ad litem* must file a report with the court in 45 days after formal notice of the commencing of the guardianship process and at least 10 days before the hearing of the petition (unless the court has granted an extension or reduction of time for good cause).[20] The report shall include the following information:[21] a description of the nature, cause, and degree of incapacity, and the basis on which this conclusion was reached; a description of the needs for care, treatment, residence, and the basis on which this conclusion was reached; an evaluation of the appropriateness of the proposed guardian with a description of the steps that the proposed guardian has taken or intends to take to meet the needs of the person; a recommendation as to whether a guardian or limited guardian should be appointed; an evaluation of the person's ability to vote and the basis on which such an evaluation was made; any expression of approval or disapproval by the person of the proposed guardianship; an identification of the persons with a significant interest in the allegedly incapacitated person's welfare; a description of how the person responded to the explanation about his or her legal rights; and, if a limited guardianship is recommended, an identification of the specific areas over which the guardian should exercise control, and the limitations to be placed upon the allegedly incapacitated person.

In addition, the guardian *ad litem* must advise the court within five days of meeting with the allegedly incapacitated person of the need for appointment of counsel to represent the person.[22] However, this step is not necessary if counsel appears before the court, or if the person communicates affirmatively a wish not to be represented after being advised of the right to representation and of the conditions under which court-appointed counsel would be available, or the person is unable to

---

17. *Id.*
18. *Id.*
19. *Id.*
20. *Id.*
21. *Id.*
22. *Id.*

communicate at all on the subject but the guardian *ad litem* is satisfied that the person does not desire counsel.[23]

During the pendency of the guardianship determination, the guardian *ad litem* may provide consent if emergency, life saving medical services are required, and the allegedly incapacitated person is unable to consent to such services.[24]

(B)(2) Guardianship Hearing

Usually the hearing is informal and may be conducted at the home of the allegedly incapacitated person. The person must be present unless this requirement is waived by the court for good cause other than mere inconvenience; if the presence of the person is waived, then the guardian *ad litem* must appear at the hearing.[25] Also, the hearing may be held in closed court. If the case is contested, the standard of proof that the person is in need of a guardian must be in the form of clear, cogent, and convincing evidence.[26]

The court disposition of the petition must be based on the findings as to the capacity, conditions, and needs of the allegedly incapacitated person and shall not be based solely on agreements made by the parties.[27] Every order appointing a guardian of the person or estate shall include[28] the amount of the bond,[29] if any, or the bond review period; when the next report of the guardian is due; whether the guardian *ad litem* should continue in that capacity; whether a review hearing is required on filing of the inventory of the estate; the extent of the authority of the guardian, if any, to invest and expend funds from the incapacitated person's estate; and the names and addresses of persons, if any, whom the court believes should receive copies of further pleadings filed by the guardian with regard to the guardianship. If the court determines that a limited guardianship is appropriate, the order should specify the limits, either by stating exceptions to the guardian authority or by stating the specific authority of the guardian.[30] Finally, the court shall consider whether the incapacitated person is capable of giving informed medical consent or of making other personal decisions and, if not, whether a guardian should be appointed for that purpose.[31]

---

23. *Id.*
24. RCW 11.88.090(7).
25. RCW 11.88.040(4).
26. RCW 11.88.045(3).
27. RCW 11.88.095.
28. RCW 11.88.095(2).
29. A *bond* is an amount of money determined by the court that the guardian must advance to a secured account while serving as a guardian.
30. RCW 11.88.095(3).
31. RCW 11.88.095(4).

(C) Authority of the Guardian

In the state of Washington, the guardian is an officer of the court, in effect an underling of the superior guardian, the court.[32] The law has specified the following powers and duties of the guardian or limited guardian:[33]

1. pay all just claims against the estate;

2. file, within three months of the appointment, a verified inventory of all property belonging to the ward including a statement about all encumbrances, liens, and other secured charges on any item;

3. file annually, within 90 days after the beginning of the appointment and within 30 days after the end of the guardianship, unless the court for good cause orders otherwise, identification of property as of the last account or initial inventory, identification of all additional property received including income by source, identification of major expenditures, adjustments to the estate to establish its fair market value, and identification of the present value of the estate's property as of the new account. The account shall also set forth the amount of bond and any other court-ordered financial protection;[34]

4. report any substantial change in income or assets within 30 days of the substantial change;

5. protect and preserve the guardianship estate, account for the financial estate of the ward with diligence, and deliver all the assets to the appropriate person at the termination of the guardianship;

6. invest the property in accordance with applicable rules for the investment of trust estates (e.g., the unconditional interest-bearing obligations of Washington or the United States);

---

32. *See* Barker and Scharf, *Washington Practice*, vol.1, § 6.19 *et seq.*
33. RCW 11.92.040 to .043.
34. If any of the ward's financial interests include payments made by the U.S. government through the Veteran's Administration, the guardian must comply with the procedures of the Uniform Veteran's Guardianship Act, Chapter 73.36 RCW.

7. apply to the court for an order authorizing any disbursements of assets on behalf of the person;

8. file, within 90 days, a personal care plan that includes a needs assessment, an assessment about the incapacitated person's ability to assist in activities of daily living, and the guardian's plans for meeting the identified needs;

9. file annually, or when an account is required, a report about the incapacitated person's status, including the person's name and address, services that he or she receives, medical and mental status, changes in abilities, activities of the guardian, recommended changes in the guardian's authority, and the identity of professionals who have assisted the incapacitated person during the period of time;

10. report to the court within 30 days any substantial change in the incapacitated person's condition or any change in the person's residence;

11. care for and maintain the incapacitated person in the least restrictive and most appropriate setting and assert the person's rights and interests;[35] and

12. provide timely, informed consent for medical treatment, if authorized by the court to do so.

The guardian's powers are limited. The guardian cannot authorize invasive mental health or medical care (for examples of such care see chapter 6.2). No guardian may involuntarily commit a ward for evaluation or treatment if the ward is unable or unwilling to provide informed consent. The exclusive procedures established by the involuntary commitment statute must be followed (see chapter 5E.4).[36] Nor can the guardian provide consent to an extraordinary, irreversible medical procedure without first obtaining court authorization, particularly for any of the following

---

35. Meeting this particular duty may require the guardian or guardian *ad litem* to petition the court for authorization to seek dissolution of the ward's marriage. The dissolution must be in the best interests of the ward, not just the heirs. Unless this course of action remained available, in certain situations, the competent party would be vested with absolute, final control over the marriage to the detriment of the incapacitated person. Marriage of Gannon, 104 Wash.2d 121, 702 P.2d 465 (1985).

36. In re Anderson, 17 Wash. App 690, 564 P.2d 1190 (1977).

procedures:[37] any procedure that induces a convulsion, psychosurgery, sterilization,[38] and other mental health procedures that restrict physical freedom of movement.[39]

(D) Termination of Guardianship

At any time after the appointment of the guardian, the court may for any good reason modify or terminate the guardianship or replace the guardian.[40] Any person, including the incapacitated person, may apply to the court for an order to modify or terminate the guardianship or to replace the guardian.[41]

The court will terminate the authority and responsibility of a guardian[42] if the person is adjudicated as no longer incapacitated; the person dies; the term of a limited guardianship has expired without a new petition seeking an extension of the term being filed and served; the guardian becomes incapacitated in some

---

37. *Id*. In cases that are expected to result in some measure of recovery, the factors that a court would weigh before authorizing an extraordinary procedure include the benefits and drawbacks of the possible treatment, the effect that the ward's present and future incompetency would have on the decision, the ward's ability to assist in pretreatment therapy, the ward's religious or moral views, and the wishes of his or her family or friends if their wishes would have been influential. A court bases its decision on what the ward would have chosen if the ward had been competent. The ward's strongly stated preference is given substantial weight if the ward has some understanding of the medical problem and possible treatments. In re Ingram, 102 Wash.2d 827, 689 P.2d 1363 (1984). In cases in which treatment merely postpones death and the incompetent is in a cognitively insapient state with no reasonable chance of recovery and if all the patient's immediate family, treating physician, and the prognosis committee agree that withdrawal of life-sustaining treatment is in the patient's best interest, the family may assent to withdrawal of life-sustaining treatment without seeking a prior appointment of a guardian. In re Colner, 98 Wash.2d 114, 660 P.2d 738 (1983). However, if no available family exists, a guardian must be appointed to act as a surrogate decision maker, like a family, to provide an objective viewpoint and evaluate the medical prognosis. Similar to the familial situation, if the treating physician, the prognosis committee, and the guardian are all in agreement, life-sustaining treatment may be ended. In re Hamlin, 102 Wash.2d 810, 689 P.2d 1372 (1984).
38. In re Hayes, 93 Wash.2d 228, 608 P. 2d 635 (1980).
39. RCW 71.05.370 (*see* chapter 5E.4).
40. RCW 11.88.120.
41. *Id*.
42. RCW 11.88.140.

manner;[43] the guardian spouse petitions for dissolution of the marriage with his or her ward;[44] and the guardian resigns.[45]

---

43. In re Shapiro's Estate, 131 Wash. 653, 230 P. 627 (1924); Guardianship of Robinson, 9 Wash.2d 525, 115 P.2d 734 (1941).
44. The general rule is that a guardian cannot maintain an action at law against a ward pending the guardianship or before the account is adjusted and settled. However, the court permitted a guardian to sue his ward for dissolving their marriage because a separate guardian *ad litem* was representing the ward's interest throughout the matter. Rupe v. Robinson, 139 Wash. 592, 247 P. 954 (1926).
45. Jorgenson v. Winter, 69 Wash. 573, 125 P. 957 (1912).

5A.2A

Conservatorship for Adults

In many states, a separate conservatorship law allows a court to appoint someone to manage the estate of a person who is no longer able to manage his or her own property or financial affairs. Washington has created no conservatorship law, but has made guardianship provisions for such cases (see chapter 5A.1).

5A.3

Annulment

Divorce dissolves a valid, functioning marriage. Annulment occurs when a marriage is declared void and held never to have legally existed. The distinction between annulment and divorce can have legal significance. For instance, a marriage that is annulled and declared void can prevent the laws of intestacy from passing an estate to a surviving spouse.[1] MHPs are not needed to testify about the grounds that would annul a marriage. However, information about annulment may be useful when working with persons who are contemplating dissolving their marriages.[2]

(A) Grounds for Annulment

The procedure for obtaining an annulment is the same as for the dissolution of a marriage (see chapter 5A.4). Marriages are void when either party is 17 years of age or younger,[3] either party has a wife or husband living at the time of their next marriage, or the parties marry a relative (called the law prohibiting consanguinity).[4]

---

1. In re Romano's Estate 40 Wash.2d 796, 246 P.2d 843 (1952).
2. Worker's compensation claims (*see* chapter 5B.2) also may be affected by whether an annulment or a divorce is pursued. A widowed spouse of a worker receives compensation benefits until the widow remarries. If a second marriage ceases by virtue of annulment rather than of divorce, presumably benefits would be regained.
3. RCW 26.04.130.
4. RCW 26.04.020; Barker v. Barker, 31 Wash.2d 506, 197 P.2d 439 (1948).

5A.4

Divorce

Washington has adopted the Uniform Marriage Act. It contains "no-fault" divorce procedures that provide for a decree of dissolution (a divorce). The process is supposed to take 90 days for uncontested cases and 150 days for contested cases (those in which the parties cannot agree to the terms of the dissolution).[1] Under the law, an agreement or litigation must focus upon spousal maintenance, property division, settlement of debt obligations, child support, and a parenting plan (see chapter 5A.5). MHPs can serve as mediators for couples contemplating or undergoing dissolution. They also may serve as evaluators and provide expert witness testimony in contested cases.

(A) Divorce Procedure

(A)(1) Who May File for Divorce

A party who is a resident of Washington or who is a member of the armed forces and is stationed in this state may petition the Superior Court to dissolve a marriage or to obtain a legal separation.[2]

(A)(2) Grounds for Dissolution

Grounds for dissolution or legal separation require only an allegation that the marriage is irretrievably broken; if the other party

---

1. RCW 26.09.030. *See* Marriage of Little, 95 Wash.2d 183, 634 P.2d 498 (1981).
2. Parties may choose to seek a legal separation because of principles of conscience or religion. Kimble v. Kimble, 17 Wash. 45, 49 P. 216 (1897).

joins in the petition or does not deny that the marriage is irretrievably broken, the court will enter a decree of dissolution.[3] If the petitioner requests the court to decree legal separation in lieu of dissolution, the court shall enter the decree in that form unless the other party objects.[4]

(A)(3) The Authority of the Court

The court has the authority to provide for the maintenance of either spouse, the disposition of property and liabilities of the parties, the residential placement of their child, the support of the child, the allocation of decision-making authority about the child, and child visitation. The court may grant temporary maintenance or child support upon a motion setting forth the facts about the need and amounts requested.[5] A temporary restraining order or preliminary injunction also may be granted to protect people within the family[6] or property of the marriage.[7]

(A)(4) Legal Process of Divorce

Family court hearings are conducted informally as a conference or series of conferences, in part, to effect the reconciliation of the parties or reach an amicable settlement.[8] If the matter is contested, the informality of the process ends.

The other party can contest the divorce on one of two grounds. If an allegation is raised that the petitioner was induced to file the petition for divorce by fraud or coercion, the court must make a finding and dismiss the petition if the facts support the allegation.[9]

A second basis for objection occurs when a party denies that the marriage is irretrievably broken.[10] The court, at the request of either party or on its own motion, may transfer the case to family court services[11] or refer the parties to another counseling service of their choice. It must request a report back from the counseling

---

3. RCW 26.09.030(1).
4. RCW 26.09.030(4).
5. RCW 26.09.060.
6. *See* chapter 5A.8, Reporting Adult Abuse.
7. RCW 26.09.060(2).
8. RCW 26.12.170.
9. RCW 26.09.030(2).
10. RCW 26.09.030(3).
11. Many of the superior courts in the various counties of the state have created family courts to provide commissioners to act as the finders of fact when children are within the household and a legal controversy may result in dissolution of the marriage, declaration of invalidity, or the disruption of the household. RCW 26.12.090.

service within 60 days[12] or continue the matter for not more than 60 days.[13]

MHPs become involved in this process whenever the court orders or recommends that the parties enter counseling.[14] If, after 60 days, the parties agree to a reconciliation, the court will dismiss the petition. If the parties have not reconciled, and either party continues to allege that the marriage is irretrievably broken, the court will enter a decree of dissolution of the marriage.

(B) An Additional Role for Mental Health Providers

MHPs also may influence and promote amicable settlements for people contemplating divorce before the parties take legal action. Parties may work out the terms of maintaining either of them, disposing of property, releasing each other from specific financial obligations, and establishing residential placement, support, and visitation of their children. Such terms may be drawn into a written separation contract.[15] Many terms are binding upon the court and shall be written into the decree of dissolution, legal separation, or declaration of invalidity, unless the court finds that the contract was unfair at the time of execution.[16]

The terms providing for the custody, support, and visitation of the children may not be binding. The court may enter a temporary custody, support, and visitation order, but retain jurisdiction to modify the order at a specified date if the best interests of the children require such action.[17] However, if the court learns from the relevant evidence that the terms are in the best interest of the children, the terms will be included in the decree, and the parties shall be ordered to comply with them.[18]

---

12. Providers can ask the judge or commissioner to protect the privacy of the parties by closing the record; the confidences may be "contrary to public policy or injurious to the interests of the children or the public morals." RCW 26.12.080.
13. RCW 26.09.030(3)(b).
14. *Id.*
15. Although the Parenting Act (*see* chapter 5A.5, Child Custody) allows counseling as a means of dispute resolution, any agreement involving property and child support arrangements should be reviewed by lawyers to assure that unfair advantage is not being taken by either party.
16. A party has a right to have the interests in the property and finances of the parties definitely and finally determined in the decree that dissolves the marriage, creates the legal separation, or declares the marriage invalid. Marriage of Little, 95 Wash.2d 183, 634 P.2d 498 (1981).
17. *Id.*
18. RCW 26.09.070(5).

Child Custody

The Parenting Act of 1987 dramatically changed how "custody" and "visitation" are decided by Washington courts. The new statutory objective is to avoid quarrels about these issues throughout the process of divorce, legal separation, or declaration of marital invalidity. Parents who act in bad faith during the negotiations or implementation of a court-approved parenting plan, fail to perform any duty in the plan, or hinder another parent from complying with the terms of the plan may suffer punitive damage awards, civil or criminal contempt, and the award of court costs and attorney fees.[1]

MHPs may become involved in the process in one of four ways:

1. providers serve as mediators with parents to develop a plan;
2. a provider may be chosen as the designated person to resolve any dispute that arises about the parenting plan;
3. providers may evaluate a parent's or child's mental health status or perform a comprehensive evaluation of the entire family that might culminate in a court appearance as an expert witness; and
4. a provider who has provided diagnostic or therapeutic services to the family or to individual family members may be subpoenaed by either party to testify in court.

---

1. RCW 26.09.160.

(A) Criteria to Establish Court Jurisdiction

The Uniform Child Custody Jurisdiction Act established the law as to the courts' jurisdictional powers over child custody matters.[2] For instance, if the child is living in Washington at the commencement of the proceeding, the court will assume jurisdiction. If, however, the child and the parents are not domiciled in Washington, then it must be shown that it is in the best interests of the child for the court to assume jurisdiction. The court will decide whether the child and at least one parent have developed significant connections with the state, and whether sufficient evidence exists in this state concerning the child's present or future care, protection, training, and personal relationships.[3] An MHP may be asked to evaluate the nature and quality of the child's relationships with the parent living in this state.

(B) Standard in Approving the Parenting Plan: Best Interest of the Child

A parenting plan must meet the following objectives:[4]

1. provide for the child's physical care;
2. maintain the child's emotional stability;
3. provide for the child's changing needs as the child grows and matures in a way that minimizes the need for future modifications to the permanent parenting plan;
4. establish the authority and responsibilities of each parent with regard to the child;
5. minimize the child's exposure to harmful parental conflict;
6. provide sufficient detail so parents meet their responsibilities established by the plan, instead of relying on judicial intervention; and
7. protect the best interests of the child.

---

2. RCW 26.27.030.
3. Id.
4. RCW 26.09.184(1).

The parenting plan must specifically allocate the parents' functions, including the time each is to spend with the child.[5]

During hearings on the Act, the mental health community identified several important parenting functions. However, in making residential provisions for the children, the court will give greatest weight to the relative strength, nature, and stability of the child's relationship with each parent, including parental performance of parenting functions.[6] Other subsidiary factors that the court will consider in determining the residential schedule for each child are

1. whether the parental plan was entered knowingly and voluntarily;

2. each parent's past and potential for future performance of parenting functions;

3. the emotional needs and developmental level of the child;

4. the child's relationship with siblings and other significant adults, as well as the child's involvement with activities within the particular physical surroundings of the existing home and school;

5. the wishes of the parents and of a sufficiently mature child; and

6. each parent's employment schedule.[7]

Each day of the year must be allocated in the residential schedule.

Ordinarily, the plan will allow both parents to be involved in the decision making. Day-to-day care and control of the child will rest with whomever the child will reside, but plans shall allocate the major decisions about the education, health care, and religious

---

5. RCW 26.09.184. Although "parent" or "party" is used throughout this section, the courts have awarded custody to a nonparent because the parent(s) is unfit and awarding custody to the nonparent would not be detrimental to the child. In re Marriage of Allen, 28 Wash. App. 637, 626 P.2d 16 (1981). *See* chapter 26.10 RCW, Nonparental Actions for Child Custody.

6. RCW 26.09.187(3).

7. *Id*. Other factors may be considered to determine the best interests of the child so long as the record clearly shows that the court considered the statutory factors: In re Marriage of Janovich, 30 Wash. App. 169, 632 P.2d 889 (1981). The court may not base residential placement solely on a young infant's need for maternal influence; Tucker v. Tucker. 14 Wash. App. 454, 542 P.2d 789 (1975); race is but one factor to consider; In re Marriage of Herden, 27 Wash. App. 566, 619 P.2d 374 (1980); a court may consider a parent's decisions and acts that are based upon a religious belief if they present a substantial likelihood of immediate or future impairment of the child's mental health or physical safety; Matter of Marriage of Cabalquinto, 100 Wash.2d. 325, 669 P.2d 886 (1983), the court considered the effect of the homosexual lifestyle of a parent and decided that homosexuality in and of itself did not bar child custody rights.

upbringing to one or both parties.[8] When mutual decision making is required but cannot be achieved, the parties must make a good-faith effort to resolve disagreements through a dispute resolution process that is specified by the plan. Dispute resolution can be performed by counseling, mediation, or arbitration through a specified individual or agency or by court action.[9] Either party may appeal a dispute resolution to the Superior Court; if the court finds that a parent has used or frustrated the dispute-resolution process without good reason, the court shall award attorney fees and financial sanctions to the prevailing parent.[10]

The plan does not require mutual decision making or a non-judicial dispute resolution process if one parent's involvement is shown to be harmful to the child's development; this would arise because of the following parental acts of misconduct:[11]

1. willful abandonment that continues for extended periods of time or substantial refusal to perform parenting functions;
2. physical, sexual, or a pattern of emotional abuse of a child; and
3. a history of acts of domestic violence[12] or of physical or sexual assault that causes grievous bodily harm or fear of such harm.

Furthermore, the court may preclude or limit any provision within the parenting plan upon a showing that a child may be adversely affected by a parent's involvement or conduct because of[13]

1. a parent's neglect or substantial nonperformance of parenting functions;
2. a parent's long-term emotional or physical impairment (including alcohol or other substance abuse) that interferes with performance of the parenting functions;
3. the absence or substantial impairment of emotional ties between the parent and the child;
4. the abusive use of conflict by the parent that creates the danger of serious damage to the child's development;
5. a parent withholding access to the child from the other parent for a protracted period without good cause; or
6. such other factors that the court finds adverse to the child's best interests.

---

8. RCW 26.09.184(4).
9. RCW 26.09.184(3).
10. RCW 26.09.184(3)(d).
11. RCW 26.09.191(1)(2).
12. RCW 26.50.010(1) (*see* chapter 5A.7, Domestic Violence).
13. RCW 26.09.191(3).

tional, alcohol or other substance, or physical impairment. Earlier judicial precedents called for assessing a parent's fitness from the present condition and not future expectations.[14]

(C) Mental Health Evaluations

When parents cannot agree about the parenting arrangements, the court is more likely to require that the parties or the children undergo comprehensive mental health evaluations. First, a court can order a mental health examination of a party whenever the mental condition is at issue.[15] If a party does not wish to participate, a court order can compel an evaluation of a party or the discovery of earlier mental health records of a party (see chapter 4.3).[16] Second, a party may request or the court on its own volition may order an investigation and report about the parenting arrangements for the child.[17]

Mental health evaluations also may be conducted on a voluntary basis.[18] This occurs when one of the parties requests a provider to evaluate a party or the children. (See chapters 4.2 and 4.3 for discussion about privilege and confidentiality and about the responsibilities and limitations that applies to providers in parenting disputes.)

---

14. RCW 26.09.191; Marriage of Wolfinder, 33 Wash. App. 326, 654 P.2d 1219 (1982). (The past sexual misconduct of a parent did not render the parent unfit for custody unless the misconduct would have a present adverse impact upon the best interest of the child).
15. Superior Court Civil Rules, 35, which permits examination of a party or person in the custody of a party: In re Marriage of Waggener, 13 Wash. App. 911, 538 P.2d 845 (1975). (The court has broad discretionary powers to inquire about any factor that may affect the best interests of the child.)
16. In re Marriage of Nordby, 41 Wash. App. 531, 705 P.2d 277 (1985).
17. RCW 26.09.220.
18. This is not recommended because of increased risk of malpractice (see chapter 6.5, Malpractice Liability).

5A.6

Reporting of Adult Abuse

The law requires MHPs to report known or suspected abuse or neglect of dependent adults and abuse, neglect, or exploitation of vulnerable adults. Violating the law can result in criminal punishment. Also, MHPs may be sued in civil court for the harm inflicted upon the person whom the reporting law is designed to protect.

(A) Terms and Definitions

Several terms in the reporting statute have legal definitions not necessarily equivalent to how they may be defined by providers. They presently are defined as follows:

1. *Adult dependent persons* are incapacitated adults not able to provide for their own protection. They are defined as persons 18 years of age or older who are adjudicated to be legally incompetent or disabled to such a degree that a guardianship has been established (see chapter 5A.2, Guardianship for Adults.) Those who may be adjudicated to be incompetent or disabled include adults who are[1] mentally ill, developmentally disabled, senile, habitually drunk, excessive users of drugs, or suffering from any other mental incapacity. Adults who are living within a nursing home,[2] or a state hospital for the mentally ill,[3] or residential treatment facility,[4] or adult family

---

1. RCW 11.88.010(1)(e).
2. Chapter 18.51 RCW and Chapter 70.124 RCW.
3. Chapter 72.23 RCW and Chapter 70.124 RCW.
4. Chapter 248-25 WAC.

home[5] also are considered disabled adults regardless of their age, incapacity, or adjudicated status.

2. *Vulnerable adult* is a person 60 years of age or older who lacks the functional, mental, or physical ability to care for himself or herself.[6]

3. *Abuse of vulnerable adults* refers to an act of physical or mental mistreatment or injury that harms or threatens a person through action or inaction by another.[7]

4. *Neglect of vulnerable adults* refers to a pattern of conduct resulting in deprivation of care necessary to maintain minimum physical and mental health.[8]

5. *Abandonment* refers to leaving a person lacking the ability to obtain food, clothing, shelter, or health care.[9]

6. *Law enforcement agency* refers to the police department, the prosecuting attorney, the state patrol, the director of public safety, or the office of the sheriff.[10]

(B) When Must a Report Be Made?

The duty to report an incident involving a dependent adult arises at the first opportunity, but never longer than 48 hours after there is reasonable cause to believe that abuse or neglect has occurred.[11] MHPs who have reasonable cause to believe that a vulnerable adult has suffered abuse, neglect, exploitation, or abandonment must make an immediate oral report to be followed by a written report to the Department of Social and Health Services (DSHS) within 10 days.[12]

Although these duties concern only past incidents, a statute imposes a duty to warn or take reasonable precautions to provide protection in cases in which future danger is threatened. If a client of an MHP communicates an actual threat of violence against a reasonably identifiable victim or victims, the provider must make reasonable efforts to communicate the threat to the victim or victims and to law enforcement personnel.[13] In addition, the MHP may begin involuntary commitment proceedings for the

---

5. Chapter 388-76 WAC.
6. RCW 74.34.020(8).
7. RCW 74.34.020(2).
8. RCW 74.34.020(5).
9. RCW 74.34.020(1).
10. RCW 26.44.020(2).
11. RCW 26.44.030(1). No report is required if no reasonable cause exists to believe that a current or potential victim is at risk; RCW 26.44.030(2).
12. RCW 74.34.030.
13. RCW 71.05.120.

client if both mental illness and a danger to another or others exists (see chapters 5A.19 and 5E.4).

(C) How a Report Must Be Made

For a dependent adult, the duty to report is met by reporting the following information, if known, to a law enforcement agency or to the DSHS:[14]

1. the name, address, and age of the victim;
2. the name and address of the guardian(s) or the address of the adult dependent person;
3. the nature and extent of the injury or injuries;
4. the nature and extent of the neglect or sexual abuse;
5. any evidence of previous injuries; and
6. any other information that may be helpful in establishing the cause of the adult dependent person's death or injuries and the identity of the perpetrator.

The duty to report harm to a vulnerable adult differs to some extent. A report must be made to the DSHS and include the following information, if known:[15]

1. identification of the vulnerable adult;
2. the nature and extent of the suspected abuse, neglect, exploitation, or abandonment;
3. evidence of previous abuse, neglect, exploitation, or abandonment;
4. the name and address of the person making the report; and
5. any other helpful information.

(D) Immunity from Liability

Any person who makes a report in good faith is immune from civil liability.[16] This language implies that gross negligence must be proven before the reporting MHP will be held civilly liable. When the MHP recklessly reports incorrect information or specifically intends to injure a particular person by making an untrue

---

14. RCW 26.44.040. An oral report may be sufficient, but if requested, it must be followed by a written report.
15. RCW 74.34.040 (both an oral and written report are required); RCW 74.34.030.
16. RCW 26.44.060(1)(a) and RCW 74.34.050.

report, the MHP may be held liable.[17] Any person who, intentionally and in bad faith or with malicious knowledge, makes a false report shall be guilty of a misdemeanor.[18]

(E) Confidentiality and Privilege

Most services provided by MHPs are confidential and privileged (see chapters 4.2 and 4.3). However, reporting harm to a dependent or vulnerable adult to the proper authorities is not a violation of confidentiality.[19]

(F) Failure to Report

A person who must make a report of abuse or neglect about a dependent person may be guilty of a gross misdemeanor when failing to do so.[20] If the charges are proven, the maximum jail term is one year, and the maximum fine may not exceed $5,000; the court may impose both imprisonment and a fine.[21] Civil liability may exist if a provider fails to comply with the duty of reporting harm inflicted on a dependent or vulnerable adult (see chapter 6.5).[22]

---

17. Spurrell v. Block, 40 Wash.App. 854, 701 P.2d 529 (1985) held that, in view of immunity from liability for reports of child abuse made in "good faith," a cause of action for defamation against the DSHS could not be supported on "a showing of mere negligence."
18. RCW 26.44.060(4); RCW 9A.20.021.
19. RCW 26.44.060(3); RCW 74.34.050(2).
20. RCW 26.44.080.
21. RCW 9.92.020.
22. Civil liability is implicitly recognized in RCW 26.44.060.

5A.7

Domestic Violence

The prevalence of domestic violence[1] in the United States is staggering. In any given year, one tenth to one fifth of all women are beaten by a man with whom they are intimately involved; during the entire course of a given relationship, an estimated one in four women will suffer abuse.[2]

The legislature has enacted several laws to prevent domestic violence and to provide its victims with protection from further abuse and physical harm. Court intervention provides three types of relief for victims of domestic violence. First, under the domestic relations statute,[3] a temporary restraining order (TRO) or a preliminary injunction can be secured against the offending party to prevent further contact. Second, the Domestic Violence Prevention Act[4] (hereafter called the Act) expands the available civil remedies. It provides a vast array of relief that includes a restraining order against further abuse, excluding the offender from the home, awarding temporary custody and visitation, ordering the offender into treatment, and ordering other relief as the court deems necessary. The court may require the offender (respondent) to pay all filing, court, and services fees and reimburse the victim (petitioner) for costs as well as attorney fees incurred in bringing the action. Finally, a criminal remedy is available that also would include a no-contact order.[5]

---

1. *Domestic violence* means physical harm, bodily assault, or the infliction of fear of imminent physical harm, bodily injury, and physical or sexual assault of one household member by another. RCW 26.50.010(1).
2. Waits, *The criminal justice system's response to battery: Understanding the problem, forging the solutions*, 60 Wash. L. Rev. 267–329 (1985).
3. Chapter 26.09 RCW; RCW 26.09.060.
4. Chapter 26.50 RCW; RCW 26.50.060.
5. Chapter 10.99 RCW; RCW 10.99.040.

MHPs may become involved by identifying an abusive or battering relationship. Providers can also advocate that victims obtain civil or criminal orders to stop the violence. The legislature has found that previous societal attitudes about domestic violence have affected the policies and practices of law enforcement agencies and of prosecutors. The new statutes stress that laws to protect the victim must be enforced and that violent domestic behavior can no longer be excused or tolerated.[6] Nevertheless, the provider also may have to intervene with law enforcement to further the clients' best interests.[7] The providers may accompany their clients during the process.

(A) Who May Obtain a Restraining Order

A TRO or preliminary injunction may be obtained by a victim who is married to the offender or who has children in common.[8] Relief provided by the Act or through filing criminal charges may be secured by family or household members. This would include "spouses, former spouses, adult persons related by blood or marriage, persons who are presently residing together, or who have resided together in the past, and persons who have a child in common regardless of whether they have been married or have lived together at any time."[9] In addition, it appears that any interested party, including an MHP, may report a criminal act of domestic violence to law enforcement authorities for investigation and prosecution.[10]

(B) How to Obtain Relief

Court intervention may be requested whenever a person requires protection. A TRO or preliminary injunction may be secured immediately whenever a person believes herself or himself to be in danger. Notice to the respondent with a copy of the petition, a copy of the temporary order for relief, and the date set for a full

---

6. Chapter 10.99 RCW.
7. *See* chapter 4.2 to determine constraints on maintaining a client's confidences.
8. RCW 26.09.050 and .060.
9. RCW 26.50.010(2); RCW 10.99.020(1).
10. A psychiatrist or psychologist must obtain a release of information from the client (victim) to avoid violating the duty to maintain confidences. Other counselors do not need a release (*see* chapter 4.2).

hearing must be served, and the hearing must be held within 14 days.[11] The court may issue the order or injunction upon a motion without requiring notice to the other party. This can occur only if it finds that irreparable injury[12] could result before a response from the other party is heard.[13] After a hearing (to be held within 14 days), the TRO or injunction may be extended for one year. Costs of proceeding with this type of action would involve a filing fee and fees to an attorney. If the client is indigent, the fee may be waived, and the client may find a legal aid attorney or another attorney who would handle the matter on a *pro bono* (free) basis.[14] Costs of filing the application and the other court-related fees including service may be waived if the petitioner is indigent.[15]

Any person may report to a law enforcement agency that a criminal act of domestic violence has occurred. A police officer may arrest a person without a warrant if the offense is committed in the presence of the officer.[16] If the investigating officer has probable cause to believe that the suspect has committed the crime, the officer is required to make a warrantless arrest and take the alleged offender into custody. The officer must make an arrest when[17]

1. the person has violated an existing civil or criminal order that restrains the person from acts or threats of violence or excludes the person from a home; or

2. the person is 18 years of age or older and within the preceding four hours has assaulted his spouse, former spouse, or a household member 18 years of age or older with whom the person resides or formerly resided. The officer must believe that a felonious assault has occurred, the assault resulted in bodily injury to the victim, and the intended victim can reasonably fear imminent serious bodily injury or death.

When any person charged with a crime involving domestic violence is released on bail or personal recognizance (see chapter

---

11. RCW 26.50.070(4).
12. *Irreparable injury* means, but is not limited to, situations in which the respondent (the alleged offender) has recently threatened the petitioner (the victim) with bodily injury or has engaged in acts of domestic violence. *See* RCW 26.50.070(2).
13. RCW 26.09.060(3).
14. RCW 26.50.040.
15. RCW 26.50.040. A determination of indigence will not include the income of the household member who is named as the respondent (the alleged offender).
16. Also, the victim may be taken to a place of safety or shelter (RCW 10.99.030(5)). Later, the court must waive any requirement that the victim's location be disclosed to anyone other than an attorney, upon a showing of the possibility of further violence. RCW 10.99.040(1)(c).
17. RCW 10.311.100(2).

5D.4), the court may prohibit contact with the victim until the trial. As a sentencing order after conviction, a no-contact order may last for the duration of probation.[18] Presumably, an affidavit or testimony by an MHP could provide the court with sufficient evidence to warrant such an order.[19] A victim or interested party would bear no financial costs for filing a criminal complaint or for its prosecution.

---

18. RCW 10.99.040(2).
19. A release of information from the client (victim) may be required (*see* chapter 4.2 and chapter 4.3).

5A.8

Reporting of Child Abuse

The law requires MHPs to report known or suspected abuse or neglect of children by any person(s), including parents, custodians, and guardians. Noncompliance may result in criminal charges or in civil liability for any harm inflicted on a child because of the provider's failure to report. Washington's reporting laws do not, however, authorize interference with reasonable child-raising practices or with discipline that does not harm a child's health, welfare, or safety.[1] Certain actions are presumed to be unreasonable methods of child discipline, and a parent or other person who employs such methods may face criminal charges.[2]

(A) Terms and Definitions

Several terms in the reporting statute have legal definitions that are different from those recognized by providers. Presently, the terms are defined as follows:

1. *Child* is any person under the age of 18 years.[3]

---

1. Physical discipline of children is not unlawful when it is reasonable and moderate and inflicted by a parent, teacher, or guardian to correct a child. Use of force against a child by any other persons is unlawful unless authorized by the child's parent or guardian. RCW 9A.16.100.
2. Actions presumed to be unreasonable include, but are not limited to, "(1) throwing, kicking, burning, or cutting a child; (2) striking a child with a closed fist; (3) shaking a child younger than three years of age; (4) interfering with a child's breathing; (5) threatening a child with a deadly weapon; or (6) doing any other act that is likely to cause or does cause bodily harm greater than transient pain or minor temporary marks." RCW 9A.16.100.
3. RCW 26.44.020(6).

2. *Child abuse or neglect* is the injury, sexual abuse, sexual exploitation, or negligent treatment or maltreatment of a child by any person under circumstances indicating harm to the child's health, welfare, and safety.[4]

3. *Sexual exploitation* includes allowing, permitting, or encouraging a child to engage in prostitution, or using a child for commercial purposes to make obscene or pornographic material.[5]

4. *Negligent treatment or maltreatment* is any act or omission that shows such a serious disregard of the consequences that it is a clear and present danger to the child's health, welfare, and safety.[6]

5. *Social service counselor* is anyone who is engaged professionally in encouraging or promoting the health, welfare, support, or education of children or in providing social services to adults or families.[7]

6. *Law enforcement agency* refers to the police department, the prosecuting attorney, the state patrol, the director of public safety, or the office of the sheriff.[8]

(B) When Must a Report Be Made?

The duty to report an incident involving a child arises at the first opportunity, but never longer than 48 hours after there is reasonable cause to believe that abuse or neglect has occurred.[9] Providers having reasonable cause to believe that a child has suffered abuse, neglect, or exploitation must make an immediate oral report, followed by a written report to DSHS, if requested.[10] However, if no reasonable cause exists to indicate that current or potential victims are at risk, no report is required.[11]

Another statute has imposed a duty to warn or to take reasonable precautions to provide protection to potential victims when future danger is threatened. If a client of an MHP communicates an actual threat of violence against a reasonably identifiable victim(s), a provider must make reasonable efforts to discuss the

---

4. RCW 26.44.020(12).
5. RCW 26.44.020(15).
6. RCW 26.44.020(16).
7. RCW 26.44.020(8). This law also applies to religious counselors and such a reporting requirement does not violate the establishment clause of the Constitution: State v. Matherwell, 114 Wash.App. 353, 788 P.2d 1066 (1990).
8. RCW 26.44.020(2).
9. RCW 26.44.030(1).
10. RCW 26.44.040.
11. RCW 26.44.030(2).

threat with the victim(s) and with law enforcement personnel.[12] In addition, the provider may begin involuntary commitment proceedings for the client if both mental illness and a danger to another exist (see chapters 5A.18 and 5E.4).

(C) How a Report is Made

In the case of child abuse or neglect, the duty to report is met by reporting the following information, if known, to a law enforcement agency or DSHS:

1. the name, address, and age of the child;
2. the name and address of the child's parents, stepparents, guardians, or other persons having custody of the child;
3. the nature and extent of the injury (or injuries), abuse, or neglect;
4. any evidence of previous injuries; and
5. any information that may be helpful in establishing the cause of a child's death, injury or injuries, and the identity of the perpetrator(s).

(D) Immunity from Liability

Any person who makes a report in good faith is immune from civil liability for reporting and testifying about the alleged child abuse or neglect.[13] The language of the reporting statute implies that gross negligence by the reporting party must be proved before he or she will be civilly liable.[14] Under this standard, a provider would not be liable unless he or she recklessly reported incorrect information or intended to make a false report to injure a particular person.

(E) Confidentiality and Privilege

Most services provided by MHPs are confidential and privileged (see chapters 4.2 and 4.3). However, reporting abuse or neglect of

---

12. RCW 71.05.120.
13. Written reports regarding children and their living conditions do not give a parent the right to sue the reporting party for defamation, even though the parent may be innocent of the reported abuse, if the reports are filed in good faith. Spurrel v. Bloch, 40 Wash. App. 854, 701 P.2d 529 (1985).
14. RCW 26.44.060.

a child to the proper authorities is not a violation of any confidentiality standards.[15]

(F) Failure to Report

A person who must report abuse or neglect of children and fails to do so may be guilty of a gross misdemeanor. The maximum sentence is one year in jail or a fine of $5,000.[16] Furthermore, a provider may be held civilly liable for any harm to a child resulting from a failure to report abuse (see chapter 6.5).[17]

15. RCW 26.44.060(3). The deposition of a victim's psychologist to discredit the victim was not allowed; Sauta v. Mount Vernon School District, 58 Wash. App.121, 791 P.2d 549 (1990).
16. RCW 26.44.080; RCW 9.92.020.
17. Civil liability is implicitly recognized in RCW 26.44.060.

5A.9

Abused and Neglected Children and Dependency Determinations

After suspected child abuse or neglect is identified, DSHS may pursue the following steps to protect the child from further harm:

1. take the child into temporary custody;
2. place the child into shelter care that could involve a preliminary shelter care hearing;
3. hold a hearing on a dependency petition; and
4. hold a hearing on an appropriate disposition.

This hierarchical process will not be pursued if one of two possibilities arises: DSHS finds that the allegations are baseless; or the parents show that they can supervise and care for the child and that it is in the child's best interest to remain with the family. MHPs may become involved in the process by evaluating the child and testifying at a dependency hearing as expert witnesses. They also may treat the child, parent, or family.

(A) Temporary Custody

Any professional that has contact with children, except lawyers, must report abuse or neglect.[1] Once a report is received and found to be credible, two possible approaches may be pursued.

Most frequently, a law enforcement agency may take a child into custody without a court order if probable cause exists indicating that the child is abused or neglected or that the child may

---

1. RCW 26.44.030(1). *See* chapter 5A.8, Reporting of Child Abuse.

be injured or disappear before obtaining a court order.[2] The child may be held in temporary custody and placed in shelter care up to 72 hours without a court order for continued shelter care.[3]

Another possible course is to obtain a court order to place the child into shelter care by filing a petition with the juvenile court alleging that the child is dependent; the child will be taken into custody if the court finds reasonable grounds to believe that the child is dependent and that the child's health, safety, and welfare will be seriously endangered.[4] The child will remain in shelter care until the dependency hearing. Whenever a child is taken into custody, the supervising agency may authorize evaluation of the child's physical or emotional condition, routine medical and dental examination and treatment, and all necessary emergency care.[5]

(A)(1) Preliminary Shelter Hearing

At the shelter care hearing, the alleged dependent must be released to the parent, guardian, or legal custodian unless the court finds reasonable cause to believe that:[6]

1. reasonable efforts to prevent or eliminate the need for removing the child from the home have not occurred, and the child has no parent, guardian, or legal custodian to provide care; or
2. the release of the child would present a serious threat or substantial harm to such a child; or
3. the parent, guardian, or legal custodian has committed a custodial interference infraction.[7]

The supervising agency or the DSHS must make reasonable efforts to advise the parents of the status of the case and inform the

---

2. RCW 26.44.050.
3. RCW 13.34.060(1); Spurrell v. Block, 40 Wash.App. 854, 701 P.2d 529 (1985). In re Brown 29 Wash.App. 744, 631 P.2d 1 (1981).
4. RCW 13.34.050. "The child of a mother who is suffering from mental illness, who does not understand the requirements of children and who is incapable of giving that child proper parental care and supplying its bare needs, is a dependent child. There is no need to wait until such a mother commits physical abuse or neglect and actually damages the child's development. . .," In re Frederickson, 25 Wash.App. 726, 610 P.2d 371, (1979). Expert testimony that the child was sexually abused, observations of the child's sexualized behavior, and evidence admitted under the child hearsay statute was sufficient to support finding that the five-year-old was sexually abused by the father, In re Dependency of S.S., 61 Wash.App.488, 814 P.2d 204, review denied, 117 Wash.2d 1011, 816 P.2d 1224 (1991). Other grounds for placing a child in shelter care arise when the child was adjudicated to be a dependent and is still subject to a dispositional order in effect; Juvenile Court Rules 2.1(b)(2): Official Rules of Court (1989).
5. RCW 13.34.060(1).
6. RCW 13.34.060(8).
7. RCW 9A.40.060 or .070, a Class C felony.

parents, guardian, or legal custodian of their rights[8] to notice about the time and place of the hearing; to representation by counsel (appointed counsel if they are indigent); to introduce evidence; to examine witnesses; and to receive a decision based solely on the evidence raised at the hearing.

(B) Dependency Hearing

DSHS will pursue filing a dependency if the child is likely to suffer further harm, and efforts to remediate the situation have failed. However, any person or agency may file a petition with the court alleging that the child is dependent because[9]

1. the child has been abandoned for an extended period as shown by statement or conduct indicating a settled intent to forego all parental rights or responsibilities;

2. the child was injured, sexually abused, or exploited, negligently treated, or maltreated under circumstances that suggest that the child's health, welfare, and safety were being harmed by the person legally responsible for the care; and

3. the child has no parent, guardian, or custodian who can care for the child without the child living in circumstances that constitute a substantial risk of damage to the his or her psychological or physical development.

The entire record of parenting may be reviewed and investigated.[10] When the rights of basic nurture, physical and mental health, and safety of the child conflict with the legal rights of the parents, the rights and safety of the child will prevail.[11] After hearing the evidence, the court makes written findings of fact concerning the dependency. If the child is not declared dependent, the child is returned to the parent.

(C) Dispositional Alternatives

If the allegations in the dependency petition are proven, the court must consider a social or predisposition study in deciding the

---

8. RCW 13.34.060; RCW 13.34.090.
9. In counties with probation officers, the allegations of the petition are to be verified by the officers in so far as possible. RCW 13.34.040.
10. In re Bennett, 24 Wash.App. 398, 600 P.2d 1308 (1979).
11. RCW 13.34.020.

disposition. The study should contain the following information:[12]

1. all social records, including facts about the child's cultural heritage;
2. what specific harm to the child should an intervention be designed to alleviate;
3. a description of specific programs (for both parents and child) needed to prevent further harm of the child, how such programs will be useful, the availability of the services, and the agency's plan for ensuring that services are delivered;
4. if removal is recommended, a full description of why the child must be removed, how any previous efforts to prevent the harm have worked, the in home treatment programs that have been considered and rejected, and the parent's attitude about removal;
5. a statement of the harm that the child may suffer because of the removal;
6. a description of the steps planned to minimize harm to the child if removal occurs; and
7. what behavior is expected before a determination can be made that supervision of the family or placement is no longer necessary.

At a subsequent dispositional hearing, the findings of the study will be considered by the court. It will determine who should receive temporary custody and what disposition is necessary. One of the following dispositions will be ordered:[13]

1. a program designed to alleviate the immediate charges relating to the child, to investigate or treat any damage that the child may have already suffered, and to aid the parents so that the child will not be endangered in the future; or
2. a placement into the custody of a relative, DSHS, or any of the residential facilities licensed by the state[14] if the court finds that reasonable efforts have failed to prevent or to eliminate the need for removing the child.

The social study and dispositional plan must be sent to the parents and their attorney for review before the dispositional hearing. They have a right to comment and, if they disagree, an

---

12. RCW 13.34.120.
13. RCW 13.34.130.
14. Foster family home or group care facility (Chapter 74.15 RCW).

alternative plan must be submitted to the court for further consideration.[15]

Wherever a child is to be removed, the agency charged with the care of the child must provide the court with a specific plan about the placement, what steps will be taken to return the child home, and what actions the agency will take to maintain parent–child ties.[16] The court supervises the application of the plan for the dependent child and reviews the status at a hearing every six months or sooner.[17] If the child is returned, close casework supervision will continue for six months, and another hearing about the need for continued intervention will occur.[18] If the child is not returned home because the reason for removal still exists, the court will document in writing that reasonable services were offered to facilitate the union; the extent to which the parents visited the child; the agency is satisfied with the parental cooperation; additional services are required; an order mandating such services, if required; and the date on which the return of the child can be expected.[19] In addition, the court, or any person or agency that has a legitimate interest in the parent–child relationship, may file a petition for termination of the parent–child relationship (see chapter 5A.10, this volume).

---

15. RCW 13.34.120(1).
16. RCW 13.34.130(2).
17. RCW 13.34.130(5).
18. RCW 13.34.130(3)(a).
19. RCW 13.34.130.(3)(b).

5A.10

Termination of Parental Rights

By law the family unit is protected unless the child's physical or mental health is jeopardized by the parents.[1] Termination of parental rights occurs infrequently, and only after rigorous due process safeguards are exercised. Once termination becomes a possibility, MHPs often undertake individual and family evaluations to help the court assess the child's emotional well-being and the parent–child relationship.

(A) Filing the Termination Petition

The DSHS, any agency, or any properly qualified adoptive parent[2] may file a petition to terminate a parent–child relationship.[3] The petition must identify the petitioner, the child, the parents, the legal guardian, and any guardian *ad litem* for a party.[4] The petition shall state why termination of the parent–child relationship is in the best interest of the child, and how the parent(s) has failed to perform parental duties under circumstances that show a

---

1. RCW 13.34.020.
2. If the child is American Indian, the Indian Child Welfare Act (ICWA) of 1978, 25 U.S.C.A. § 1903 *et seq.*, applies. *See* chapter 5A.13, this volume, for more discussion.
3. RCW 26.33.100(1).
4. When termination is being sought because of a legal or mental parental incapacity, the court must appoint a guardian *ad litem*. Any recommendations made to the court by the guardian *ad litem* are subject to the court's discretion; In re Santore 28 Wash.App. 319, 623 P.2d 702 (1981), *rev. denied* 95 Wash.2d 1019 (1981).

substantial lack of regard for the parental obligations.[5] The petition may be filed even before a child's birth.[6]

(B) Prehearing Requirements

After the petition is filed, the notice of a hearing is served on the petitioner, the parents who do not consent to the termination of their parental rights, any legal guardian or guardian *ad litem* of a party, and if, the child is an American Indian or an Alaska Native, the child's tribe or clan.[7] The notice will inform the nonconsenting parents that they have a right to an attorney, that counsel will be appointed if an indigent parent requests it, and that failure to respond to the termination action within 20 days of service is in itself sufficient ground for termination.[8]

To aid the court in reaching its decision, a written social study about the situation must be produced. A copy of the social study and proposed service plan must be sent to the parents and their lawyer at least 10 working days before the hearing. The parent(s) may submit an alternate plan to correct the problems.[9]

(C) Termination of Parental Rights

Before termination is ordered, all evidence must be presented in open court and subjected to cross examination.[10] If the child has been declared dependent, it must be shown beyond a reasonable doubt that there is little likelihood that conditions will be remedied or that the child can be returned to the parent in the future.[11] If the child is American Indian or Alaska Native, no termination may occur unless the evidence supports beyond a reasonable doubt that the child is likely to suffer further emotional or physical damage (including testimony from expert witnesses).[12]

If the termination arises from the adoption statutes, clear, cogent, and convincing evidence must be presented showing that

---

5. RCW 26.33.100(2).
6. RCW 26.33.100(3).
7. RCW 26.33.110(2). As to notice to the child's tribe, *see* 25 U.S.C. § 912(a).
8. RCW 26.33.110(2)(b).
9. RCW 13.34.120. The court is required to hold a hearing only if the facts in the dependency are in dispute; In re Dependency of L.S., 62 Wash.App. 1, 813 P.2d 133 (1991).
10. In re McGee, 36 Wash.App. 660, 679 P.2d 933 (1984).
11. RCW 13.34.190.
12. 25 U.S.C. § 1912(f); In re Fisher, 31 Wash.App. 550, 643 P.2d 887 (1982). The court was entitled to consider the child's attachment to the grandmother and half-brother; In re A.V.D., 62 Wash.App. 562, 815 P.2d 277 (1991).

it is in the best interest of the child for the termination to occur and that the parents have disregarded their parental obligations.[13] Commonly understood obligations of parenthood entail the following minimum attributes:[14]

1. expressed love and affection for the child;

2. expressed personal concern over the health, education, and general well-being of the child;

3. the ability to supply the necessary food, clothing, and medical care;

4. the ability to provide an adequate domicile; and

5. the ability to furnish social and religious guidance.

Substantial failure to meet these minimum parental attributes must occur before parental rights are terminated.[15]

Also, the court may consider the child's need for permanent placement through adoption when weighing the child's interests against parental rights.[16] Many scenarios exist in which the courts of Washington have found that the right to a parental relationship is subordinate to the moral, intellectual, and material welfare of the child. The following are typical scenarios:

1. *Abandonment of the child.* A parent's nearly complete disregard for the child following a marital dissolution, coupled with a failure to provide support for the child, form a substantial lack of regard for parental obligations.[17]

2. *Child abuse or neglect.* This is typified by injuries, sexual abuse, sexual exploitation, or negligent treatment that suggests a substantial lack of regard for the child's health, welfare, and safety.[18]

3. *Parental mental incapacity.* An intractable mental condition of the parent impairs the ability of the parent to care for the child's health, welfare, and safety.[19]

---

13. RCW 26.33.120(1).
14. In re Adoption of Lybbert, 75 Wash.2d 671, 453 P.2d 650 (1969).
15. A finding that termination would lead to an "atmosphere of stimulation, intellectually and emotionally" for the children was not sufficient; In re Hendrickson, 7 Wash.App. 485, 499 P.2d 908 (1972).
16. In re Clark, 26 Wash.App. 832, 611 P.2d 1343 (1980).
17. In re Adoption of Lybbert, 75 Wash.2d 671, 453 P.2d 650 (1969); In re Maypole, 4 Wash.App. 672, 483 P.2d 878 (1971).
18. RCW 26.44.020(12). In re Dunagan, 74 Wash.2d 807, 447 P.2d 87 (1968) (beating); In re Nuller, 40 Wash.2d 319, 242 P.2d 1016 (1952) (brutality); In re Warren, 40 Wash.2d 342, 243 P.2d 632 (1952) (poverty alone is not sufficient grounds); In re Dodge, 29 Wash.App. 486, 628 P.2d 1343 (1981) (a parent's unmanageable psychotic condition caused delusions that might lead to physical abuse or death of the child).
19. In re Dodge, 29 Wash.App. 486, 628 P.2d 1343 (1981); In re Mosely, 34 Wash.App. 179, 660 P.2d 315 (1983).

4. *Parental felony and imprisonment.* The parent's incarceration is only one factor to be considered. Other factors include the nature of the crime committed, the identity of the victim, the parent's conduct before and during imprisonment (e.g., the parental obligations such as love and affection, personal concern, financial support, and social and religious guidance).[20]

(D) Effect of Termination

A termination order divests the parent and child of all legal rights, privileges, duties, and obligations with regard to each other, including inheritance and support rights.[21]

---

20. In re Sego, 82 Wash.2d 736, 513 P.2d 831 (1973); In re Adoption of Dobbs, 12 Wash. App. 676, 531 P.2d 303 (1975); In re Pawling, 101 Wash.2d 392, 679 P.2d 916 (1984).
21. The court may order a guardianship as an alternative to parental termination. A parent whose parental rights are terminated is not allowed visitation rights; In re A.V.D., 62 Wash.App.562, 815 P.2d 277 (1991).

5A.11

Guardianship for Minors

A guardian is typically appointed for a minor when the custodial parent is unable to care for the child because of the parent's death, legal termination of parental rights or of the child's dependency, or the minor's estate must be managed or protected. MHPs may become involved in this type of case during the selection of the guardian or during the treatment of a ward.

(A) Application and Preparation for the Guardianship Hearing

Three methods exist by which guardians are appointed for a minor in the state of Washington. The first two methods are found in the statutes that regulate guardianship for adults and for children.[1] One of the methods does not involve the detailed preparation and application process described earlier (see chapter 5A.2, Guardianship for Adults). Instead, a testamentary appointment (accomplished through a will) establishes a guardian(s) for the child, or the estate, or both.[2] Upon the death of both parents, before letters of guardianship are issued, the guardian(s) must appear before a Superior Court to subscribe to and file a bond (unless ruled unnecessary by the court).[3] The guardian then acquires the same powers and must perform the same duties, with

---

1. Chapter 11.88 RCW.
2. RCW 11.88.080. The court shall confirm the appointment, unless the court finds, based on the evidence presented at a hearing on the matter, that the individual appointed is not qualified to serve.
3. RCW 11.88.100.

regard to the minor child and the estate, as described in chapter 5A.2.

The second method found within the statute regulating guardianship differs little from the procedures described for adults (see chapter 5A.2). Any person or entity interested in the child's welfare may petition the Superior Court to establish a guardianship. A difference arises in the application process: Notice need not be given about a hearing on a guardianship petition if[4]

1. the petition is requested by a parent who wishes to become the guardian or limited guardian, and the child is younger than 14 years of age;

2. the petition is accompanied by a consent of the child 14 years of age or older, and the child agrees to the appointment; or

3. the petition is filed by a nonresident guardian of a child (e.g., the ward and guardian have moved to Washington, and guardianship was granted by another jurisdiction).

The third method arises when any person or entity files a petition in juvenile court alleging that a child is dependent (see chapter 5A.9). Often, the petition will request that a guardianship be created. In this type of case, the petition must be verified[5] and contain a statement of fact that the child is dependent because of being[6]

1. abandoned, when the child's parent, guardian, or other custodian by statement or conduct has avoided all parental rights and responsibilities in spite of an ability to pursue them;

2. abused or neglected, as defined by Chapter 26.44 RCW (see chapter 5A.8);

3. inadequately cared for because of the danger of substantial damage to the child's psychological or physical development; or

4. developmentally disabled, as defined by RCW 71.20.016, and the parent, guardian, or custodian along with the DSHS determine that services appropriate to the child's needs cannot be provided in the home.

---

4. RCW 11.88.040(4).
5. RCW 13.34.040.
6. RCW 13.34.030(2).

(B) The Guardianship Hearing

A hearing about the testamentary appointment of a guardian or appointment of a guardian through Chapter 11.88 RCW does not differ from the process described earlier about adults, nor do the rights and duties differ if the appointment is made. However, a striking distinction exists between pursuing guardianship through Chapter 11.88 RCW or guardianship for a dependent child through Chapter 13.34 RCW. If the matter is contested by any interested party under chapter 11.88 RCW, the burden of proof is much greater (clear and convincing evidence is needed) than it is for the process under chapter 13.34 RCW (only a preponderance of evidence is needed). Most guardianship actions involving children and coming to the attention of MHPs are likely to arise through the dependency process. The goal of a dependency action is to determine the welfare and best interests of the child.[7] To justify a guardianship, the court needs to find only by a preponderance of the evidence that[8]

1. the child was dependent as defined earlier;
2. a dispositional order was filed under RCW 13.34.130;
3. the child was removed from the custody of the parent for at least a period of six months;
4. the services ordered by the court to correct parental deficiencies within the foreseeable future were provided;
5. there is little likelihood that the conditions will improve so that the child can return to the parent in the near future; and
6. a guardianship, rather than a termination of the parent–child relationship (see chapter 5A.10) or a continuation of the child's current dependent status, is in the best interest of the family.

If the evidence supports the establishment of a guardianship for the child, the court orders the appointment of a person or agency to serve as guardian and specifies the rights and responsibilities regarding the custody and control of the child. These may include the appropriate frequency of parent–child visitation and the amount and nature of continued involvement by the supervising agency.[9]

---

7. In re Hansen, 24 Wash.App. 27, 599 P.2d 1304 (1979).
8. In re Hansen, 24 Wash.App. 27, 599 P.2d 1304 (1979).
9. RCW 13.34.232. The court may order the establishment of a guardianship as an alternative to the termination of parental rights (*see* chapter 5A.10); In re A.V.D., 62 Wash.App. 562, 815 P.2d 277 (1991). The statute does not allow an award of visitation rights to a parent whose parental rights have been terminated. *Id.*

(C) Termination of the Guardianship

A guardian's authority and responsibility end upon the guardian's death, resignation, or removal or upon the child's death, adoption, or reaching 18 years of age.[10] Any person or entity interested in the welfare of the child may petition for removal of the guardian if the best interest of the child is in question.[11] After a hearing to determine whether to terminate the existing guardianship, a new guardian may be appointed if necessary.

---

10. RCW 11.88.140; *see* termination of an adult guardianship (chapter 5A.2) for more extensive discussion and citations that presumably apply to wards who are children.
11. RCW 11.88.120; RCW 11.92.150.

5A.12

Foster Care

Foster care is a 24-hour per day substitute care for children whose parents cannot or will not provide normal family care for them. Care may be provided by either a licensed foster family home or a group care facility.[1] MHPs may become involved in the licensing of a home, in training foster family licensees,[2] and in providing assessment and therapeutic services to those placed in foster care.[3]

(A) Licensing Requirements

Persons or organizations must apply for a license or certification to provide foster care services through the DSHS. The DSHS checks for convictions of child abuse within the potential foster family and for any other crime involving physical harm. The criminal history checks are run on each person in the family who will have unmonitored access to children, to expectant mothers, or to developmentally disabled persons.[4] Applicants for a license must be at least 18 years of age and demonstrate that they possess "the understanding, ability, physical health, emotional stability and personality suited to meet the physical, mental, emotional

---

1. WAC 388-70-012.
2. WAC 388-73-302. The DSHS is required to provide ongoing foster parent training; this includes contracting for a variety of support services to reduce feelings of isolation and stress, and to increase skills and confidence. RCW 74.14B.020.
3. The department is mandated in the legislature to provide therapeutic day care and day treatment, and counseling for children who have been abused or neglected. RCW 74.14B.040; RCW 74.14B.050.
4. WAC 388-73-022.

and social needs of persons under care."[5] If both foster parents in a two-parent home (or the single foster parent in a one-parent home) are employed outside the home, the DSHS must give written approval; approval is based on the needs of the persons to be cared for.[6] The foster parents must have sufficient regular income to maintain their own family without resorting to the payments made for the persons in their care.[7]

(B) Placement of People in Foster Homes

Except in an emergency,[8] a person shall be placed into foster care only with written consent from parents or under court order.[9] The following circumstances warrant such a placement:[10]

1. temporary residential care is required when the child is taken into custody after running away;[11]

2. the child requires shelter care because probable cause suggests that abuse or neglect has occurred and that the child would be injured if not placed there;[12]

3. the child is declared dependent by the court and the court's order of disposition removes the child from home to placement into foster care;[13]

4. the court has terminated the parent and child relationship and has placed the custody of the child with the DSHS;

5. the DSHS may make a group care placement if it has assessed the child's and family's need and determined that it is the most appropriate placement option; or

6. the child's parents or legal guardians have voluntarily requested placement of the child into foster care.

A foster family home may provide care to expectant mothers or developmentally disabled persons as well.

---

5. WAC 388-73-030.
6. WAC 388-73-306.
7. *Id.*
8. *See* chapter 5A.9, Abused and Neglected Children and Dependency Determinations: Temporary Custody. RCW 26.44.050.
9. WAC 388-73-212(4).
10. WAC 388-70-013.
11. Chapter 13.32A RCW, Runaway Youth Act.
12. RCW 13.34.050. *See* chapter 5A.9, Abused and Neglected Children and Dependency Determinations.
13. *Id.*

If the person is not to return home, the agency must place the person with a foster family or in a group home that will meet his or her physical, emotional, and cultural needs. A written social study of each person eligible for foster care services serves as the basis for selecting the particular foster care option. The social study includes the child's school records, any copies of psychological or psychiatric evaluations, a narrative description of the background of the case, an identification of the person's interpersonal relationships, the problems and type of behavior that require care away from the person's home, and previous placement history.[14]

To make an informed decision about accepting the person into their home, the DSHS provides the foster parents with sufficient information about the person, such as, his or her behavioral and emotional problems, and the person's history with the family of origin.[15] Before the actual placement, the DSHS prepares both the person to be placed and the foster family.[16] After the placement, the frequency of the caseworker's contact with the child and foster family is determined by the needs, but each active foster home is visited not less than once every 90 days.[17]

Special requirements exist for placement of American Indian children.[18] An important requirement is that potential placements be considered in the following order:[19] relatives; an Indian family of the same tribe as the child; an Indian family of a Washington tribe of a similar culture; any other family that can provide a suitable home for an Indian child, such suitability decided through consultation with a local Indian child welfare advisory committee. Depending on the extent of the tribe's sovereignty, the tribe's child welfare advisory committee and the tribal court may exercise exclusive jurisdiction over the matter.

A person may reside in a foster home for as little as one night or as long as several years. This determination is based on the needs of the person placed and on whether the weaknesses of the person's family are addressed.

---

14. WAC 388-73-076.
15. WAC 388-73-212(6).
16. WAC 388-73-212(3). This remains very general but presumably could involve MHP services.
17. WAC 388-73-212(7).
18. WAC 388-70-091 to -095; WAC 388-70-600 to -640; WAC 388-73-044.
19. WAC 388-73-044(6).

5A.12A

Conservatorship for Minors

In many states, a separate conservatorship law allows a court to appoint someone to manage the estate or financial affairs of a minor. Washington has created no conservatorship law. Guardianship provisions may apply to certain cases (see chapter 5A.11).

Adoption

The purpose of adoption is to provide stable homes for children while protecting the rights of all parties.[1] MHPs may contribute to the evidence required by the court during the adoption proceedings. Preplacement and postplacement adoption evaluations must be filed before the court can render its decision.[2]

(A) Adoption Requirements

Any person who is legally competent and is 18 years of age or older may become an adoptive parent.[3] A child cannot be placed with a prospective adoptive parent until a preplacement report is filed with the court.[4] A potential adoptive parent may request an agency,[5] the DSHS, an individual approved by the court, or a qualified court employee to prepare a preplacement report.[6] The report must contain a recommendation about the fitness of the person as an adoptive parent. Also, it must document the investigation about the home environment, family life, health, facilities, and resources of the potential adoptive parent.[7] The petitioner

---

1. RCW 26.33.010.
2. RCW 26.33.180 to .200.
3. RCW 26.33.140(2).
4. RCW 26.33.180. Unless ordered by the court, such a report is unnecessary if the petitioner seeks to adopt the child of the petitioner's spouse or if the adoptee is 18 years of age or older (RCW 26.33.220).
5. *Agency* means any public or private association, corporation, or individual licensed or certified by the DSHS as a child-placing agency under Chapter 74.15 RCW.
6. RCW 26.33.190(2).
7. RCW 26.33.190(2).

must give to the person responsible for writing the report three days' written notice of any proceeding at which the report will be considered; the reporting person may testify or waive the right to participate in the proceeding.[8]

Any person may be adopted in Washington in spite of age or residence.[9] When the petition for adoption is filed, the court will require a postplacement report to determine the adequacy of the placement. The report will address whether the placement remains in the best interest of the child.[10] The report must be filed within 60 days of the court's request and contain all available information about the physical and mental conditions of the child; if relevant, information about the child's membership in any American Indian tribe;[11] the home environment, family life, health, facilities, and resources of the petitioner(s); and any other facts and circumstances relating to the advisability of the adoption.[12]

(B) Petition for Relinquishment

Often, rights to a child are relinquished at birth by both parents, and they consent to the child being adopted. A parent, DSHS, or an agency may file, with the court, a petition to relinquish a child to DSHS or to an agency.[13] The consent of the parent(s) to the adoption must accompany the petition.[14] If written consent of the prospective adoptive parent(s) is not filed with the petition, DSHS or another agency must provide consent.[15] The petition with the written consent to adoption may be filed before the child's birth. However, if the child is American Indian, neither document can

---

8. RCW 26.33.230.
9. RCW 26.33.140(1).
10. RCW 26.33.200(1).
11. Under the Indian Child Welfare Act of 1978, a number of laws exist that regulate child custody proceedings, including termination of the child–parent relationship and any action that results in a final decree of adoption. 25 U.S.C. § 1903(1). An *Indian child* is any unmarried person under the age of 18 years who is either a member of an American Indian tribe or is eligible for membership in an American Indian tribe and is the biological child of a member of a tribe; 25 U.S.C. § 1903(4). Under state law, in any adoptive placement of an Indian child, preference shall be given, in the absence of good cause to the contrary, to placement with (a) a member of the child's extended family; (b) other members of the child's tribe; or (c) other American Indian families; 25 U.S.C. § 1915(a).
12. *Id*. The preparer(s) of the report must be licensed or certified by the DSHS for child placing under Chapter 74.15 RCW.
13. RCW 26.33.080.
14. *Id*.
15. *Id*.

be signed until 10 days after the child's birth, and both must be recorded before a court of competent jurisdiction.[16]

(B)(1) Hearing on Petition for Relinquishment

The court will set the time and place for the hearing, which may not be held sooner than 48 hours after the child's birth or the signing of the necessary consents, whichever is later.[17] The court may enter a temporary order giving custody of the child to the prospective adoptive parent if a preplacement report is filed;[18] otherwise, temporary custody of the child will be given to DSHS or to an agency. Notice of the hearing must be served on any relinquishing parent or alleged father, DSHS, or the child placing agency, as specified by statute.[19]

For any proceeding under the adoption chapter,[20] the court must appoint a guardian *ad litem* for a parent or alleged father under 18 years of age.[21] Also, the court may appoint a guardian *ad litem* for a child adoptee or for any incompetent party involved in any proceeding. The guardian *ad litem* will represent the interests of the parent and must report to the court whether the written consent to adoption or petition for relinquishment was signed voluntarily, with an understanding of the consequences.[22]

If the court approves the petition for relinquishment, it may award custody of the child to the prospective adoptive parent who is appointed legal guardian; if no adoptive parent is available, then the DSHS or the child-placing agency is appointed legal guardian and ordered to place the child with an adoptive parent.[23]

(C) Petition for Adoption

An adoption proceeding is initiated by filing with the court a petition of adoption, written consent to adoption, and a preplacement report.[24] In addition to information identifying the

---

16. *Id.*; Indian Child Welfare Act of 1978, 25 U.S.C. § 1913(a). If the tribe has exclusive jurisdiction over its matters concerning children, the tribal court must consent to the relinquishment.
17. RCW 26.33.090(1). If the child is American Indian, the time requirement is 10 days.
18. *Id.* If the child is American Indian, the requirements of voluntary foster care also must be met; 25 U.S.C. § 1913(a).
19. RCW 26.33.310.
20. Chapter 26.33 RCW.
21. RCW 26.33.070.
22. *Id.*
23. RCW 26.33.090(4).
24. RCW 26.33.150.

petitioner(s) and the adoptee, the petition must contain a statement stating whether the child is covered under the Indian Child Welfare Act.[25] The following types of consents to an adoption are required by

1. the adoptee, if 14 years of age or older;
2. the parents of an adoptee under 18 years of age;
3. an agency or DSHS to whom the adoptee has been relinquished; or
4. the legal guardian of the adoptee.

Generally, consent to adoption may not be revoked after court approval. However, within one year after the approval, the consent may be revoked if fraud or duress occurred[26] or if the consenting parent lacked mental competency at the time.[27]

(C)(1) Hearing on Petition for Adoption

After receiving all documents, the court must schedule a hearing on the petition and provide notice of the date, time, and place of the hearing to the petitioner; any person or agency whose consent was required, unless it was waived; the child's tribe, if the child is American Indian; and the preparer(s) of the preplacement report(s).[28] At the hearing, the court will enter a decree of adoption if it is in the best interest of the child. The court's decision is based on the petition, the preplacement and postplacement reports, other evidence introduced at the hearing, and all necessary con-

---

25. *Id.*
26. In re Infant Child Perry, 31 Wash.App. 268, 641 P.2d 178 (1982). Undue influence and overreaching are types of fraud that involve unfair persuasion. In determining whether it has occurred, the court will consider the fairness of the resulting bargain, the availability of independent advice, and the susceptibility of the person persuaded. In re Adoption of Baby Girl K, 26 Wash.App. 897, 615 P.2d 1310 (1980). A lack of full understanding about the consequences of surrendering parental rights, together with inexperience, emotional stress, and uncertainty, are insufficient to find that fraud, deceit, or coercion has occurred. In the case of an American Indian child, consent may be withdrawn for any reason before entry of the final decree of adoption and for fraud or duress within two years after the decree is issued. *See* 25 U.S.C. § 1913(a); RCW 26.33.160(4)(g).
27. RCW 26.33.160(3).
28. RCW 26.33.240.

sents.[29] If the court finds that the adoption is not in the best interest of the child, it must make appropriate provision for the care and custody of the child (see chapter 5A.9).[30]

(D) Effect of Adoption

The effect of entering a decree of adoption is to divest any parent of all legal rights and obligations with regard to the adoptee, except past-due child support obligations; the adoptee becomes the child, legal heir, and lawful issue of the adoptive parent.[31] A decree will not disentitle a child to any benefit due from a third party, agency, state, or the United States.[32] Adoption will not affect any rights or benefits that the child has acquired by descending from a member of an American Indian tribe.

---

29. *Id.* For an American Indian child, 25 U.S.C. requires that the court either adopt a preferential placement or find good cause why that should not be done: In re the Adoption of M v. Navajo Nation, 832 P.2d 518 (1992). Good cause is a matter of judicial discretion, and the court must exercise its discretion in light of many factors, including the best interest of the child (25 U.S.C. § 1902, In re Interest of Bird Head, 213 Neb. 741, 331 N.W.2d 785), the suitability of persons preferred for placement (*Id.*), the wishes of the biological parents (25 U.S.C. § 1915(c)), the child's ties to the tribe (In re Appeal in Maricopa County, Juvenile Action No. A-25525, 136 Ariz. at 534, 667 P.2d at 234), and the child's ability to make any cultural adjustments necessitated by a particular placement (In the Interest of J.R.I I., 358 N.W.2d at 321-22).
30. *Id.*
31. RCW 26.33.260.
32. RCW 26.33.270.

5A.14

Family in Conflict

(A) Incorrigibility Standard Abandoned

The law for families in conflict established a means for providing social services before parental abuse, neglect, or abandonment of the child become perilous, or before the children are driven by severe family conflict to run away.[1] Incorrigibility determinations no longer label children in the state of Washington. If parents and their children are unable to live together, the law provides for temporary removal of the children without transferring any of the legal rights or duties of the parents. The goal is to sustain the family unit despite very serious family conflict that a less restrictive alternative, such as counseling or crisis intervention services, has failed to remedy. MHPs are likely to become involved by providing family reconciliation services. Such services develop skills and supports within the family to resolve conflicts without resorting to more serious interventions, such as termination of parental rights (see chapter 5A.10).

---

1. In 1977 and again in 1979, the legislature repealed many of the statutes that applied to minors, including incorrigibility determinations. The Juvenile Court Act replaced the repealed statutes and established several procedures, proactively addressing a number of problems involving minors. These statutes changed procedures regarding (1) children who are runaways and who face conflict in their families (Chapter 13.32A RCW; Chapter 74.13 RCW); (2) children who are abused, neglected, or abandoned by their parents (Chapter 13.34 RCW); and (3) children who commit crimes (Chapter 13.34 RCW).

(B) Terms and Definitions

Before considering how the statutes operate, it is necessary to understand the legal meanings of the terms used:

1. *child* or *minor* means any person under the chronological age of 18 years;[2]

2. *parent* means the legal custodian(s) or guardian(s) of a child;[3]

3. *family reconciliation services* may include, but are not limited to, referral to services for suicide prevention, psychiatric or other medical care or to psychological, welfare, legal, educational, or other social services;[4]

4. *crisis residential center* means an agency operating under contract with the DSHS to provide temporary, protective care to children in a facility or specialized foster home operated in a way that assures that minors placed there will not run away;[5]

5. *unlawful harboring* of a minor refers to the crime committed when a person provides shelter to a minor without the consent of a parent. In addition, after the person knows that the minor has run away, the person breaks the law if he or she intentionally fails to release the minor to a law enforcement officer, fails to reveal the location of the minor to the officer, obstructs the officer from taking the minor into custody, or helps the minor in avoiding the custody of the officer.[6]

(C) Identification of Conflict

Families who are in conflict may request family reconciliation services from the DSHS (e.g., the parent advises the agency that the child is absent without consent).[7] More frequently, a law enforcement agency will become involved first (e.g., an officer finds a child in dangerous circumstances considering the child's age, location, and time of day). A law enforcement officer must take the child into custody in either situation. In addition, the

---

2. RCW 13.32A.030(1).
3. RCW 13.32A.030(2).
4. RCW 13.32A.040.
5. WAC 388-73-014(a). Yet, the child must not be locked up or physically restrained unless restraint is necessary to protect others from physical injury, to obtain possession of a weapon, or to protect property from serious damage (WAC 388-73-012(10) and WAC 388-73-048)).
6. RCW 13.32A.080. Presumably, any private person may lawfully provide shelter to the minor absent from a home in all other instances without notifying the authorities or the parent(s).
7. RCW 13.32A.040.

child will be taken into custody if an agency who is supervising a child notifies the police that the child has run away, or if the juvenile court finds that probable cause exists to believe that the child has violated a court-placement order.[8]

Once in custody, the child must be informed of the reason and, at the officer's discretion, transported to one of the following destinations:[9]

1. to the child's home unless (a) the child indicates distress at the prospect of being returned; (b) the officer believes some type of neglect or abuse is occurring; (c) it is not practical to take the child home; or (d) no parent is available to accept custody;

2. to the home of a responsible adult (other than the child's parent) where the officer reasonably believes that the child will be provided with adequate care and supervision, and the child will remain at that home until a placement can be agreed to;

3. to a designated crisis residential center; or

4. to a juvenile detention center if the child has violated a court-placement order.

Once a child is taken into custody, DSHS must offer services to the family in an attempt to reconcile the differences between the parent(s) and the child.[10] If reconciliation cannot be achieved, DSHS must find a living situation for the child that is agreeable to both parents and child.[11]

If either the parents or the child do not agree with the placement, the parents, the child, or the DSHS may petition the juvenile court for an alternate residential placement.[12]

(D) Juvenile Court Hearing

When a petition is filed with the juvenile court, the court must[13]

1. schedule a date for a fact-finding hearing;

2. notify the parent(s) and child of such date;

3. appoint legal counsel for the child;

4. inform the child and the parent(s) of the legal consequences of the court approving or disapproving the petition; and

---

8. RCW 13.32A.050.
9. RCW 13.32A.060.
10. RCW 74.13.031(4).
11. RCW 74.13.031(4).
12. RCW 13.32A.140 and RCW 13.32A.150.
13. RCW 13.32A.160(1).

5. notify all parties of their right to present evidence at the hearing.

Before the hearing, the child may remain at home or be placed in a crisis residential center, foster family home, group home, with a responsible adult other than the parent, or any other suitable home found by DSHS.[14] Upon the request of the child or parent, any temporary placement must be reviewed by the court within three court days.[15]

At the conclusion of a fact-finding hearing, the court may issue an order placing the child in a residence other than the home of the parent(s) only if it is established, by a preponderance of the evidence, that[16] the petitioner has made a reasonable effort to resolve the conflict; the conflict cannot be resolved while the child continues to live in the parental home; and reasonable efforts have been made to prevent or eliminate the need for removing the child from the parental home. If the court denies a petition for alternative placement, the court may require that the child stay with the parent(s).[17]

(E) Disposition

If out-of-home placement is approved, the DSHS must submit within 17 days a disposition plan about a three-month, alternate residential placement of the child designed to reunite the family and resolve the family conflict.[18] The court may modify the plan. The court's dispositional order must specify the person or agency with whom the child will be placed. The order will delineate those parental powers temporarily awarded to the person or agency (e.g., the right to authorize medical, dental, and optical treatment, and parental visitation rights).[19] Family reconciliation services will continue during this period, and the placement may continue as long as there is agreement by the child and the parent(s). A review hearing may be held every three months to approve or disapprove the continuation of the placement. The court must decide whether reasonable efforts have been made to

---

14. RCW 13.32A.160(2).
15. RCW 13.32A.160(3).
16. RCW 13.32A.170(1).
17. RCW 13.32A.170(4). If a child fails to comply with a court order to stay at home, contempt proceedings can be pursued by the court 90 days after its order; RCW 13.32A.170(6). A child found in contempt shall be imprisoned only in a secure juvenile detention facility; RCW 13.32A.250(3).
18. RCW 13.32A.170(2)(3).
19. RCW 13.32A.180. The disposition cannot be made to secure residence but must be made to other types of residential placements.

reunite the family. If out-of-home placement is continued, the court may modify the dispositional plan.

The procedures reviewed in this chapter permit the minor child to be removed from a parental home if the family is experiencing a conflict so severe that removal of the child is the only feasible means to assist the family, and if the conflict cannot be remedied by a less restrictive alternative, such as counseling or crisis intervention services. An alternate residential placement does not violate due process even when the parents can care for the child.[20] This action by the state does not infringe upon parental rights as severely as does a finding of dependency (see chapter 5A.9) or termination of parental rights (see chapter 5A.10). Although such a placement alone cannot serve as a basis for termination of parental rights, the next step of a dependency action leads to the termination of parental rights. Ultimately, a dependency action may result in a full termination of parental rights if the parents do not correct their objectionable behaviors.

---

20. In re Sumey, 94 Wash.2d 757, 621 P.2d 108 (1980).

5A.15

Juvenile Offenders

The juvenile court hears the complaints filed against juveniles who are alleged to have broken the criminal law. A person who is younger than 18 years of age and has not been transferred to adult court for an earlier offense will appear before the juvenile court. Although MHPs may become involved at all stages of the process, they are employed most frequently during the dispositional phase.

(A) Legal Capacity

The law holds that children under the age of eight years are incapable of committing a crime.[1] A child 8 to 11 years of age is presumed to be incapable of committing a crime and the state has the burden of rebutting the presumption of incapacity;[2] the purpose of creating this presumption is to protect those individuals who are unable to appreciate the wrongfulness of their behavior. Competent evidence upon the question of age can be presented by physicians.[3] Once a determination of capacity is made, the prosecution still must prove beyond a reasonable doubt that the juvenile possessed the intent (*mens rea*) to commit the crime (see chapter 5D.7, Mens Rea).

---

1. RCW 9A.04.050.
2. *Id.*; State v. Q.D., 102 Wash.2d 19, 685 P.2d 557 (1984).
3. *Id.* Presumably, other MHPs could be qualified to serve as experts, although the statute mentions only physicians.

(B) Taking the Juvenile into Custody

A juvenile may be taken into custody[4]

1. if the juvenile court finds that probable cause exists to believe that the juvenile has committed an offense or has violated the terms of a dispositional or release order;

2. without a court order, by a law enforcement officer, if probable cause exists to believe that the juvenile has committed an offense;

3. by a court order, if the juvenile is to be held as a material witness; or

4. if the DSHS suspended the parole of the offender.

A juvenile taken into custody may not be held in detention unless there is probable cause to believe that an offense has been committed, or that a term of a dispositional order has been violated. This finding can be coupled with one of the following:[5] it is unlikely that the juvenile will appear for further proceedings; detention is required to protect the juvenile from himself or herself; the juvenile is a threat to community safety; the juvenile will intimidate witnesses or is a material witness; the juvenile has another case pending; the juvenile is a fugitive from justice; or the juvenile's parole has been suspended or modified. MHPs may be called upon to evaluate whether the juvenile is a danger to self or others. If mental illness is not severe and the juvenile is dangerous, the juvenile will be held in detention. Presumably, involuntary commitment would be pursued if the juvenile is mentally ill and a danger to self or others.

When a juvenile is taken into custody and held in detention, the juvenile must be released within 72 hours (weekends and holidays are excluded). This must occur unless an injunction is filed, or the juvenile court holds a hearing about a community supervision modification, termination of diversion, or parole modification.[6]

Many procedural due process rights exist for juveniles. These include notice about the time, place, and purpose of a hearing and the right to counsel or appointed counsel if the juvenile is indigent.[7]

---

4. RCW 13.40.040(1).
5. RCW 13.40.040(2).
6. RCW 13.40.050(1)(a).
7. RCW 13.40.050(2); RCW 13.40.140.

(C) Filing Information

Within 72 hours after the prosecutor has filed an information (a concise statement of the essential facts forming the offense), a detention hearing as described earlier must be held. The court determines whether the case is properly before it, whether it should be treated as a diversion case, or whether the juvenile should be released.[8] The court can release the juvenile on his or her personal recognizance[9] if detention is not required, or order any combination of the following conditions:[10] place the juvenile in the custody of a designated person agreeing to supervise the juvenile; place travel restrictions upon the juvenile; require regular reporting to the court; or enforce any condition other than detention to assure appearance at later hearings.

(D) Diversion Agreement

The prosecutor may divert a case without filing any information if the alleged offense is a misdemeanor or gross misdemeanor, and if the present offense does not combine with any past offenses to exceed three offenses, provided that none of those was a felony.[11] Prosecution for more serious offenses also may be diverted, but only after the court has considered information concerning these offenses and has ordered diversion.[12]

The diversion agreement is considered to be a contract between the juvenile and a diversionary unit. The juvenile agrees to fulfill certain conditions instead of prosecution. The agreement is limited to the following constraints:[13]

1. community service not to exceed 150 hours;
2. restitution limited to the amount of actual loss incurred by the victim but not to exceed the amount that the juvenile has the means or potential to pay;
3. attendance of up to 2 hours of counseling or up to 10 hours of educational or informational sessions at a community agency; and
4. a fine, not to exceed $100.

---

8. RCW 13.40.050(4).
9. RCW 13.40.050(5).
10. RCW 13.40.050(6).
11. RCW 13.40.070(6).
12. RCW 13.40.050(4).
13. RCW 13.40.080(2).

This agreement may not exceed a period of six months for any type of misdemeanor or one year for a felony; it may extend beyond the 18th birthday of the divertee.[14]

(E) Adjudication Hearing

If diversion is an inadequate remedy and the court has not declined jurisdiction (see chapter 5A.18, Transfer of Juveniles to Stand Trial as Adults), the court will advise the defendant of the allegations and require a plea to be entered.[15] Either party may make preliminary motions before the plea (e.g., the juvenile is incompetent to stand trial, see chapter 5A.16). If the defendant pleads guilty, the court may proceed with disposition or continue the case for a dispositional hearing; if the plea is not guilty, a hearing date is set.[16]

At the hearing, the prosecution must prove guilt beyond a reasonable doubt. Juveniles are entitled to all the usual due process rights except a right to a jury trial.[17] If the defendant is found not guilty, he or she must be released from detention. If found guilty, the court may either proceed immediately to disposition or continue the case. Typically, the court may request a predisposition study to aid it in evaluating matters about the disposition, including the juvenile's mental or physical condition. Often MHPs will provide evidence about the existence and effect of a mental or physical condition that has significantly reduced the juvenile's culpability.

(F) Disposition

Both the prosecution and defense counsel may submit recommendations to the court for disposition. Several factors must be considered by the court in determining the disposition.[18] These could include specific mitigating factors.[19] Providers may evaluate the juvenile and testify about the existence and effect of a mental or physical condition that has reduced the juvenile's culpability, but

---

14. RCW 13.40.080(4).
15. RCW 13.40.130(1)
16. RCW 13.40.130(2).
17. RCW 13.40.140, right to an attorney, right to confront witnesses, the privilege against self-incrimination, and suppression of evidence obtained illegally; State v. Lawley, 91 Wash.2d 654, 591 P.2d 772 (1979), no right to jury trial.
18. RCW 13.40.150.
19. State v. Fellers, 37 Wash.App. 613, 683 P.2d 209 (1984).

not sufficiently to establish a defense (see chapter 5A.17, Nonresponsibility Defense).[20]

Although the legislature has enacted determinate sentences, the court has some discretion in imposing a sentence.[21] Generally, sentences within the standard range are based upon the age, seriousness of the crime, and criminal history of the offender. Nevertheless, upon a finding of "manifest injustice" supported by clear and convincing evidence, the court may impose a disposition outside the standard range.[22] Never will the term of confinement exceed what an adult would serve for the same offense, nor may the sentence continue beyond the juvenile's 21st birthday, unless he or she was tried as an adult.[23]

(G) Maintenance, Access, and Confidentiality of Records

Agencies involved with the juvenile are responsible for the accuracy, completeness, and security of their records.[24] In general, the maintenance, access, and release of information about a juvenile, even a juvenile offender, are quite circumscribed.[25] Information released during juvenile court proceedings remains available as an open record, but it can be sealed, two years after discharge from the supervising agency or after entry of the dispositional order whichever occurs last.[26] Any information not revealed at the trial about the juvenile or the family cannot be released unless it is lacking any identifying characteristics.[27] Finally, all juvenile offender records can be destroyed if the court finds that[28]

1. two years have elapsed since the completion of a diversion agreement, the offender is 18 years of age or older, and has acquired no other criminal history except the one referral for diversion; or

2. the offender is at least 23 years of age, has not subsequently been convicted of a felony nor found guilty of a serious offense, and no current criminal proceeding is pending.

---

20. RCW 13.40.150(2)(h).
21. RCW 13.40.160.
22. *Id.*; State v. Rhodes, 92 Wash.2d 755, 600 P.2d 1264 (1979). The opinions of experts will provide evidence for the court to find manifest injustice. State v. P., 37 Wash.App. 773, 686 P.2d 488 (1984); State v. Taylor, 42 Wash. App.74, 709 P.2d 1207 (1985).
23. RCW 13.40.160(7).
24. RCW 13.50.010(3).
25. RCW 13.50.010.
26. RCW 13.50.010(11).
27. RCW 13.50.050(5).
28. RCW 13.50.050.

5A.16

Competency of Juveniles to Stand Trial

The Juvenile Justice Act of 1977 is silent on whether a juvenile criminal defendant has the right to be aware of and participate in the proceedings. Presumably, if there is reason to suspect that a juvenile is incompetent,[1] the court must follow the procedure for adult criminal defendants (see chapter 5D.5, Competency to Stand Trial).[2]

---

1. *Incompetent* means that the person lacks the capacity to understand the nature of the proceedings or to assist in the defense as a result of mental disease or defect; RCW 10.77.010(6).
2. Washington's Supreme Court applied a statute of the criminal code to juveniles availing themselves of the infancy defense. This statute is not set forth within the Juvenile Justice Act of 1977 (*see* chapter 5A.15, Juvenile Offenders—Legal Capacity); the principles of construction that may apply suggest that the court would permit incompetency procedures for juveniles; State v. Q.D., 102 Wash.2d 19, 685 P.2d 557 (1984).

5A.17

Nonresponsibility Defense

Language within the Juvenile Justice Act of 1977 suggests that minors have a right to raise a diminished capacity defense, the insanity defense, or a defense of duress to a criminal charge. The courts will apply the same procedures established for adult prosecutions (see chapter 5D.8, Diminished Capacity; and chapter 5D.9, Criminal Responsibility).

5A.18

Transfer of Juveniles to Stand Trial as Adults

Under certain circumstances, the law permits the juvenile court to decline jurisdiction and transfer the minor to stand trial for the criminal charges as an adult in the Superior Court. The juvenile court, the prosecuting attorney, or the defense attorney may turn to an MHP to evaluate the juvenile. The evaluation may be used as evidence at the decline hearing.

(A) Initiation of the Decline Hearing

Before a hearing on the charges, the parties, their counsel, or the court itself may request transfer of the juvenile for adult prosecution. In a few specified instances, a mandatory decline hearing must be held unless waived by the court, the parties, and their counsel.[1] A decline hearing is unnecessary if a juvenile has been transferred to adult court on an earlier offense. After that, the juvenile is treated as an adult for all future offenses.[2]

---

1. RCW 13.40.110(i). This will occur if the juvenile is 16 or 17 years of age and the information alleges a Class A felony or an attempt to commit a Class A felony; the juvenile is 17 years of age and the information alleges a Class A felony, such as assault in the second degree, extortion in the first degree, indecent liberties, kidnapping in the second degree, rape in the second degree, or robbery in the second degree.
2. State v. Mitchell, 32 Wash.App. 499, 648 P.2d 456 (1982); State v. Sharon, 100 Wash.2d 230, 668 P.2d 584 (1983).

(B) Decline Hearing

In determining whether to decline jurisdiction, the juvenile court must consider all relevant evidence presented by the parties. The written decision is based upon balancing the best interest of the juvenile with the interest of protecting the public.[3] The case law in Washington has established many factors that are to be evaluated in making the decision:[4]

1. the seriousness of harm caused by the alleged offense to the community, and whether protection of the community requires transfer to adult court;

2. whether the alleged offense was committed in a violent, premeditated, or willful manner;

3. whether the alleged offense was against persons or against property, greater weight being given to offenses against persons, especially if personal injury resulted;

4. the prosecutory merit of the complaint;

5. the desirability of trial and disposition of the entire offense in one court when the juvenile's associates in the alleged offense are adults;

6. the sophistication and maturity of the juvenile as determined by a review of his or her home life, emotional attitude, and pattern of living;

7. the record and previous history of the juvenile; and

8. the prospect for protecting the public and rehabilitating the juvenile by using the procedures, services, and facilities currently available to the juvenile court.

Often MHPs will evaluate and testify about the juvenile's sophistication and maturity. Also, whether the juvenile will remain a threat to the public.[5] However, expert opinions are not binding on the court and are considered to be only part of the evidence; to reach its decision, the court will apply the specific

---

3. RCW 13.40.110(2).
4. State v. Holland, 98 Wash.2d 507, 656 P.2d 1056 (1983) citing to a U.S. Supreme Court holding that limits the discretion permitted by the statutes to the eight "determinative factors." Kent v. United States, 383 U.S. 541 (1966).
5. State v. Holland, 98 Wash.2d 507, 656 P.2d 1056 (1983). If adjudicated as a juvenile, often the sentences would be shorter. Protection of the public interest alone is a factor that permits declination under RCW 13.40.110. State v. Toomey 38 Wash.App 831, 690 P.2d 1175 (1984), *cert. denied*, 471 U.S. 1067, *rev. denied* 103 Wash.2d 1012 (1985). However, if the difference in maximum sentences between the juvenile and adult systems is minimal, the public is deemed adequately protected if the juvenile is tried by the juvenile court. State v. Foltz, 27 Wash.App. 554, 619 P.2d 699 (1980).

criteria to facts about the juvenile that are established by a pre-ponderance of the evidence.[6]

(C) Disclosure of Evaluations after Declination Hearing

After a juvenile is transferred to adult court for criminal prosecution, and the juvenile takes the stand to testify in his or her own defense[7] or raises the insanity defense,[8] testimony of the MHPs who assisted the defendant at the juvenile decline hearing may be admitted into evidence without violating the attorney–client privilege, privilege against self-incrimination, or presumable provider–client privilege. Providers evaluating the defendant should appraise the juvenile of this possibility during the informed consent process (see chapter 6.1, Informed Consent for Services).

---

6. State v. Toomey, 38 Wash.App. 831, 690 P.2d 1175 (1984), *cert. denied*, 471 U.S. 1067, *rev. denied* 103 Wash.2d 1012 (1985).
7. State v. Holland, 98 Wash.2d 507, 656 P.2d 1056 (1983). The prosecution can use the defendant's earlier statements to the provider to impeach the defendant's credibility if the statements satisfy the trustworthiness standards.
8. State v. Bonds, 98 Wash.2d 1, 653 P.2d 1024 (1982). All available evidence of the defendant's mental condition at the time of the crime will be admitted.

5A.19

Voluntary Admission and Civil Commitment of Minors

The legislature enacted Chapter 71.34 RCW to ensure that minors in need of mental health care would receive appropriate treatment. Minors are protected from needless hospitalization and deprivation of liberty by the law.[1] The legislation also established that a minor has the legal capacity to provide consent for obtaining mental health services and restricted the right of the parent(s)[2] to participate in the decision or be informed about confidences that arise during the treatment (see chapter 5A.21, Consent, Confidentiality, and Services for Minors). MHPs may become involved in the evaluation and treatment of minors both as voluntary or involuntary patients.

(A) Voluntary Admission and Civil Commitment of Minors

A minor may be admitted for inpatient evaluation and treatment when three conditions are met:[3]

---

1. RCW 71.34.010.
2. Throughout this chapter, *parent* means a biological or adoptive parent having legal custody of the child or a person or agency judicially appointed as legal guardian of the child.
3. RCW 71.34.030(2); WAC 275-54-030(2).

1. the professional person in charge of the facility finds that the minor is in need of inpatient treatment because of a mental disorder;[4]

2. the facility can provide the type of evaluation and treatment required for the minor; and

3. it is not feasible to treat the minor in a less restrictive setting or in the minor's home.

If these conditions are met, consent must be obtained. A minor younger than 13 years of age may be admitted with just the consent of the parent.[5] A minor older than 12 years of age may be admitted with the consent of the parent but only if accompanied by the minor's written consent, knowingly and voluntarily given[6] (see chapter 6.1, Informed Consent for Services). However, parental consent is not necessarily required for minors older than 12 years of age. If the minor acquired agreement about the need for inpatient treatment from the professional in charge of the facility, the law permits admission without parental consent.[7] Notice of the admission must be given by the facility to the parent(s) in the following manner:[8]

1. it must be provided in the form most likely to reach the parent(s) within 24 hours and advise them of the admission;

2. it must include the location and telephone number of the facility; and

3. it must convey the name of the staff person designated to discuss the minor's need for inpatient treatment.

If the minor has been admitted without parental consent, the minor must be released upon the parent's request unless a Superior Court sustains the minor's consent to voluntary inpatient treatment (see chapter 5A.21, Consent, Confidentiality, and Services for Minors).

---

4. *Mental disorder* means any organic, mental, or emotional impairment that has substantial adverse effects on an individual's cognitive or volitional functions. The presence of alcohol abuse, drug abuse, juvenile criminal history, antisocial behavior, or mental retardation alone is insufficient to justify a finding of "mental disorder." RCW 71.34.010(12); WAC 275-54-010(13). It is unclear whether minors may be admitted to inpatient facilities for other characterological disorders. Outpatient services may be requested and received with or without the parents' consent for the disorders mentioned earlier (*see* chapter 5A.21).
5. RCW 71.34.030(2)(a); WAC 275-54-030(2)(a).
6. RCW 71.34.030(2)(b); WAC 275-54-030(2)(b).
7. RCW 71.34.030(2)(c); WAC 275-54-030(c).
8. RCW 71.34.030(2)(c); WAC 275-54-030(2)(c).

Once the minor is admitted, the multidisciplinary treatment team[9] must develop an individualized treatment plan within 14 days after a complete assessment has been conducted; the assessment must include but is not limited to an assessment of physical, psychological, chronological age, developmental, family, educational, social, cultural, environmental, recreational, and vocational needs of the minor.[10] After implementation, the plan must be reviewed and evaluated in writing by the team at least every 30 days.[11] The plan must also include a written discharge plan.[12]

A written request from the parent of a minor under the age of 13 years will result in immediate discharge from the facility.[13] A minor older than 12 years of age may give written notice of the intent to leave any time.[14] The staff member dates the notice, records the existence of the notice, and sends copies of it to the minor's attorney, if any, the county-designated mental health professional (CDMHP), and the parent.[15] The minor must then be discharged within 24 hours of the notice unless the CDMHP files a petition for initial detention on the next judicial day after the minor's request to leave.[16] If a minor is released, it must be to the parent(s) or to a person authorized by the parent(s) to take custody of the minor. If the parents refuse either alternative, the minor must be referred and released to the appropriate juvenile authority for necessary dependency action.[17]

(B) Involuntary Civil Commitment

To be involuntarily evaluated or treated, a minor who is 13 to 18 years of age must meet criteria similar to those of adults (see chapter 5E.4, Involuntary Civil Admission of Mentally Ill Adults). If the minor suffers from a mental disorder[18] and presents a

---

9. This team must include a physician, a psychologist, a nurse, a social worker, an occupational therapist, and a recreational therapist. A child psychiatrist must be available for consultation if not present on the staff. All must have documented skills and experience in working with impaired youth; WAC 248-23-030(4).
10. WAC 248-23-030(3)(b).
11. WAC 248-23-030(3)(b)(iii).
12. WAC 248-23-030(3)(b)(iv).
13. RCW 71.34.030(3)(a); WAC 275-54-030(2)(f)(i).
14. RCW 71.34.030(3)(b); WAC 275-54-030(2)(f)(ii).
15. RCW 71.34.030(3)(c); WAC 275-54-30(2)(f)(iii).
16. RCW 71.34.030(3)(d); WAC 275-54-030(2)(f)(iv).
17. WAC 275-54-120(1); RCW 71.34.170 appears to permit release to any responsible person without parental authorization.
18. *Supra,* note 4.

likelihood of serious harm,[19] or is gravely disabled,[20] the CDMHP may take the minor into custody for evaluation and treatment at an inpatient facility.[21] A minor 13 years of age or older may also enter the involuntary treatment process by being brought to an inpatient facility or an emergency room for immediate mental health services.

If the minor suffers from a mental disorder, requires immediate inpatient treatment, and remains unwilling to consent to a voluntary admission, the minor could be detained for up to 12 hours to be evaluated by a CDMHP.[22] Within the 12-hour period, the CDMHP must serve on the minor a copy of the petition for initial detention, notice of initial detention, and a statement of rights;[23] the CDMHP must also advise the minor both orally and in writing that a commitment hearing will be held within 72 hours (this excludes weekend and holiday hours) because probable cause exists to commit the minor, and that the right exists to talk immediately with an attorney to prepare for the hearing.[24] The admitting facility must take reasonable steps to notify immediately the minor's parent(s) of the admission unless it is determined that this notification would be seriously detrimental to the minor's condition or treatment.[25] This initial 72-hour treatment period must not be exceeded unless the minor's good faith application for voluntary treatment is accepted, or a petition for a 14-day commitment is filed.[26]

A petition urging a 14-day commitment must be signed by the physicians or by one physician and one MHP who have examined the minor.[27] Unless a continuance is requested by the minor or the minor's attorney, a 14-day commitment hearing in

---

19. *Likelihood of serious harm* means that a substantial risk of physical harm will be inflicted by the minor either on his or her own person, as evidenced by threats or attempts to inflict physical harm on oneself; on another, as evidenced by behavior having caused such harm or placed another person or persons in reasonable fear of sustaining such harm; or on the property of others, as evidenced by behavior having caused substantial loss or damage to property of others. RCW 71.34.020(11); WAC 275-54-020(12).
20. *Gravely disabled* refers to a minor who, as a result of a mental disorder, is in danger of serious physical harm because of a failure to provide for his or her essential human needs of health or safety, or who manifests severe deterioration in routine functioning evidenced by repeated and escalating losses of cognitive or volitional control over his or her actions and is not receiving such care as is essential for his or her health or safety. RCW 71.34.020(8); WAC 278-54-020(8).
21. RCW 71.34.050(1); WAC 275-54-050(1).
22. RCW 71.34.040; WAC 275-54-040.
23. WAC 275-54-290.
24. RCW 71.34.050; WAC 275-54-050.
25. RCW 71.34.060(3); WAC 275-54-040(7).
26. RCW 71.34.060(4); WAC 275-54-040(9).
27. RCW 71.34.070; WAC 275-54-060(2).

Superior Court must be held within 72 hours after the minor's admission.[28]

At the hearing, the minor's rights include being represented by an attorney, presenting evidence on his or her behalf, questioning persons testifying in support of the petition, and the court being informed about the probable effects of medications taken within the last 24 hours.[29] The court must find by a preponderance of the evidence that the minor suffers from a mental disorder, presents a likelihood of serious harm or is gravely disabled, requires inpatient treatment (or less restrictive alternative treatment), and refuses to consent to voluntary treatment.[30] If the court decides that the minor does not meet the criteria for the 14-day commitment, the minor must be released.[31] If committed, the minor must be released before or at the end of the period unless a petition for 180 commitment days is pending before the court.[32]

An additional period of commitment may be required beyond the 14-day period. Additional commitment periods of 180 days are possible to obtain if more rigorous procedural or due process safeguards are met. The petition, hearing, and commitment process differs from a 14-day commitment in the following manner:

1. the petition must be signed by two examining physicians, one of whom shall be a child psychiatrist, or by one physician and one MHP who specializes in treating children;[33] and

2. the Superior Court must find by clear, cogent, and convincing evidence that the minor is suffering from a mental disorder and presents a likelihood of serious harm or is gravely disabled and is in need of further treatment that can be provided only in a 180-day commitment.[34]

If the minor meets the criteria for continued commitment and a less-restrictive alternative is not appropriate or available, the court may order hospitalization.[35] If the minor does not meet the criteria for continued commitment, the minor must be released.[36] Successive 180-day commitments are permitted on the same grounds under the same procedures as the original 180 days of commitment.[37]

---

28. RCW 71.34.080(1).
29. RCW 71.34.080(6); WAC 275-54-070(2).
30. RCW 71.34.080(9); WAC 275-54-070(1)(a).
31. RCW 71.34.080(10); WAC 275-54-070(4).
32. RCW 71.34.080(12); WAC 275-54-070(5).
33. RCW 71.34.090(3); WAC 275-54-080(2)(f).
34. RCW 71.34.090(6); WAC 275-54-080(8).
35. RCW 71.34.090(7); WAC 275-54-080(9).
36. RCW 71.34.090(7); WAC 275-54-080(11).
37. RCW 71.34.090(8); WAC 275-54-080(12).

During the commitment periods, as would occur for a voluntary commitment explained earlier, the multidisciplinary treatment team must develop and implement an individualized treatment and discharge plan. It must be reviewed and reevaluated in writing by the team every 30 days.

Finally, the records and files created in any court proceeding are confidential and available only to the minor, the minor's parent(s), and the minor's attorney. The confidences divulged during either voluntary or involuntary treatment remain confidential, and the privilege is qualified quite narrowly (see chapters 5A.21, Consent, Confidentiality, and Services for Minors).

5A.20

Education for Handicapped and Highly Capable Children

Washington law states that all children, whatever their cognitive or physical abilities, must be provided with an appropriate educational program. This applies to every disabled student between the ages of 3 and 21 years as well and for whom free special education services may consist of specially designed instruction, physical education, career development, vocational education, audiology, occupational therapy, orientation and mobility instruction, physical therapy, communication disorder services, social work services, psychological services, medical services, and parent counseling and training services.[1] MHPs may be called upon to evaluate the child, to consult with school staff in planning programs to meet special needs as suggested by the assessment results, and to manage a program of counseling for the student and parents.

(A) Terms and Definitions

Before discussing how a child may obtain special education services, it is necessary to understand the legal meanings of the terms that are within the statutes:

1. *Handicapped children* are children under the age of 21 years who are physically, emotionally, or mentally disabled, or suffer from specific learning and language handicaps that are caused by perceptual–motor disabilities, including problems in visual

---

1. WAC 392-171-315.

and auditory perception and integration.[2] The disabilities can be temporary or permanent. To control excessive costs, extensive functional definitions and eligibility criteria exist for the disabling conditions:[3]

a. *Developmentally delayed students* are those who, for their age, test below a specific statistical cutoff for certain areas of developmental functioning. The areas include delays in cognitive, communication, fine motor, gross motor, or social and emotional functioning.[4]

b. *Orthopedically impaired students* are those who lack the normal function of muscles, joints, or bones because of a congenital anomaly, disease, or permanent injury, and such a condition adversely affects their educational performance.[5]

c. *Health impaired students* are those who have chronic or acute health problems, such as congenital heart defect or other congenital syndrome(s), disorders of the cardiorespiratory systems, disorders of the central nervous system including epilepsy or neurological impairment, autism, or other profound health circumstances or degenerative conditions, any of which adversely affect their educational performance.[6]

d. *Learning disabled students* suffer from a deficit in one or more of the basic psychological processes involved in understanding or using spoken or written language. Such a disorder may include problems in visual and auditory perception or integration. Or it may result in an impaired ability to think, speak clearly, read well, write legibly and with meaning, and perform mathematical calculations accurately, including those involving reading. The disorder involves intellectual functioning above that specified for mental retardation, coupled with a severe discrepancy between intellectual ability and academic achievement.[7]

e. *Mentally retarded students* are those who demonstrate significantly subaverage general intellectual functioning that exists concurrently with deficits in adaptive behavior.

---

2. RCW 28A.13.010.
3. *Id.* Providers are urged to refer to the complete statutory language of each functionally defined condition as it becomes relevant for providing evaluation or treatment services. Legal definitions of handicaps often are more narrowly defined than medical or social science definitions. Evaluation standards are established for each condition within the statutes.
4. WAC 392-171-382 to -391.
5. WAC 392-171-396.
6. WAC 392-171-401.
7. WAC 392-171-406.

These are manifested during the developmental period and adversely affect educational performance.[8]

f. *Multi-handicapped students* are those who suffer from two or more handicapping conditions each of which is so severe as to warrant a special program because these students cannot be accommodated in a regular special education program designed for only one of the impairments.[9]

g. *Hearing impaired students* are those who suffer from a documented hearing deficit that is so severe that the student is impaired in processing verbal communications, with or without amplification, and that it adversely affects educational performance.[10]

h. *Visually impaired students* are those who are so visually handicapped that even with correction their educational performance is adversely affected.[11]

2. *Consent* means that the parent or adult student has been fully informed about the activity for which consent is sought in his or her native language or other mode of communication. The information must be understood before being agreed to in writing. The writing must describe the activity to be conducted and list the records that will be released and to whom. It must be understood that the consent is granted voluntarily and may be revoked at any time (see chapter 6.1, Informed Consent for Services);[12]

3. *Highly capable students* are those students who have been assessed to have superior intellectual ability. Determinations must be based on cognitive ability defined by intelligence test results; academic achievement measured by achievement test results; and exceptional creativity demonstrated by unique or outstanding creative products or problem-solving ability.[13]

(B) Identification Procedures

Local school districts must conduct activities to identify students with suspected handicapping conditions. Students from birth to 21 years of age are eligible. Activities may include but are not

---

8. WAC 392-171-421.
9. WAC 392-171-432.
10. WAC 392-171-436.
11. WAC 392-171-446.
12. WAC 392-171-311(4).
13. WAC 392-170-040.

limited to[14] preschool developmental screening, local media informational campaigns, liaison with public health and other medical and social agencies (public or private), questionnaires for first-time enrolling students, screening of district-wide group standardized test results, and in-service education to teaching staff. Any source, including MHPs, parents, medical personnel, school district personnel, community agencies, and interested persons may initiate an evaluation to determine a student's need for special education.[15]

As soon as the school authorities suspect that the student bears a handicapping condition,[16] they must provide written notice to the parent(s).[17] Within the next 15 days, school personnel must review existing school, medical, and other records within their possession to determine whether the student requires an assessment; the decision shall be written and signed by the authority.[18] If the student requires further assessment, the parent(s) must first provide consent to permit the school, other agencies, and professionals to exchange information.[19] If consent is given, the school district must fully assess the student within 35 days; if consent is refused, the assessment must be completed in three days if the refusal is overridden by an administrative hearing officer.[20]

The process for identifying highly capable students is less formal. Nominations may be received from any source.[21] Each nominee is screened by district authorities to determine whether clear, current evidence exists that the student would meet the eligibility criteria.[22]

(C) Assessment Procedures

An assessment for a handicapping condition must meet the minimum required statutory procedures, but the breadth of the evaluation can be as broad as a multidisciplinary team judges necessary.[23] The team must be composed of licensed, registered,

---

14. WAC 392-171-336. This section is titled *Childfind*.
15. WAC 392-171-341(1).
16. WAC 392-171-341(2).
17. Written notice would be sent to an adult student or to that person's legal guardian. Hereafter, the reader should note this possibility wherever parent is mentioned.
18. WAC 392-171-341(3).
19. WAC 392-171-341(5).
20. WAC 392-171-341(4).
21. WAC 392-170-045.
22. WAC 392-170-050.
23. WAC 392-171-346.

or certified professionals to include at least one special education teacher, the school psychologist, and the student's regular education teacher; in addition, at least one person qualified to conduct individual diagnostic assessment in the area of the suspected disability must serve if the school psychologist is not qualified.[24]

Detailed procedures for conducting the assessment are specified in the administrative regulations. Assessment data are to be summarized in writing, dated, and signed; they must identify the procedures and instruments used, the results obtained, how the findings relate to the student's instructional program, including a description of the factors that interfere with the student's performance, and the special education and related services required to assist the student in his or her educational placement.[25] If the parent(s) disagrees with the assessment results obtained by the school district an independent educational assessment may be obtained.[26]

The assessment process for selecting highly capable students is managed by a multidisciplinary committee[27] that makes the determination from the following criteria:[28]

1. the student scores in the top 10% in cognitive ability as proven by a standardized ability test;

2. the student scores in the top 5% in one or more academic achievement areas; or

3. the student shows behavioral characteristics of exceptional creativity.

Each student selected as highly capable must be provided with an educational opportunity that considers the student's unique needs and capabilities.[29]

---

24. WAC 392-171-351(1). A physician must be added to the team whenever a health problem may affect the educational program. WAC 392-171-361.
25. WAC 392-171-351(8); WAC 392-171-366.
26. WAC 392-171-371. If the school district does not initiate an administrative hearing for the impartial review of its evaluation process, and the hearing officer does not approve of the process, it must provide the funds for an independent evaluation. The parents still have the right to an independent evaluation at their own expense if the hearing officer approves of the school's process.
27. The team must consist of at least a classroom teacher with training and experience in teaching highly capable students, a psychologist or other provider trained to interpret cognitive and achievement test results, and a district administrator with responsibility for supervising the program for these students; WAC 392-170-070.
28. WAC 392-170-055.
29. WAC 392-170-080.

(D) Placement in a Special Education Program

Within 30 days after the student's assessment is completed, a meeting must be held to develop an individualized education program (IEP).[30] The school district initiates and conducts the meeting, which will include[31] a school district supervisor of the special education and related services, the student's regular teacher or therapist, one or both parents, a member of the assessment team(s); and other individuals at the discretion of the district or parent(s). From the assessment analysis and parental advice, each student's IEP must be developed to include[32]

1. a physician's review of the student's health status to interpret any medical implications to be considered during planning for orthopedically or health impaired students;

2. a statement regarding the present level of educational performance;

3. special annual goals stated in terms that provide for measurement of progress, expected levels of performance, and schedules for their accomplishment;

4. an identification of specific special educational and related services required by the student, including physical education;

5. career development and vocational education goals and short-term instructional objectives for students older than 13 years of age;

6. projected dates for beginning and ending the services, including the number of school days and hours per day; and

7. appropriate objective criteria, evaluation procedures, and schedules for determining, at least on an annual basis, whether short-term instructional objectives are being met.

A copy of the IEP must be given to the parents.[33] Consent must be obtained before placement and services begin.[34]

The placement and services are to be provided within a regular educational environment, if possible, or with non-handicapped students to the maximum extent appropriate to the needs of the student.[35] The continuum of placements includes

---

30. WAC 392-171-456(1).
31. Id.
32. WAC 392-171-461(1).
33. WAC 392-171-461(2).
34. WAC 392-171-466(2).
35. WAC 392-171-471.

instruction in regular classes, special classes, special schools, home instruction, or instruction in hospitals or institutions.[36]

A full reassessment by the multidisciplinary team must occur, at least once every three years or upon request from the parent(s), a teacher, or the IEP committee.[37]

The administrative regulations do not define clearly how to provide an education to meet the unique needs and abilities of highly capable students,[38] other than the program must recognize the limits of the resources provided by the state and options available to the district.[39]

(E) Due Process Rights

Notices to the parents of suspected handicapped children, including a full explanation of all the procedural safeguards available, must be provided in the native language or other mode of communication of the parent.[40] The notices must describe the actions proposed or refused (screening, assessment, and IEP) by the school district, provide an explanation of why the district proposes or refuses to take action, identify any options that the district considered and the reasons why they are rejected, and describe each assessment result, other factors, or reports used as the basis for the proposal or refusal.[41]

Either the parent or the school district may initiate an administrative hearing to challenge or to show the appropriateness of a proposed action when the other refuses to proceed with any part of the special education process, including the identification and screening of the student, the full assessment, and the provision of individualized special education and related services.[42] Also, an administrative hearing is available for highly capable students. The hearing must be held upon written request by the parents or the school district to the Office of the Superintendent of Public Education.[43] If the parents request such a hearing, the school must advise them of any free or low-cost legal services available in their area.[44]

---

36. WAC 392-171-476.
37. WAC 392-171-512. The reassessment process is detailed in WAC 392-171-514 to -519.
38. WAC 392-170-080.
39. Id.
40. WAC 392-171-526.
41. Id.
42. WAC 392-171-531.
43. Id.
44. WAC 392-171-536.

The hearing must be conducted by a qualified, impartial person selected by the chief administrative law judge.[45] At the hearing the parties have the right to present evidence, including expert testimony, cross examine, and compel attendance by witnesses, prohibit the introduction of any evidence that has not been disclosed to that party at least five days before the hearing, and obtain a written transcript of the hearing.[46] The parents can invoke the additional right of opening the hearing to the public and of having the child present.[47] After the hearing, the hearing officer will make a decision on the issue in controversy and document the findings of fact and conclusions of law. The decision is final unless modified or overturned on appeal by a court of law.[48]

45. *Id.*
46. WAC 392-171-551.
47. *Id.*
48. WAC 392-171-561.

5A.21

Consent, Confidentiality, and Services for Minors

The state of Washington has enacted progressive new laws that encourage minors to seek alcohol, drug, and mental health care and treatment without the complications of parental involvement. The law concerning the minor's capacity to give consent and the scope of confidentiality permits treatment decisions to be made in response to clinical needs. Parental rights[1] to participate in and be informed of treatment decisions are restricted so that minors will be encouraged to seek treatment. Health care providers could be held civilly liable for failing to obtain appropriate consent before providing services and to maintain confidential information provided by the minor during treatment.

(A) Consent

Outpatient alcohol or drug services may be provided to any consenting person 14 years of age or older[2] or upon application by a parent, a legal guardian, or other legal representative.[3] Unless the legally responsible adult joins in the consent for outpatient alcohol or drug services, he or she will not be liable for payment of the care.[4] Any minor 13 years of age or older may request and receive mental health services without the consent of the parents or

---

1. Throughout this chapter, *parent* means a biological or adoptive parent having legal custody of the child or a person or agency judicially appointed as legal guardian of the child.
2. RCW 70.96A.095.
3. RCW 70.96A.110.
4. RCW 70.96A.095.

guardian.[5] Parental authorization is required for any type of outpatient service if the minor is younger than the specified ages.[6]

Voluntary inpatient or residential alcohol or drug services cannot be provided without parental notification,[7] however, a minor 14 years of age or older can consent to receiving such services.[8] Unless the legally responsible adult joins in the consent for outpatient alcohol or drug services, the child will not be liable for payment of the care.[9]

For mental health inpatient services, a minor younger than 13 years of age may be admitted upon application by the minor's parents.[10]

A minor older than 12 years of age may be voluntarily admitted by an application from the parents that is accompanied by the written consent, knowingly and voluntarily given by the minor (see chapter 6.1, Informed Consent for Services).[11] In addition, a minor older than 12 years of age may be admitted voluntarily into the facility without parental consent.[12] The facility must provide the type of evaluation and treatment services needed by the minor, and the professional in charge must find it unfeasible to treat the minor in a less restrictive setting.[13] Notice must be given by the facility to the minor's parents in the following manner:[14] It must be provided in the form most likely to reach the parents within 24 hours of the admission and must advise the recipient that the minor has been admitted to inpatient treatment; the location and telephone number of the facility must be conveyed; and the name of the staff person designated to discuss the minor's need for inpatient treatment must be included.

(B) Gaining Release of Minor Admitted Voluntarily to a Mental Health Inpatient Facility

If the minor has been admitted without the parent's consent, the minor must be released upon the parent's request unless the

---

5. RCW 71.34.030(1); WAC 275-54-030(1).
6. RCW 70.96A.095 (alcohol and drug services); RCW 71.34.030(1) and WAC 275-54-030(1) (mental health services).
7. RCW 70.96A.120 (6).
8. RCW 70.96A.095.
9. Id.
10. RCW 71.34.030(2)(a); WAC 275-54-030(a).
11. RCW 71.34.030(2)(b); WAC 275-54-030(b).
12. RCW 71.34.030(2)(c); WAC 275-54-030(c).
13. RCW 71.34.030(2); WAC 275-54-030(2).
14. RCW 71.34.030(2)(c); WAC 275-54-030(2)(c).

facility files a petition with the Superior Court.[15] The petition signed by the person in charge of the facility must state why the minor requires inpatient treatment and that release would threaten the minor's health and safety,[16] that the minor has provided informed consent to such treatment,[17] and that a less restrictive alternate treatment is unavailable or is not in the best interests of the minor.[18] A copy of the petition must be served upon the minor and sent to the minor's attorney and the minor's parents.[19]

A hearing must be held within three days of filing the petition.[20] At the hearing, the facility must prove by a preponderance of the evidence the three substantive allegations within the petition.[21] The parents may apply to the court for separate counsel to represent them if they cannot afford counsel.[22] If the court rules for the facility, the parent will not have the right to demand immediate release until the next renewal of voluntary admission.[23] The minor's need for continued inpatient treatment must be reviewed and documented at least each 180 days.[24]

(C) Confidentiality

If a client of authorized age consents to alcohol or drug care services, client confidences are subject to disclosure only when the patient provides a release,[25] for good cause upon the court approving the issuance of a subpoena to compel production of records or testimony;[26] to comply with state laws mandating the reporting of suspected child abuse or neglect;[27] when a patient commits a crime on the program premises, or against program personnel, or threatens to do so;[28] to medical personnel to the extent necessary to meet a medical emergency;[29] and for research and audit purposes if specific protections are followed.[30]

---

15. RCW 71.34.030(c); WAC 275-54-030(2)(c)(iii).
16. RCW 71.34.030(c)(ii); WAC 275-54-030(2)(c)(iii).
17. RCW 71.34.030(c); WAC 275-54-030(2)(c)(iv)(E).
18. WAC 275-54-030(2)(c)(iv)(F).
19. WAC 275-54-030(c)(v).
20. RCW 71.34.030(1)(c)(v); WAC 275-54-030(c)(vi).
21. RCW 71.34.030(1)(c)(vii); WAC 275-54-030(c)(vii).
22. RCW 71.34.030(iv); WAC 275-54-030(c)(ix).
23. WAC 275-54-030(c)(x).
24. WAC 275-54-030(d).
25. RCW 70.96A.150 (1)(a).
26. RCW 70.96A.150 (1)(b); 42 C.F.R. § 2.61(a).
27. RCW 70.96A.150 (1)(c).
28. RCW 70.96A.150 (1)(d).
29. 42 CFR § 2.51.
30. 42 CFR § 2.53.

Confidentiality must be maintained when mental health services are provided to minors. Information may be disclosed only in the following instances:[31]

1. in communications between mental health or medical professionals for providing services to the minor or in making appropriate referrals;
2. during guardianship or dependency proceedings;
3. if a *bona fide* release is provided by the minor or by the parent in the instances in which the parent is legitimately acting for the minor;
4. to the extent necessary to make a claim for financial aid, insurance, or medical assistance;
5. to the courts as necessary (e.g., involuntary treatment, transferring a minor from a juvenile correctional institution to a treatment facility, ruling upon a petition for voluntary consent of a minor to be admitted for inpatient treatment that the parent contests);[32]
6. to law enforcement officers or public health officers as necessary to carry out their responsibilities. The information must be limited to the facts, dates of admission and discharge, the name and address of the treatment provider, and the last known address of the client;
7. to law enforcement officers, public health officers, and relatives if a minor has escaped from custody but then only such information as may be necessary to provide for public safety or assist in apprehending the minor may be disclosed; and
8. to appropriate law enforcement agencies and to a person whose health and safety have been threatened, or who is known to have been threatened or repeatedly harassed by the minor.

Whenever disclosure of information is made, the date and circumstances, the name(s) to whom the disclosure was made, the relationship to the minor, and the information revealed must be entered in the minor's clinical record.[33]

---

31. RCW 71.34.200; WAC 275-54-300.
32. *See* Chapter 71.34 RCW.
33. RCW 71.34.220; WAC 275-54-300(15).

5A.22

Consent for Abortion

In 1991, Washington voters approved Initiative 120, the Reproductive Privacy Act.[1] The law guarantees the right to an abortion for any woman to protect her life or health. She also may obtain an abortion if the fetus has not achieved viability. The fetus will not be viewed as "a viable fetus" unless, in the physician's judgment, the fetus has a "reasonable likelihood" of survival outside the uterus without resorting to extraordinary medical measures. The law also requires that the state pay for an abortion for any woman eligible for state-funded maternity services.

---

1. The Act was codified in Chapter 9.02 RCW.

5A.23

Evaluation and Treatment of Children at the Request of a Noncustodial Parent

MHPs may be asked to provide evaluation and treatment services to a child at the request of a noncustodial parent.[1] Under the Parenting Act of 1987, either parent may make "emergency decisions" affecting the health and safety of the child.[2] In addition, the court may modify a parenting plan if the facts show that a substantial change in the child's environment is detrimental to his or her physical, mental, or emotional health or if material facts were unknown to the court when the plan was ordered.[3] Providers may be subpoenaed as experts to provide evidence as to changes or to previously unknown material facts (e.g., the drug abuse of the custodial parent).

Whenever a provider's services are sought for a child by a known noncustodial parent whose child cannot provide legal consent, and the health and safety of the child do not permit a valid emergency decision, the custodial parent must provide consent.[4] However, a noncustodial parent may encourage the child to seek and provide his own consent to evaluation and treatment. So long as the minors possess the legal capacity to provide their own consent for services, they do not need either of the parents' permission (see chapter 5A.21, Consent, Confidentiality, and Services for Minors).

---

1. Throughout this chapter, *custodial parent* means a biological or adoptive parent having legal custody of the child or a person or agency judicially appointed as legal guardian of the child.
2. RCW 26.09.08(4)(a).
3. RCW 26.09.19(1).
4. RCW 71.34.030. Before the enactment of Chapter 71.34 RCW in 1985 that established the laws for mental health services of minors, no statute or other authority prohibited the noncustodial parent from consenting to mental health services. McDaniel v. McDaniel 14 Wash.App. 194, 539 P.2d 699 (1975).

Other Civil Matters

5B.1

Mental Status of Licensed or Certified Professionals

Washington laws include provisions concerning the mental status of licensed or certified professionals. Some professions have established formal programs to deal with impaired members of those professions. Competency or fitness to carry on a profession is often a prerequisite to licensure or certification. Provisions concerning mental status generally arise during the regulation of the licensed providers (e.g., discipline, suspension or revocation of license). These provisions are of concern because MHPs may be asked to evaluate professionals and to testify before licensing and credentialing boards or a court concerning the mental status of a professional and his or her ability to fulfill the responsibilities of the profession.

As noted earlier (see chapter 1 and the relevant subchapter for the particular profession), nearly all licensure or certification statutes provide for suspension or revocation of a license if the individual is not competent to carry on a practice. This chapter discusses only the laws that refer specifically to the mental status of a professional.

(A) Uniform Disciplinary Act

The provisions of the Uniform Disciplinary Act[1] apply to many of the health and health-related professions.[2] The provisions of the Act address directly the mental capacity of applicants and license holders. If the disciplining authority believes that a license holder or applicant may be unable to practice with reasonable skill and safety to consumers by reason of any "mental or physical condition,"[3] notice is given to the professional, and a hearing on the issue will be held. The disciplining authority may require the individual to submit to a mental or physical examination, and the individual may submit evidence of similar examinations at his or her own expense. If the individual is found unable to practice with probable skill and safety, at reasonable intervals, he or she has the right to demonstrate the ability to resume competent practice.

The Uniform Act also provides that an individual, by applying for a license, practicing, or filing a license renewal, is deemed to have given consent to submit to a mental, physical, or psychological examination when directed in writing by the disciplinary authority and to have waived all doctor–patient privileges regarding his or her mental or physical condition.[4]

(B) Attorneys

The Board of Governors of the Bar Association may withhold permission to take the bar examination until completion of an inquiry into an applicant's character and fitness. Unlike some

---

1. Chapter 18.130 RCW.
2. The Uniform Disciplinary Act applies to dispensing opticians, drugless healers, midwives, ocularists, massage operators and businesses, dental hygienists, and acupuncturists; to the podiatry board, chiropractic disciplinary board, dental disciplinary board, board of funeral directors and embalmers, optometry board, board of osteopathic medicine and surgery, medical disciplinary board, board of physical therapy, board of occupational therapy practice, examining board of psychology, board of practical nursing, board of nursing, and veterinary board of governors; and to the certification and registration of social workers, mental health counselors, and marriage and family therapists. RCW 18.130.040.
3. RCW 18.130.170. There is no specified test by which this determination may be made. However, the Act states that a determination by a court of competent jurisdiction that a "license holder or applicant is mentally incompetent or mentally ill is presumptive evidence of the license holder's or applicant's inability to practice with reasonable skill and safety."
4. RCW 18.130.170(3).

other states,[5] applicants are not required to certify their mental and physical competency to practice law. Once licensed, an attorney is subject to discipline for any "conduct demonstrating unfitness to practice law."[6]

(B)(1) Disability Inactive Status

The Rules of Lawyer Discipline also provide two mechanisms for automatic and discretionary transfer of an attorney to "disability inactive status." Automatic transfer occurs when an active lawyer has

1. been found to be incapable of assisting in his or her own defense in a criminal action;
2. been acquitted of a crime on the ground of insanity;
3. had a guardian (but not a limited guardian) appointed for his or her person or estate upon a finding of incompetency; or
4. been found to be incapable mentally of conducting the practice of law in any other jurisdiction.

Discretionary transfer to disability inactive status occurs when, following a hearing, it appears to a review committee that there is reasonable cause to believe that an active attorney is unable to practice law adequately because of insanity, mental illness, senility, excessive use of alcohol or drugs, or other mental or physical incapacity.

For both automatic and discretionary transfers, the standard used to decide whether a criminal defendant is competent to stand trial is applied. The attorney must be capable of properly understanding the nature of the proceedings and of assisting legal counsel in defense of the proceedings.[7]

(B)(2) Reinstatement to Active Status

A lawyer on disability inactive status may petition for reinstatement to active status by setting forth the facts demonstrating that the disability has been removed; the lawyer has the burden of showing that the disability has been removed in fact. The filing of a petition for reinstatement is deemed a waiver of any professional–patient privilege with regard to any treatment received by the lawyer during the period of disability. The lawyer will be required to reveal the name of each psychiatrist, psychologist,

---

5. For example, the state of Arizona requires that an applicant for the bar file a certificate by a licensed physician stating that he or she is mentally and physically able to engage in the active and continuous practice of law. 17A A.R.S. Sup.Ct.Rules, Rule 34(b)(7).
6. Rules of Lawyer Discipline, Rule 1.1, Grounds for Discipline.
7. In re Meade, 103 Wash.2d 374, 693 P.2d 713 (1985).

physician, or other person and each hospital or other institution in which the lawyer was examined or treated since transfer to disability inactive status. The Washington State Bar Association (WSBA) Lawyers' Assistance Program can provide evaluation and treatment of a disabled lawyer at no or low cost. Because the program is run by WSBA, the credibility of its treatment providers is great and can result in less scrutiny of treatment records.

The criteria to be used in determining whether an attorney on disability inactive status can be reinstated are whether the attorney is presently able to represent clients competently; able to conduct him or herself in a manner reflecting no discredit on the profession; and able to maintain the standards of the profession.[8]

(C) Pharmacists

As a prerequisite to licensure, applicants must be able to demonstrate that they are not unfit or unable to practice because of mental disability.[9] Pharmacy licensure may be refused or a licensed pharmacist may be disciplined if the individual exhibits mental impairment.[10]

(D) Physicians

Physicians (and physician's assistants) are subject to the provisions of the Uniform Disciplinary Act.[11] In addition, the Medical Disciplinary Board has established an impaired physician program for the detection, intervention, and monitoring of impaired physicians. The program is intended to address the problems raised by the presence of the "diseases of alcoholism, drug abuse, or mental illness."[12] In furtherance of this goal, the program can

1. receive and evaluate reports of suspected impairment from any source;
2. intervene in cases of verified impairment;
3. refer impaired physicians to treatment programs;
4. monitor the treatment and rehabilitation of impaired physicians; and

---

8. *Id.*
9. RCW 18.64.080.
10. RCW 18.64.160(5) and (8).
11. RCW 18.71.019; RCW 18.71A.025.
12. RCW 18.72.301(3).

5. provide posttreatment monitoring of and support to rehabili-
tated physicians.

The program must report to the medical disciplinary board any impaired physician who refuses to cooperate with the program, who refuses to submit to treatment, or whose impairment is not alleviated through treatment; and who, in the opinion of the program, is unable to practice medicine with reasonable skill and safety. However, impairment alone shall not give rise to a presumption of inability of the individual to practice medicine with reasonable skill and safety.[13]

---

13. RCW 18.72.371(4).

5B.2

Industrial Insurance

The industrial insurance law provides employees with protection against treatment costs and income losses resulting from work-related accidents or disease. The legislature abolished the jurisdiction of the courts over industrial insurance because remedies resulting from adjudication were uncertain, slow, and inadequate.[1] Injuries at work occur frequently The judicial process remedies often resulted in little of the cost of the injuries being borne by the employer while injured workers suffered and the expense to the public was great.[2] As a result, the employer now purchases compensation insurance (or is self-insured)[3] to provide the benefits for its workers. The administrative process now provides fixed and certain compensation for work-related accidents or disease, regardless of fault, at the expense of the industries that employ the workers.[4] Civil actions by the worker against the employer are not permitted.[5] Unlike other states, no employer or worker can exempt him or herself from the burdens or waive the

---

1. RCW 51.04.010.
2. *Id.*
3. Chapter 51.14 RCW.
4. Favor v. Department of Labor & Industries, 53 Wash.2d 698 (1959).
5. RCW 51.04.010. However, an employer is free to agree to indemnify a third party for an employee's injury that has the effect of making the employer wholly liable. In addition, an injury from an intentional assault by a coemployee is actionable beyond the limits of workers' compensation. The Industrial Insurance Act provides a remedy for harm resulting from injuries suffered in the work place. Unlike the law against discrimination (*see* chapter 5B.12), it does not permit remedies for nonphysical injuries (e.g., dignitary injuries). Reese v. Sears, Roebuck & Co., 107 Wash.2d 563, 731 P.2d 497 (1987).

benefits of workers' compensation. Any such agreements are void.[6]

The workers' compensation laws apply to psychologists and psychiatrists[7] in two ways: (a) an injured worker may consult a psychologist or psychiatrist after an injury,[8] and (b) the Department of Labor and Industries (DLI) may request that an injured worker undergo a psychiatric examination.[9] In this regard, psychologists and psychiatrists play an important role in classifying unspecified, permanent partial disability,[10] and in evaluating the issue of permanent bodily impairment.[11] Other MHPs may play a role in treating the injured employee.

(A) Scope of the Coverage

Benefits are payable for accidents or disease that occur during employment.[12] To qualify, the worker must be acting at the employer's direction or in the furtherance of the business.[13]

(A)(1) Injuries

Workers' compensation benefits are paid for injuries[14] arising during employment.[15] For an injury to be compensable, there must be proof that the injury[16]

1. is one defined by statute;

---

6. RCW 51.04.060.
7. *See* WAC 296-20-01001 and -02002. *See also* WAC 296-21-050. Note that medical fees under WAC 296-21-050 include payment for medical hypnotherapy.
8. RCW 51.28.020 and WAC 296-20-020. However, a physician is required to assist in filing a workers' compensation claim.
9. However, the DLI must show good cause for making such a request. Tietjen v. Department of Labor and Industries, 13 Wash.App. 86, 534 P.2d 151 (1975).
10. WAC 296-20-200.
11. WAC 296-20-210 and -220. Although only a physician can make a determination of permanent bodily impairment, that determination requires an assessment of loss of mental functioning and is within the purview of psychiatrists and psychologists. WAC 296-20-330 contains the rules for evaluation of permanent impairment of mental health.
12. RCW 51.04.090.
13. RCW 51.08.013. Going to and from work at the job site will be viewed as acting during employment because this time is immediate to the actual time in which the worker is engaged in the work process.
14. RCW 51.04.010. *Injury* means a sudden and tangible happening of a traumatic nature, producing an immediate or prompt result, and occurring from without, and such physical conditions as result therefrom. *See* RCW 51.08.100.
15. *In the course of employment* means that the employee was acting at his or her employer's direction or in furtherance of the employer's business. RCW 51.08.013.
16. RCW 51.08.100.

2. occurred during employment;

3. was a sudden and tangible happening;

4. is of a traumatic nature; and

5. produced an immediate result.

There must be a causal connection between the injured worker's physical condition and his or her employment.[17] The sudden and tangible happening requires causation between the employment and the physical injury; in effect, but for the event at work, the injury would not have occurred.[18] Repetitive traumas resulting from years of work do not satisfy this standard.[19]

If the injury of the worker occurred because of the deliberate intention of the employer or of the employer's agent to produce such an injury, a cause of action at law, such as a negligence claim, can be maintained by the worker. In addition, a claim for industrial insurance can be filed.[20] A third person, who is not employed with the worker but injures the worker, is liable for the worker's injuries. The worker may elect to seek damages from the third person.[21] An election not to proceed against the third person acts as an assignment of the cause of action to the DLI. Any subsequent recovery by the DLI must be advanced to payment of the legal costs incurred, the injured worker,[22] the DLI for benefits distributed to the worker, and the worker for the remaining balance.[23]

If injury or death occurs because the worker is deliberately self-destructive or engaged in felonious behavior, neither the worker nor his or her beneficiaries shall receive compensation.[24] However, no deliberate intention will be found if the "suicidal death occurs from uncontrollable impulse, delirium or frenzy without conscious volition to produce death, irresistible impulse, or delirium caused by injury related to drugs, pain and suffering, and/or other forms of acute dementia."[25]

(A)(2) Disease

For an occupational disease to be compensable, it must be shown that the disease:[26]

---

17. Garrett Freightlines v. Department of Labor and Industries, 45 Wash.App. 335, 725 P.2d 463 (1986).
18. *Id.*
19. *Id.*
20. RCW 51.24.020; Hardy v. State, 38 Wash.App. 399 (1984).
21. RCW 51.24.030.
22. The worker is entitled to 25% of the settlement or judgment.
23. RCW 51.24.050.
24. RCW 51.32.020.
25. Schwab v. Department of Labor and Industries, 76 Wash.2d 784 (1969).
26. RCW 51.08.140.

1. is work-related;

2. arises proximately[27] out of the employment; and

3. arises naturally out of employment because

   a. it arises "as a matter of course because of or incident to the distinctive conditions of [the worker's] particular employment,"

   b. the "work conditions more probably caused the disease or disease-related disability than conditions in everyday life. . .," and

   c. the conditions that caused the disease were conditions of employment, as opposed to conditions occurring coincidentally in the work place.[28]

(B) Workers' Compensation and Mental Stress Disorder

Washington law has recognized the compensability of mental injuries under workers' compensation since Peterson v. Department of Labor and Industries in 1934.[29] The Peterson court noted that

> The effects of an accident are at least two-fold; they may be merely muscular effects . . . and there may also be, and very frequently are, effects that one may call mental, nervous and hysterical. . . . The effects of this second class, as a rule, arise as directly from the accident that the worker suffered as the muscular effects do; and it seems . . . entirely a fallacy to say that a man's right to compensation ceases when the muscular mischief is ended, but the nervous and hysterical effects still remain.[30]

Nevertheless, claims that are based on mental conditions or disabilities caused by job stress are difficult to prove.[31]

---

27. This requires "competent medical testimony which shows that the disease is probably, as opposed to possibly, caused by the employment." Dennis v. Department of Labor and Industries, 109 Wash.2d 467, 477 (1987).

28. For example, conditions of the work place rather than conditions of employment were found when an employee suffered from emotional symptoms resulting from not receiving training and placement in a special position; believing that one supervisor was hostile and the other alcoholic; and fearing job loss. Kinville v. Department of Labor and Industries, 35 Wash.App. 80, 664 P.2d 1311 (1983).

29. 78 Wash. 15, 33 P.2d 650 (1934).

30. Id.,18–19 (quoting Sykes v. Republic Coal Co., 94 Mont. 239, 22 P.2d 157).

31. RCW 51.08.142; Kinville v. Department of Labor and Industries, 35 Wash.App. 80, 664 P.2d 1311 (1983). Worker exhibited schizophrenic symptoms before starting job. She failed to show that "the occupational disease" arose naturally out of her employment because that environment exposed her to a greater risk of developing the mental condition than employment in general or remaining unemployed.

(B)(1) Injuries

Proof in cases involving mental injuries may be easier to sustain. One of the issues in Price v. Department of Labor and Industries[32] was whether the expert testimony of a psychologist in a mental injury claim must have some objective basis to be presented. The court noted that the objective–subjective distinction was not appropriate in cases involving mental injuries because medical and psychological opinions derived from psychiatric examinations are often based on conversations with the injured individual and are, thus, necessarily subjective. The court admitted the evidence. However, the case for compensation would be strengthened if objective evidence existed as to the origin and extent of the mental disability. For instance, neuropsychological assessment often can provide evidence as to the extent of the cognitive deficits brought on by a head injury and the extent of the recovery from such injuries.

(B)(2) Disease

Whether a mental condition may be caused by an occupational disease is less clear. Although mental injuries are otherwise compensable as arising from a sudden traumatic occurrence, it is more difficult to prove that such injuries arise from an occupational disease.[33] The disease must be caused by the employment, and it must be shown that, but for the employment, the disease would not have arisen. The disease need not be the sole proximate cause of the worker's disability.[34]

(C) Processing a Claim

Whenever an accident occurs to any worker, the worker must report the accident to the employer or the employer's agent. The employer is obligated to report the accident to the DLI, and the DLI must immediately forward to the worker and his or her beneficiaries or dependents a statement, in nontechnical language, of the rights under the law.[35]

---

32. 101 Wash.2d 520, 682 P.2d 307 (1984).
33. The test for whether a mental injury arises naturally out of employment is controlled by the following reasoning: "Competent medical testimony...[must show]... that the disease is probably, as opposed to possibly, caused by the employment." Dennis v. Department of Labor and Industries, 109 Wash.2d 467, 477 (1987).
34. City of Bremerton v. Shreeve, 55 Wash.App. 334 (1989).
35. RCW 51.28.010. There is no well-defined time limit for such reporting because each case is be decided on its own merits.

The worker must file the claim with the DLI, together with a certificate from the physician who attended to the injury.[36] In case of death of the worker, beneficiaries must apply for benefits and provide proof of death.[37] No application about an injury shall be valid or enforceable unless it is filed within one year after the day upon which the injury occurred.[38] Claims for occupational disease must be filed within two years following the date on which the worker obtained written notice from a physician about the existence of the disease or from the date of death.[39] The department may suspend any action on a worker's claim or deny any compensation for the following reasons: the worker refuses to submit to a medical examination, persists in injurious practices that impair recovery, refuses to submit to medical treatment essential to the recovery, or obstructs an evaluation for vocational rehabilitation and fails to cooperate with the rehabilitation.[40]

The physician has a duty to inform the worker of his or her rights under the law and to lend all necessary assistance in making an application for compensation and in providing proof of the injury or occupational disease.[41] Within five days of the date of treatment, the physician must specify the condition of the injured worker at the time of the treatment, provide a description of the treatment given, and suggest an estimate of the probable duration for recovery from the injury. Any physician who fails, neglects, or refuses to file such a report may be subjected to a civil penalty not to exceed $250.[42] An attending physician's failure to perform the statutory duty of informing the worker about his or her rights and lending all necessary assistance in applying for compensation does not excuse the worker from filing a claim within one year.[43]

The DLI determines the disability and the amount of payments.[44] The employer's insurance carrier (or the employer, if self-insured) must make allowable payments promptly to the injured worker.[45]

If a claimant is not satisfied with the decision of the DLI, he or she may request a mediation session before an authorized indus-

36. RCW 51.28.020.
37. RCW 51.28.030.
38. RCW 51.28.050.
39. RCW 51.28.055.
40. RCW 51.32.110.
41. *Id.* A physician may be deemed liable for negligence by not performing this statutory duty. Wilbur v. Department of Labor and Industries, 38 Wash. App. 553 (1984).
42. RCW 51.48.060.
43. Wilbur v. Department of Labor and Industries, 38 Wash.App. 553 (1984).
44. RCW 51.04.020(2).
45. RCW 51.32.210.

trial appeal's judge. If no final agreement is reached, appeals may be made to the Board of Industrial Insurance Claims.[46]

(D) Workers' Compensation Benefits

When the injury to the worker is so serious as to require transportation to a place of treatment, the DLI will reimburse the employer for the transportation.[47]

Death benefits will provide compensation for the expenses of a burial. In addition, various other lump-sum distributions or monthly benefit payments may be paid out. The amounts depend on the marital status of the worker and on who the survivors are (children or parents).[48]

Determination of permanent total disability benefits does not occur until the worker's condition becomes constant, and he or she is not able to return to a condition of self-support as an able-bodied worker.[49] During the period of permanent disability, the worker shall receive[50] monthly benefit payments that depend on the marital status, the number of children, and the amount established under the law for various permutations; the services of an attendant, if the worker is physically disabled and requires such services; and the pension to which the worker was entitled from the job. If the worker dies after first being declared permanently disabled, the amount of the death benefits will depend on whether the cause of death was related to the injury and on the various permutations of payments that either the worker elected to receive or that are established by the law.[51]

Permanent partial disability payments will be made depending on the particular loss of a body part and on the amount established by law for the loss of such a part.[52] If permanent partial disability is followed by permanent total disability, the monthly compensation shall be reduced by the lump sum paid out for the loss of the particular body part.[53] When a preexisting disease delays or prevents recovery, the effects of the injury must

---

46. *See generally* Chapter 51.52 RCW that delineates the appeals process, including the timing of appeals, burdens of proof, and channels for subsequent appeals to the courts. The board is also responsible for appeals of attending professionals for payment for services rendered to injured workers. RCW 51.52.050.
47. RCW 51.36.020.
48. RCW 51.32.050.
49. RCW 51.32.055.
50. RCW 51.32.060.
51. RCW 51.32.067.
52. RCW 51.32.080.
53. *Id.*

be ascertained as to their role in producing the permanent partial disability and appropriate compensation shall be awarded.[54]

Temporary total disability provides monthly benefits and attendant services up to the time when the worker is able to return to work. Payments will continue until the new earnings restore that which existed before the injury or disease.[55] The worker's physician shall decide whether the worker is physically able to perform the work; in case of any dispute as to worker's ability to perform the available work offered by the employer, the DLI shall make the final determination.[56]

Rehabilitation services shall be provided to return the worker to gainful employment.[57] After evaluation of eligibility for such services, but before a declaration is made of the worker's permanent disability, the DLI at its sole discretion and consistent with the worker's physical and mental status, may approve services to restore the worker to gainful employment[58] (see chapter 5B.3 for a full discussion of these services).

Every worker who loses the use of a body part will be provided proper artificial substitutes or visual or hearing aids to correct the loss.[59] Mechanical devices such as crutches and modification of the worker's vehicle and home will be provided by the department at the established rates of reimbursement.[60]

(E) Audits of Health Care Professionals

The department has the authority to examine all records, including patient records, during an audit provided that such disclosures would not subject the provider to any liability for breaching the confidential relationship between provider and patient.[61] No original records may be removed from the premises of the health care professional.

---

54. RCW 51.32.100.
55. RCW 51.32.090.
56. *Id.*
57. RCW 51.32.095.
58. *Id.*
59. RCW 51.36.020.
60. *Id.*
61. RCW 51.36.110.

Vocational Disability Determinations

Washington law provides for two separate vocational rehabilitation programs. The first is associated with the workers' compensation program and is operated by the DLI Office of Rehabilitation Services and focuses on training or retraining of injured workers (see chapter 5B.2). This program is nearly exclusively within the purview of vocational rehabilitation counselors.[1] The second program is operated by the Department of Social and Health Services (DSHS) and provides mostly for the vocational training of individuals receiving public assistance. Both programs are aimed at creating gainful employment for individuals consistent with their physical and mental status.

MHPs may provide evaluation, consultation, or therapeutic services to people engaged in these programs. Sometimes, the programs will incorporate such services in the self-sufficiency plans described below.

(A) Department of Labor and Industries

The main purpose of this program is to enable the injured worker to be trained and placed in gainful employment.[2] The DLI is directed to use the services of professionals, both in the public

---

1. The educational and experience requirements for counselors are contained in WAC 296-18A-510.
2. RCW 51.32.095(1). *Gainful employment* means any occupation, not to exclude self-employment, that allows a worker to be compensated with wages or other earnings. WAC 296-18A-420(2).

and private sector and to provide vocational rehabilitation that will lead to a job that is compatible with the worker's physical and mental status. In obtaining this objective, the following priorities for placing the worker are to be followed:[3]

1. return to the previous job with the same employer;
2. modify the previous job with the same employer to include a transitional return to work;
3. find a new job with the same employer in keeping with the worker's limitations or restrictions;
4. modify the previous job with a new employer;
5. find a new job with a new employer or develop self-employment based upon transferable skills; and
6. provide short-term retraining and job placement.

The costs of vocational rehabilitation under this program may include

1. books, tuition fees, supplies, equipment, transportation, child or dependent care, and other necessary expenses not to exceed $3,000 in any 52-week period;
2. the cost of continuing the temporary, total disability compensation while the worker is actively and successfully undergoing a formal program of vocational rehabilitation; and
3. training fees for on-the-job training and the cost of furnishing tools and other equipment necessary for self-employment or reemployment.[4]

The latter two categories of funding are authorized only for 52 weeks. Upon written order of the DLI, funding can be extended for another 52 weeks.

(A)(1) Service Monitoring

The DLI has established criteria to monitor the quality and effectiveness of rehabilitation services, and referrals are made to vocational rehabilitation services based on the following performance criteria:[5]

1. objective criteria, including
    a. the cost to the medical aid fund, including fees paid to vocational or other providers at the request of the vocational rehabilitation counselor;

---

3. RCW 51.32.095(2).
4. If the worker is required to reside away from his or her customary residence, the reasonable cost of board and lodging can also be paid.
5. RCW 51.32.095(4); WAC 296-18A-460.

b. the cost to the accident fund, including time loss compensation, loss of earning power payments, and training costs paid while vocational rehabilitation services are provided;

c. the cost to the second injury fund because of approved job site modifications;

d. the length of services provided, from time of referral to date of issuance of closing reports; and

e. the ratio of referrals to completed reports.

2. subjective criteria, including

a. the ability of the vocational rehabilitation provider and counselor to comply with applicable laws and regulations; and

b. the adequacy of the vocational rehabilitation provider's facilities.

Providers who wish to contract with the DLI for vocational rehabilitation services are selected through a request for proposal process. Proposals are to be evaluated and referrals made on the basis of the criteria listed above.

(A)(2) Vocational Rehabilitation Process

After a determination by a referral source[6] that vocational rehabilitation is both necessary and likely to enable the injured worker to become employable, the worker will be referred to a vocational rehabilitation provider.[7] The provider will create a vocational rehabilitation plan to be approved by the DLI. The plan must contain the following information:[8]

1. assessment of the skills and abilities made on the basis of the physical capacities and mental status, aptitudes, and transferable skills of the injured worker;

2. the services necessary to enable the injured worker to find gainful employment;

3. labor market information showing the employability of the injured worker at plan completion;

4. an estimate of the cost and the time necessary for plan completion;

---

6. A referral source can be either the state through the workers' compensation program or a self-insured employer. WAC 296-18A-420(8).

7. A provider is any vocational rehabilitation counselor or firm that has a vendor number to bill, for services, the Washington Department of Labor and Industries. WAC 296-18A-420(4).

8. WAC 296-18A-450.

5. a direct comparison of the injured worker's skills with potential types of employment to show a likelihood of success;

6. if necessary, a job analysis of the injured worker's previous occupation, including earnings, may be included; and

7. any other information that will significantly affect the plan.

The plan must also address each priority, described earlier,[9] with a justification given about why each preceding priority was not used. The plan must be signed by the vocational rehabilitation counselor and the injured worker.

(A)(3) Required Reports

The following reports are required from the vocational rehabilitation provider during the conduct of the plan:[10]

1. *Contact report.* Contact with the injured worker must be reported to the DLI within 21 days of referral to the provider. Notification is to be made on a form provided by the DLI.

2. *Progress report.* A progress report must be made upon the request of the DLI on an approved form. The DLI must be informed immediately of factors affecting plan completion or changes of status or in anticipated plan costs.

3. *Closing report.* Upon completion of the formal program, a closing report must be submitted to the DLI. It must contain at least the following information:

   a. assessment of the injured worker's employability status at the time of completion of vocational services;

   b. whether the injured worker has returned to work; and

   c. any remaining barriers to the injured worker finding gainful employment.

(A)(4) Disputes[11]

The object of the dispute resolution process is to avoid delay in the rehabilitation process by quickly addressing problems brought by injured workers and employers. The process focuses on the employability determination or the final vocational rehabilitation plan. The DLI must receive notice of a dispute in writing and including the reasons for the dispute. This must occur within 15 days of receiving the determination notice that is sent to both the injured worker and the employer. To resolve the dispute, the DLI may initiate an investigation involving any or all parties. The

---

9. RCW 51.32.095(2); WAC 296-18A-450(2).
10. WAC 296-18A-400.
11. WAC 296-18A-470.

DLI must notify all parties of any decision within 30 days after receiving the notice of the dispute.

(A)(5) Responsibilities of the Parties

Each party involved in the vocational rehabilitation process has specific responsibilities.[12]

The attending physician

1. must maintain open communication with the injured worker's assigned vocational rehabilitation counselor and the DLI;
2. must respond to any requests for information in a timely fashion;
3. must do all that is possible to hasten the vocational rehabilitation process, including making an estimate of physical capacities or restrictions;
4. may review the vocational rehabilitation plan, and if he or she feels that the injured worker is not physically capable of carrying out the plan or that the plan is unnecessary, he or she must notify the DLI immediately stating the reasons for such opinion.

The claims unit within DLI must

1. notify the employer of the referral to a vocational rehabilitation provider;
2. send the employer a copy of the closing report; and
3. give written notice to an injured worker if a complaint of noncooperation has been made.

The employer must

1. assist the vocational rehabilitation counselor in any way necessary to collect data regarding the former gainful employment of the injured worker; and
2. assist the vocational rehabilitation counselor and attending physician in finding out whether a modified job could be made available for the injured worker.

The injured worker must cooperate with all reasonable requests from all responsible parties in determining the extent of the disability and in developing the rehabilitation process.

The vocational rehabilitation provider shall

1. develop a formal program to assist the eligible injured worker to become employable;

---

12. WAC 296-18A-480.

2. maintain accurate records that will be reviewed periodically by the DLI;

3. notify the DLI of noncooperative behavior by the injured worker; and

4. keep all parties informed of the progress and development of the formal rehabilitation program.

(B) Department of Social and Health Services

The DSHS administers a vocational rehabilitation program funded jointly by the state and federal governments. The program assists persons who are disabled either physically or mentally when that disability prevents them from obtaining or maintaining employment.[13] In addition, vocational and mental health services related to vocational rehabilitation are authorized for the developmentally disabled,[14] the visually handicapped,[15] and people on public assistance.[16] The DSHS provides vocational rehabilitation through its continuing general assistance program (GAP).[17] This program provides for the needs of persons who are either pregnant or incapacitated and unable to maintain gainful employment.[18]

---

13. Chapter 74.29 RCW

14. Chapter 71A.10 RCW; see chapter 5E.6.

15. Chapter 74.18 RCW; DSHS must provide vocational rehabilitation to this population to develop skills necessary for self-support and self-care. People are eligible for this program if they have no vision or limited vision that constitutes a substantial handicap to employment and can reasonably be expected to benefit from vocational rehabilitation services to gain employment.

16. Chapter 74.21 RCW. The Family Independence Program was established to break the cycle of poverty and dependence by providing readiness training, job training, education, and work opportunities while providing a basic level of financial and medical assistance and other incentives for pursuing self-sufficiency. Chapter 74.25 RCW. The Job Opportunities and Basic Skills Training Program is another program established to provide the full range of necessary education, training, and supportive services, including child care, adequate transportation, and appropriate counseling, to assist people in achieving self-sufficiency.

17. RCW 43.20A.030; WAC 388-37-010. The DSHS is the authorized authority for receipt of federal funds for vocational rehabilitation. RCW 43.20A.300.

18. WAC 388-37-010(1). The remainder of this chapter focuses on the latter category (i.e., those incapacitated and not capable of gainful employment).

(C) Vocational Rehabilitation Recipient Eligibility Requirements

Such services are provided to persons who are disabled physically or mentally. This includes behavioral disorders characterized as "deviant social behavior" or impaired abilities to maintain normal relationships with family and community.[19] However, the services must be expected to render the person fit to engage in a gainful employment consistent with the person's capacities and abilities.[20]

When other terms of eligibility are fulfilled, GAP becomes available to incapacitated individuals.[21] They must be physically, emotionally, or mentally unable to work because of a condition expected to continue for at least 60 days from the date of application.[22] To continue receiving GAP, an incapacitated individual must accept and follow through on required available medical treatment that can be expected to render him or her able to work. In deciding eligibility because of incapacity, the DSHS must[23]

1. consider medical and other related evidence of the incapacitating condition and make a decision confirming or denying the existence of eligibility within 45 days of application;

2. request additional information when necessary;

3. ascertain the probable duration of incapacity;

4. require available medical treatment that can be expected to render the client able to work; and

5. recommend available medical services provided under the state-financed medical care services program.

A determination of eligibility will not be made if an applicant fails to cooperate in any part of the documentation process.

(C)(1) Determining Incapacity[24]

The primary source of evidence for physiological incapacity will be a written report from a physician, a certified registered nurse, or the chief of medical administration of the Veterans' Administration. The primary source of evidence for a mental incapacity

---

19. RCW 74.29.010.
20. *Id.*
21. In this context, incapacity refers to the individual's capacity to earn income by employment. WAC 388-37-030.
22. WAC 388-37-030(1). Persons incapacitated by alcoholism or drug addiction are not included in this definition, but an alcoholic or drug addict who is incapacitated because of other mental or physical conditions may be eligible for general assistance. WAC 388-37-030(1).
23. WAC 388-37-032.
24. WAC 388-37-35.

will be a report from a psychiatrist, licensed clinical psychologist, or mental health professional designated by a local community mental health agency.[25] When it appears that an individual may have a developmental disability, such persons may be referred to a medical professional who is skilled in identifying developmental disabilities. Supplemental evidence may be obtained from other treating practitioners, including chiropractors, nurses, physician's assistants, or the DSHS institutions and agencies from which the individual has received services.

Medical findings must show that a medical condition is present that could be expected to produce the reported symptoms of the incapacity. Clear, objective medical information, including professional observation and relevant medical history must be present. The determination of incapacity will be made on the basis of the facts of each case. This requires evaluation of the severity of the impairment and its effect on the individual so that it can be decided whether there remains any capacity to engage in gainful employment. Although the primary reason for incapacity must be a medical impairment, vocational factors, such as age, education, and work skills, may also be considered.

Severity of a medical impairment is defined as the degree to which an individual is restricted in his or her ability to perform basic work-related activities. This is measured on a scale from one to five (01 means that no impairment has been identified and 05 means that the ability to perform one or more of the basic work-related activities is absent). Ratings of 01 and 02 mean that the individual is considered capable of gainful employment and not eligible for GAP. Ratings of 03 and 04 may or may not indicate incapacity, depending on further assessment of functional capacities and vocational factors. Finally, a rating of 05 indicates incapacity and clear eligibility for GAP.

(C)(2) Progressive Evaluation Process

The DSHS determines the existence, severity, and duration of incapacity for GAP using a step-by-step evaluation process called the Progressive Evaluation Process (PEP).[26] Each step of the PEP is evaluated sequentially until a decision to approve or deny has been made. The seven steps in the PEP are

1. Review of medical evidence to ensure that requirements are met.[27] The medical report required for a Step 1 determination must be written by an authorized medical professional.

---

25. At the discretion of DSHS, a physician can also evaluate an individual's mental condition. WAC 388-37-035(2).
26. WAC 388-37-100.
27. WAC 388-37-115.

2. Assignment of total mental severity rating.[28] If a mental impairment is claimed, the severity of the disorder must be determined on the basis of psychosocial and treatment history, clinical findings, results of special tests, and professionally observed symptoms that indicate impairment of the ability to perform basic work-related activities.

3. Assignment of physical severity rating.[29] If a physical impairment is claimed, the severity rating must be determined from current medical evidence that provides an objective description of an individual's medical condition.

4. Assignment of one total severity rating for each individual when a combination of impairments exists.[30]

5. Determination of the present mental and physical functional capacities of the individual. The functional capacities of persons with mental impairments with an overall severity rating of 03 or 04 are evaluated in terms of two factors:

   a. cognitive factors that include the ability to understand, remember, and follow instructions; learn new tasks; exercise judgment and make decisions; and perform routine tasks without undue supervision; and

   b. social factors that include ability to relate appropriately to co-workers and supervisors, interact appropriately in public contacts, tolerate the pressures of a work setting, care for self, and maintain appropriate behavior in a work setting.

   For individuals with a physical impairment with a severity rating of 03 or 04, functional capacities are assessed on the basis of the individual's exertional, exertionally related, and nonexertional physical limitations.[31]

6. Review of the possibility that the individual can still do some type of relevant past work.[32] Before considering age and educational factors, the ability of an individual to perform relevant past work is assessed in relation to current functional capacities. All of the individual's relevant past work will be evaluated to decide exertional and skill requirements for each job.

7. Assessment of the ability of the individual to perform other work when the individual is not capable of doing any relevant

---

28. WAC 388-37-120. The regulations provide detailed guidelines for rating the severity of mental retardation, organic brain damage, and functional or nonfunctional psychotic disorders.
29. WAC 388-37-130.
30. WAC 388-37-140.
31. WAC 388-37-160.
32. WAC 388-37-180; WAC 388-37-170.

past work and is less than 55 years of age.[33] Individuals with severity ratings of 03 or 04, whose incapacity has not yet been determined by means of Step 6, are assessed for possible referral for an administrative review.

(C)(3) Redetermination of Eligibility

GAP recipients must have their eligibility redetermined at least once every six months.[34] Before a determination that the person is no longer incapacitated, at least one of the following conditions must be met:[35]

1. new evidence must show a clear improvement in the medical condition; or[36]

2. it can be established that the previous decision was based on faulty or insufficient information or erroneous procedure.

GAP recipients will be screened to decide the appropriateness of a referral to other agencies (e.g., the Social Security Administration, Supplemental Security Income, Department of Vocational Rehabilitation, or Veterans' Administration). This will be done if it can reduce their need for assistance. The state of Washington also benefits by having to spend less of its money.

---

33. WAC 388-37-190; WAC 388-37-170. These regulations describe a complicated set of factors for determining eligibility.
34. WAC 388-37-050.
35. WAC 388-37-050(2).
36. WAC 388-37-050(2). Clear improvement means that, since the last decision, the physical or mental impairments upon which the decision was based have decreased in severity, or the effect of that impairment has been significantly diminished (through therapy, medication, rehabilitation, etc.) to the point where the individual is capable of gainful employment.

Emotional Distress as a Basis for Civil Liability

Emotional distress, also known as mental suffering, may be the basis for specific civil tort actions (personal injury lawsuits) or damages may be awarded for mental suffering as part of another cause of action. MHPs may be asked to evaluate the person who claims to have suffered the distress and to testify as to its etiology, severity, duration, and methods to treat it.

(A) Intentional Infliction of Emotional Distress

Many actions involving emotional distress are brought under the tort of outrage.[1] The cause of the distress, the nature of the injury, and the motivations of the injuring person determine whether a suit can stand by itself or be part of another cause of action. To establish such a claim, the plaintiff must show that severe emotional distress was inflicted intentionally or recklessly through the outrageous or extreme conduct of the defendant. The conduct must be so extreme in degree so as to exceed the bounds of decency. It is regarded as atrocious and utterly intolerable in a

---

1. For a general overview of Washington law on the tort of outrage, *see* Robins v. Hasum, 733 F.2d 1004 (1985).

civilized community, with the plaintiff or the plaintiff's immediate family members[2] being present as the object of the conduct.[3]

In deciding whether reasonable minds could differ on whether the conduct was sufficiently extreme and outrageous to result in liability, the court must consider[4]

1. the position occupied by the defendant (e.g., the power differential of the relationship between the plaintiff and the defendant was greater for the defendant);

2. whether the plaintiff was peculiarly susceptible to emotional distress (such a plaintiff would be less likely to recover under this cause of action);

3. whether the defendant's conduct may have been privileged under the circumstances (e.g., an MHP testifying at an involuntary commitment hearing);

4. the degree of the emotional distress must constitute much more than a mere annoyance, inconvenience, or the embarrassment that normally occurs in a confrontation between two parties;

5. proof that the defendant was aware of the high probability that the conduct would cause severe emotional distress; and

6. proof that the defendant proceeded in conscious disregard of this possibility.

Whether the conduct under question is extreme or outrageous is a question for the jury.[5]

Damages may be awarded for actual emotional distress; in such an action, physical symptoms need not accompany such a trauma.[6] However, to be compensable, mental suffering must at least be manifested in objective symptoms.[7]

---

2. Immediate family members who are permitted to bring wrongful death actions include spouses, children, stepchildren, parents, and siblings. Strickland v. Deaconess Hosp., 47 Wash.App. 262, 735 P.2d 74 (1987).
3. Browning v. Slenderella Sys., 54 Wash.2d 440, 341 P.2d 859 (1959); Grimsby v. Samson, 85 Wash.2d 52, 530 P.2d 291 (1975); Deeter v. Safeway Stores, Inc., 50 Wash.App. 67, 747 P.2d 1103 (1987); Rice v. Janovich, 109 Wash.2d 48, 109 P.2d 1230 (1987).
4. Spencer v. King County, 39 Wash.App. 201, 692 P.2d 874 (1984); Phillips v. Hardwick, 29 Wash.App. 382, 628 P.2d 506 (1981).
5. Jackson v. Peoples Federal Credit Union, 25 Wash.App. 81, 604 P.2d 1025 (1979). Before the question will go to the jury, the trial court must make an initial determination that a cognizable claim has been made by the plaintiff (i.e., whether reasonable minds can differ on whether the conduct was sufficiently extreme and outrageous).
6. Browning v. Slenderella Sys., 54 Wash.2d 440, 341 P.2d 859 (1959).
7. Corrigal v. Ball & Dodd Funeral Home, Inc., 89 Wash.2d 959, 577 P.2d 580 (1978).

(B) Negligent Infliction of Emotional Distress

Washington law permits legal action for negligent infliction of emotional distress. To maintain this cause of action, the following elements must be shown:[8] the defendant had a duty to avoid negligent infliction of emotional distress; the duty was owed to those individuals who were foreseeably endangered; the resulting emotional distress must be manifested by objective symptoms;[9] and the reaction of the plaintiff must have been reasonable.[10]

As with intentional infliction of emotional distress, a defendant is liable only to a plaintiff who is placed in peril by the defendant's negligent conduct. Liability also extends "to family members present at the time who fear for the one imperiled."[11]

(C) Emotional Distress as an Element of Damages

Both intentional and negligent infliction of emotional distress require the presence of emotional distress. However, there are other claims that do not require emotional distress for the defendant to be liable. Yet, the trauma of the emotional distress may be compensated as an element of damages.

Psychological problems that are causally connected to the defendant's conduct may be considered by the jury when evaluating damages.[12] Washington case law liberally construes damages for emotional distress as being available upon proof for other intentional torts (e.g., wrongful employment termination;[13] injury to reputation and personal humiliation;[14] wrongful birth;[15] nui-

---

8. Hursley v. Giard, 87 Wash.2d 424, 553 P.2d 1096 (1976).
9. Hursley, id., leaves open the question of whether liability exists under this cause of action when there is emotional distress but no physical symptoms.
10. The question of reasonable reaction is one of fact for the jury to determine.
11. Cunningham v. Lockard, 48 Wash.App 38, 45, 736 P.2d 305 (1987).
12. Note, however, that Washington unlike many other jurisdictions does not allow damages for emotional distress (mental anguish) in wrongful death actions. Pike v. United States, 652 F.2d 31 (1981).
13. Cagle v. Burns and Roe, Inc., 106 Wash.2d 911, 726 P.2d 434 (1986).
14. Rasor v. Retail Credit Co., 87 Wash.2d 516, 726 P.2d 1041 (1976).
15. Harkeson v. Parke-Davis, Inc., 98 Wash.2d 460, 656 P.2d 483 (1983).

sance;[16] breach of contract;[17] indecent or sexual assault;[18] and certain cases under the Washington Consumer Protection Act).[19]

16. Wilson v. KeyTronic Corp., 40 Wash.App. 802, 701 P.2d 518 (1985).
17. Cooperstein v. Van Natter, 26 Wash.App. 91, 611 P.2d 1332 (1980).
18. Raymond v. Ingram, 47 Wash.App. 781, 737 P.2d 314, *review denied* (1987).
19. Keyes v. Bollinger, 31 Wash.App. 286, 640 P.2d 1077 (1982).

5B.5

Wrongdoers Who Are Mentally Ill and Civil Liability

A person's mental status may affect the outcome of civil litigation. For instance, this may occur because a person's mental status at the time of the personal injury can preclude damages being paid from insurance policies. MHPs may be asked to evaluate people who are involved in civil litigation. They may testify as to the person's mental status when the injuries occurred or at the time of the trial.

(A) Liability of a Mentally Ill Person

A person who is mentally ill will be held liable civilly for the injuries caused to others or to property. For instance, a mentally ill person was held liable civilly for the knife assault on another with whom he was incarcerated.[1] The Restatement of Torts followed by our jurisdiction when other law is silent also holds a mentally ill person liable for injuries caused to others or to property.[2]

(B) Mental Illness and Insurance

Many liability, death, and accident insurance policies preclude claiming benefits if the injury was caused by intentionally inflicting harm. This is also true for committing suicide or a suicidal attempt whether or not the person was mentally ill. The exclusion

---

1. Kusash v. McCorkle, 100 Wash. 318, 170 P. 1023 (1918).
2. Restatement (Second) of Torts § 282(B).

also may extend to covering the costs of legal representation. However, in a case in which a closed head injury resulted from an accident, the court found that the accident was the direct cause of a suicidal death.[3] The exclusionary clause did not apply to this claim and benefits were paid in spite of the suicide.

(C) Procedural Rights of Mentally Ill Persons

Unless the person has been declared incompetent and a guardian was appointed (see chapter 5A.2), no different procedural rights would apply during any civil litigation.

---

3. Norbeck v. Mutual of Omaha Ins. Co., 3 Wash.App. 582, 476 P.2d 546 (1970).

5B.6

Competency to Contract

The lack of mental capacity to contract will not relieve any obligation unless the person has been declared incompetent, and a guardian has been appointed. Even a person who is involuntarily committed for mental illness may dispose of property and sign contracts validly.[1] MHPs who evaluate and treat people who lack capacity to dispose of property and contract should consider obtaining a formal ruling of incompetency to protect the best interests of their clients (see chapter 5A.2, Guardianship for Adults).

(A) The Effect of Incompetency

After the person has been declared incompetent, the guardian has a duty to pay all just claims against the estate which arose before the guardianship was declared.[2] An order may be sought from the court having jurisdiction over the guardianship to compel performance of the contract even if the ward had become incapacitated before the performance was necessary.[3]

If adjudicated incompetent, the guardian alone may contract on behalf of the ward; the ward will lack capacity to incur any further contractual duties.[4] However, the ward may bind the guardianship assets contractually during a lucid interval while

---

1. RCW 71.05.370.
2. RCW 11.92.035.
3. RCW 11.92.130.
4. United Pacific Ins. Co. v. Buchanan, 52 Wash.App. 836, 765 P.2d 23 (1988).

contracting with a party who is unaware of the existence of the guardianship, if it is shown that the guardian enabled such an action through dereliction of his or her duties.[5]

---

5. *Id.*

5B.7

Competency to Sign a Will

A person who makes a will or amends an existing one must have a *sound mind* or testamentary capacity.[1] If testamentary incapacity is shown, the testator's estate will be distributed according to the terms of a previously valid will.[2] MHPs may provide testimony about having evaluated or treated the testator during the time in which the will was made (but see chapters 4.2 and 4.3 for limitations on revealing confidential information). They also may provide an opinion about the person's mental status at the time the will was signed on the basis of reports from other witnesses.

(A) Test of Testamentary Capacity

The test of whether the testator was of sound mind at the time in which the will was signed[3] requires proof that the testator knows the nature and extent of his or her property, who are his or her relatives and heirs, and who will receive the property ("recollect the objects of his bounty").[4]

Testamentary capacity is presumed when the will is executed in legal form and apparently rational in its construction.[5] If it can be established that the testator's mental capacity was intact

---

1. RCW 11.12.010.
2. If no valid will exists, the estate will be distributed through the intestacy statutes of the state of Washington.
3. Capacity of a person to make a will must be determined as of the time at which it is made. Gwinn Estate, 36 Wash.2d 583, 219 P.2d 591 (1950).
4. Roy Estate, 113 Wash. 227, 193 P. 682 (1920); Dean v. Jordan, 194 Wash. 661, 79 P.2d 331 (1938); Reilly Estate, 78 Wash.2d 623, 479 P.2d 1 (1970).
5. Reilly Estate, 78 Wash.2d 623, 479 P.2d 1 (1970).

shortly before executing the will, the presumption of testamentary capacity arises and continues unless overcome by clear, cogent, and convincing evidence.[6]

(B) Proving Testamentary Incapacity

Serious illness,[7] senile dementia,[8] insanity,[9] eccentricity,[10] unusual religious beliefs,[11] cruelness,[12] or addiction to intoxicants[13] or narcotics[14] do not necessarily lead to a finding of incapacity. Even someone who is committed for involuntary treatment[15] may meet the test of testamentary capacity. The party attempting to overturn the will must show that, at the time in which the will was created, the test of testamentary capacity could not be met.

---

6. Proof of clear, cogent, and convincing evidence was met when witnesses testified that the testator could talk about everyday matters and gardening (Mitchell Estate, 41 Wash.2d 326, 249 P.2d 385 (1952)); attorneys familiar with the testator testified that, in their professional opinions, the testator was unable to understand the legal document and unable to recollect the objects of his bounty. Matter of Estate of Eubank, 50 Wash.App. 611, 749 P.2d 691 (1988).
7. Testator suffered from epileptic dementia for at least 15 years before execution of the will. The "mental derangement" prevented the testator from meeting the test of testamentary capacity as testified to by witnesses to the signing of the will and by physicians who had examined the testator. Hartley v. Lord, 38 Wash. 221, 80 P. 433 (1905).
8. A testator who willed all her property to her attorney did not have testamentary capacity because evidence showed that, at the time of making the will, she suffered from senile dementia that caused delusions and prevented her from transacting business as usual. Adams Estate, 164 Wash. 64, 1 P.2d 840 (1931).
9. To invalidate a will because testator was laboring under delusions, evidence must show that the delusions affected the person to whom the property was left in the will. Meagher Estate, 60 Wash.2d 691, 375 P.2d 148 (1962).
10. Mental incapacity was not shown because the testator was eccentric in dress, remained an ardent suffragist, and believed that she was being persecuted for her beliefs, but because her business abilities to amass and manage a fortune were intact up to her death. Converse v. Mix, 63 Wash. 318, 115 P. 305 (1911).
11. Belief in spiritualism does not incapacitate a person from making a valid will. Hanson Estate, 87 Wash. 113, 115 P. 264 (1915). When religious beliefs are produced by a mental disorder, testamentary capacity may be doubted. Ingersoll v. Gourley, 78 Wash. 406, 139 P. 207 (1914).
12. Testator may make an unjust, cruel will based on an unexplained dislike for a relative although such actions alone do not suggest the presence of delusional thinking that would nullify the will. Gwinn Estate, 36 Wash.2d 583, 219 P.2d 591 (1950).
13. Incapacity will not be found if the testator was mentally capable of transacting business, even if the testator was frequently under the influence of intoxicants. Weatherall v. Weatherall, 63 Wash. 526, 115 P. 1078 (1911).
14. Testatrix was competent to sign will, even though at times delirious and under the influence of drugs, although she appeared to those in attendance to understand her property and who would benefit from the bequests. Geissler Estate, 104 Wash. 452, 177 P. 330 (1918).
15. WAC 275-55-241; Lundgren Estate, 189 Wash. 33, 63 P.2d 438 (1936).

5B.8

Competency to Vote

The right to vote cannot be denied or revoked unless the person has been declared mentally incompetent by judicial process (see chapter 5A.2, Guardianship for Adults) or if a person has been convicted of an infamous crime and his or her civil rights have not been restored.[1]

---

1. Constitution of the state of Washington, Article VI, Elections and Elective Rights, [4,06] 3.

5B.9

Competency to Obtain a Driver's License

The Department of Motor Vehicles (DMV) shall not issue a driver's license to a person who has been evaluated, by a Department of Social and Health Service's approved program, for alcoholism and drug abuse (see chapter 5E.5);[1] a person who has previously been adjudged mentally ill (see chapter 5E.4) or incompetent because of mental disability or disease (see chapter 5A.2);[2] and a person whom the DMV has concluded would not operate a motor vehicle safely because of substantial evidence of physical or mental disability.[3] A person who is viewed as disabled by DMV has a right to prove that, in spite of the disability, he or she can drive a motor vehicle safely. MHPs may become involved with the case at this point if they are called upon to evaluate the effect of the disability.

(A) Certificate to Remove Disability

The DMV can require that a certificate, "showing his or her condition," be signed by a licensed physician or other proper

---

1. RCW 46.20.031(4). A license may be issued if the department determines that such a person has been granted a deferred prosecution (see Chapter 10.05 RCW) or is satisfactorily participating in or has completed an alcohol or drug treatment program and has established control of his or her alcohol or drug abuse problem.
2. RCW 46.20.031(5). No person so adjudged shall be denied a license to drive if the Superior Court should find him or her able to operate a motor vehicle during the incompetency.
3. RCW 46.20.031(8). Such a decision by the DMV is subject to review by a court of competent jurisdiction.

authority designated by the DMV.[4] Once the certificate is obtained, the person may apply for a license. The certificate may not be offered as evidence in any court except when an appeal occurs after a license has been refused, suspended, or revoked.[5]

---

4. RCW 46.20.041. Such a certificate could not be used to avoid liability by an epileptic driver who was attempting to defend against an injured plaintiff's action. The law shields the professional who provided the certificate from later civil liability. Tumelson v. Todhunter, 105 Wash.2d 596, 716 P.2d 890 (1986).
5. *Id*. In addition, the certificate may be provided to the director of the Department Retirement Systems for determining eligibility for continuing disability benefits.

5B.10

Product Liability

Product liability is a legal term that describes an action for personal injuries arising out of the use of a product.[1] Although a product liability claim may be based on several principles, including negligence[2] or warranty,[3] this chapter focuses on a claim based on strict tort liability. The central element of this claim is that the product was unreasonably dangerous to the user when it left the manufacturer's control.[4] MHPs, who have developed a special expertise in human factors,[5] may evaluate the dangerousness of a product and testify in court about whether the product is dangerous to an extent beyond that contemplated by an ordinary consumer.[6]

---

1. *See* Chapter 7.72 RCW.
2. *Negligence* means that the wrongdoer failed to meet a duty established by law (either statute or case law) toward the person or property injured, and that the wrongdoer's conduct fell below what would be expected from a reasonably prudent person under these particular circumstances.
3. A *warranty claim* alleges that the product did not work as promised or as represented by the seller or manufacturer.
4. Davis v. Globe Mach. Mfg. Co., Inc., 102 Wash.2d 68, 684 P.2d 692 (1984). Strict liability focuses on the product and on the consumer's expectation about the product, whereas negligence focuses on whether the conduct of the sellers or manufacturers was reasonable.
5. This is an interdisciplinary field that focuses on the interrelationship among peoples' abilities and the requirements of a product's design within a specified environment.
6. Lenhardt v. Ford Motor Co., 102 Wash.2d 208, 683 P.2d 1097 (1984). Strict liability focuses attention on the product and on the buyer's expectations, not on the actions of the seller.

(A) Elements of a Product Liability Claim

A product manufacturer is subject to strict liability[7] if the claimant's harm was proximately caused by the fact that the product was not reasonably safe in construction,[8] or not safe because it did not conform to the manufacturer's express warranty[9] or to the implied warranties established by Chapter 62A RCW.

To recover under the theory of strict liability, the plaintiff need not prove that the product is defective as a separate matter. Rather, the plaintiff need only prove that the product is dangerous to the extent beyond that contemplated by an ordinary consumer. The consumer has an expectation of buying a product that is reasonably safe, and if there is something in the design that does not meet that expectation, then the design is necessarily defective.[10] A manufacturer generally has no duty to warn as to obvious or known dangers.[11]

Two types of evidence that may be introduced to prove strict liability are[12] state of-the-art evidence that relates to the technological feasibility of alternate, safer designs in existence when the product was originally manufactured;[13] and evidence of industry practice regarding a particular design or manufacturing technique used by most manufacturers in that industry.[14]

---

7. RCW 7.72.030(2).
8. A product is not reasonably safe in construction if the product deviates in some material way from the design specifications or the performance standards of the manufacturer or deviates in some material way from otherwise identical units of the same product line.
9. An express warranty fails if part of the basis of the bargain includes material facts concerning the product that prove to be untrue.
10. Lenhardt v. Ford Motor Co., 102 Wash.2d 208, 683 P.2d 1097 (1984).
11. Davis v. Globe Mach. Mfg. Co., Inc., 102 Wash.2d 68, 684 P.2d 692 (1984). The worker knew about the danger before the injury; in a strict liability claim, this type of assumption of risk operates to reduce damages rather than to bar liability.
12. Historical, medical, and scientific evidence about the dangers of a particular product may be considered by the trier of fact. It is considered to be state-of-the art evidence or evidence about custom in the industry. Lenhardt v. Ford Motor Co., 102 Wash.2d 208, 683 P.2d 1097 (1984); Crittenden v. Fibreboard Corp., 58 Wash.App 649, 794 P.2d 554 (1990). Such evidence may suggest what an ordinary consumer expects in the way of product safety. Falk v. Keene Corp., 113 Wash.2d 645, 782 P.2d 974 (1989).
13. Davis v. Globe Mach. Mfg. Co., Inc., 102 Wash.2d 68, 684 P.2d 692 (1984). Evidence of manufacturer's postsale manufacture of safety improvements for the product may be proof of the product's safety defects at the time of the sale.
14. Lenhardt v. Ford Motor Co., 102 Wash.2d 208, 683 P.2d 1097(1984). Alternative designs or customs of the industry may not be admissible for evaluating the expectations of an ordinary consumer unless the plaintiff introduces such evidence.

A product seller may be subject to strict liability for harm caused by a product used beyond its useful safe life if the product seller has warranted that the product may be used safely for a longer period of time, or has intentionally misrepresented or concealed facts about the product.[15] If the harm was caused more than 12 years after the time of delivery, a presumption arises that the injury occurred after the useful safe life of the product had expired.[16] No product liability action may be brought more than three years from the time at which the claimant discovered or, in due diligence, should have discovered the harm it caused.[17]

---

15. RCW 7.72.060.
16. *Id.*
17. *Id.* This also is subject to the applicable provisions of Chapter 4.16 RCW pertaining to the tolling and extension of a statute of limitation.

5B.11

Unfair Competition

Unfair methods of competition and unfair or deceptive acts or practices in the conduct of any trade or commerce are unlawful under the Consumer Protection Act.[1] MHPs may provide evidence as to the effects of a type of marketing that attempts to confuse the consumer into believing that one's business products or services were produced by another. Empirical research, such as consumer surveys, may help determine whether the defendant's business practices resulted in such confusion.

(A) Legal Test of Unfair Competition

The elements of a private cause of action under the Consumer Protection Act that must be proven include[2] that (a) the defendant's act was unfair or deceptive;[3] (b) it occurred during the conduct of trade or commerce;[4] (c) such an act or practice affects the public interest;[5] (d) it caused injury to the plaintiff's business

---

1. RCW 19.86.020.
2. Howell v. Spokane & Inland Empire Blood Bank, 114 Wash.2d 42, 785 P.2d 815 (1990).
3. Proof that the defendant's act or practice is unfair or deceptive is demonstrated by showing that it can deceive a substantial portion of the public. Saunders v. Lloyd's of London, 113 Wash.2d 330, 779 P.2d 249 (1989).
4. Trade or commerce shall include the sale of assets or services and of any commerce directly or indirectly affecting the people of the state of Washington. RCW 19.86.010.
5. To prove unlawful practice, the court must consider whether the practice occurred during the defendant's conduct of business; the practice was a generalized pattern of conduct; repeated acts occurred before business was transacted with the plaintiff; repetition of the practice will occur; or if it was only a single transaction, whether many consumers were affected. Mason v. Mortgage America, Inc., 114 Wash.2d 842, 792 P.2d 142 (1990).

or property;[6] and (e) a causal connection exists between the unfair or deceptive practice and the injuries suffered.[7] It is not necessary to prove intent to deceive, proof of a specific party being deceived, or the possibility of future deception by the defendant.[8]

(A)(1) Trademark Confusion

A *trademark* means "any word, name, symbol, designation, character name, distinctive feature used in advertising, slogan, or device or any combination of the above that is adopted and used by a person or business to identify goods made or sold and to distinguish them from goods made or sold by others or used to identify the services of one person or business to distinguish those services from the services of others."[9] Trademarks are typically registered under federal law, but they also may be registered under Washington law.[10] In either event, registration is not determinative of whether the person or business has established a trademark.

In determining whether a trademark imitation has caused confusion, mistake, or deception used in association with goods or services, the court must consider all relevant factors including, but not limited to, the following:[11] the similarity of the marks in their entireties as to appearance, sound, meaning, connotation, and commercial impression; the similarity of the goods or services and the nature of the goods and services; the similarity of the trade channels; the conditions under which sales are made and buyers to whom sales are made; the fame of the marks; the number and nature of similar marks in use on similar goods or services; the nature and the extent of any actual confusion; the length of time during and conditions under which there has been concurrent use without evidence of actual confusion; the variety of goods or services on which the marks are used; and the nature and extent of potential confusion.

---

6. Proof of this element is shown if the consumer's property interest or money is reduced because of the conduct, even to a small extent. Mason v. Mortgage America, Inc., 114 Wash.2d 842, 792 P.2d 142 (1990).
7. If the state sues to enforce the Consumer Protection Act on behalf of the public, consumer reliance need not be shown to prove that a misrepresentation was deceptive or unfair as long as it is possibly deceptive or unfair; but in a private action, the plaintiff must establish that, but for the defendant's deceptive or unfair act, the injury would not have occurred. Nuttall v. Dowell, 31 Wash.App. 98, 639 P.2d 832 (1982).
8. State v. A.N.W. Seed Corp., 116 Wash.2d 39, 802 P.2d 1353 (1991).
9. RCW 19.77.010(4).
10. RCW 19.77.030.
11. RCW 19.77.140.

5B.12

Employment Discrimination

The Washington legislature has found that practices of discrimination against any of its inhabitants because of race, creed, color, national origin, gender, marital status, age or that the presence of any sensory, mental, or physical handicap are a matter of state concern. Such discrimination threatens not only the rights and proper privileges of its inhabitants but menaces the institutions and foundation of a free democratic state.[1] As employers or agents of employers, MHPs must not engage in the unfair practice of discrimination when involved in personnel selection, discharge, and promotion. Providers also may need to have knowledge about the law because of their roles in industrial consultation and test construction.

(A) Who Is Affected by Employment Discrimination Law

The law applies to any person acting in the interest of an employer who employs eight or more persons. The law does not apply to any religious or sectarian organization not organized for private profit;[2] nor does it apply to federal employees, American Indian tribal employees, or private membership club employees when the clubs are exempt from taxation.[3]

---

1. RCW 49.60.010.
2. RCW 49.60.040.
3. *See* Section 501(c) of the Internal Revenue Code of 1954.

(B) Unlawful Employment Practices

Employers or their agents cannot discriminate against an employee because of age, gender, marital status, race, creed, color, national origin or because of the presence of any sensory, mental, or physical handicap.[4] An employer engages in unfair employment practices when, because of such discrimination, a person was[5] not hired on the basis of the characteristics listed above rather than on the basis of *bona fide* lack of occupational qualifications;[6] discharged[7] or barred from employment on the basis of one of the characteristics;[8] and discriminated against with regard to salary compensation or to other terms or conditions of employment on the basis of one of the characteristics.[9] In addition, the printing of any statement, advertisement, publication, or application form for employment must not express any discrimination on the basis of any one of the characteristics.[10]

Any person injured by such discrimination[11] shall have a civil action to enjoin further violations and to recover actual damages sustained. The plaintiff also may be entitled to be refunded

---

4. Alcohol abuser was not viewed as handicapped because the disease was not arrested nor was it amenable to treatment. Phillips v. City of Seattle, 51 Wash.App. 415, 754 P.2d 116, *affirmed* 111 Wash.2d 903, 766 P.2d 1099 (1988). A separate statute establishes unfair practices with regard to HIV infection, *see* RCW 49.60.172.
5. RCW 49.60.180.
6. Requiring employees to take a lie detector test is unlawful and can lead to criminal and civil penalties (*see* chapter 5C.3).
7. To establish a case of racially motivated discharge, the plaintiff must show that he was a member of a protected class replaced by someone not in a protected class, he was discharged after having done satisfactory work, and employer's evidence showing that discharge occurred for nonracial reason was only a charade. Jones v. Kitsap County Sanitary Landfill, Inc., 60 Wash.App. 369, 803 P.2d 841 (1991).
8. To prove handicapped discrimination, handicapped employee did not have to prove that the municipal corporation intentionally engaged in outrageous and extreme conduct to recover damages for emotional distress (*see* chapter 5B.4). Dean v. Municipality of Metropolitan Seattle-Metro, 104 Wash.2d 627, 708 P.2d 393 (1985). The employer had a duty to provide the employee, who had become handicapped from a work-related injury, with an alternative position for which the employee might have been qualified. Reese v. Sears, Roebuck & Co., 107 Wash.2d 563, 731 P.2d 497 (1987).
9. Two female employees recovered damages for physical, emotional, and mental suffering (*see* chapter 5B.4) when they proved that the employer knew or should have known that a male co-worker's unwelcomed physical and verbal sexual advances were creating an offensive work environment. The employer took no corrective action for more than two years after becoming aware of the situation. Glasgow v. Georgia-Pacific Corp., 103 Wash.2d 401, 693 P.2d 708 (1985).
10. *Id.*
11. Any act violating Chapter 49.60 RCW.

the expenses of the law suit, including attorney's fees,[12] or other remedies authorized by the United States Civil Rights Act of 1964,[13] including punitive damages.[14]

---

12. A prevailing party can recover costs of travel, copying, telephone, depositions, and attorney's fees that were necessary expenditures in preparation and trial of case, even if the remedy sought was only an injunction; Blair v. Washington State University, 108 Wash.2d 558, 740 P.2d 1379 (1987). However, the plaintiff was not allowed to recover expert witness fees in excess of compensation paid to an ordinary witness; Shannon v. Pay 'N Save Corp., 104 Wash.2d 722, 709 P.2d 799 (1985).
13. 42 U.S.C.A. § 2000a *et seq.*
14. RCW 49.60.030. For punitive damages, *see* Miles v. F.E.R.M. Enterprises, Inc., 29 Wash.App. 61, 627 P.2d 564 (1981).

Civil/Criminal Matters

5C.1

Jury Selection

A jury is a body of persons temporarily selected from among the qualified inhabitants of a particular district. It is invested with the power to present and indict a person for a public offense (a grand jury) or to try a question of fact (a petit jury).[1] Each county auditor compiles a list of registered voters from which a list of prospective jurors is randomly selected.[2] The Superior Court will impanel a grand jury of 12 persons to hear, examine, and investigate evidence concerning criminal activity and corruption.[3] Petits juries are bodies of 12 persons or less[4] selected for matters (either criminal or civil) tried before the Superior Court. They consist of six people for courts of lesser jurisdiction. Jurors are drawn by lot from those present at the court for a particular session.[5] The attorneys may prevent particular people from remaining on a jury. MHPs may be involved in rejecting potential jurors by conducting pretrial surveys, constructing questions to ask potential jurors, and evaluating jurors based on the results of pretrial surveys or of in-court observations.

---

1. RCW 2.36.010.
2. RCW 2.36.055 to .065, a right to inspect the random selection process exists. Excluding a potential juror on the basis of a clerk's subjective knowledge about the juror's relationship with a defendant was an abuse of discretion. State v. Tingdale, 117 Wash.2d 595, 817 P.2d 850 (1991).
3. RCW 2.36.010.
4. The jury shall consist of 6 persons unless the parties, in their written demand for jury, request a jury of 12 in number or consent to a lesser number. RCW 4.44.120.
5. RCW 2.36.010.

(A) Juror Qualifications

A person shall be competent to serve as a juror unless that person is[6] less than 18 years of age; not a citizen of the United States; not a resident of the county in which he or she has been summoned to serve; or convicted of a felony and has not had his or her civil rights restored. Eligible jurors are notified that they will be called to serve as a juror, as needed, from the first Monday of the month to the last Saturday of the month. Sometimes, the jury term is extended by the court if necessary for the administration of justice.[7]

(B) Excuse of Unfit Persons

No person may be excused from jury service by the court except[8]

1. if the person does not meet the qualifications to serve as a juror;
2. if a showing is made by the potential juror of undue hardship, extreme inconvenience,[9] or public necessity;[10]
3. if the person has served on jury duty during the last two years;
4. if the judge finds any other reason deemed sufficient; or
5. if the judge believes that the person has manifested unfitness to serve as a juror by reason of bias, prejudice, indifference, inattention, or any other physical or mental defect or conduct disorder that is incompatible with efficient jury service.

---

6. RCW 2.36.070.
7. RCW 2.36.010. A person summoned for jury duty who intentionally fails to appear as directed may be prosecuted for committing a misdemeanor. RCW 2.36.170.
8. RCW 2.36.100 to .110.
9. RCW 2.36.165. Employers must provide employees with sufficient leave to serve as a juror. Any employer who threatens, coerces, harasses, or denies the employee promotional opportunities because the person attempts to serve as a juror may be prosecuted for committing a misdemeanor, and a civil cause of action may be brought by the employee for damages and reinstatement to the job with attorney's fees being allowed if the employee prevails.
10. Officers of the United States and of the state of Washington, attorneys at law, school teachers, practicing physicians, licensed embalmers, active members of the fire and police departments, and all persons older than 60 years may be excused because of necessity. Failing to request the excuse is not a cause for challenge as to competency to serve. RCW 2.36.080 and RCW 4.44.200.

Either party may challenge a potential juror with each party having three peremptory challenges[11] and an unlimited number of challenges for cause.[12]

The process during which the challenges are made is called *voir dire*. It begins with the judge identifying the parties and briefly outlining the nature of the case. The plaintiff and then the defendant examine the potential jurors as to their qualifications to serve as jurors while the judge supervises. Causes of challenge belonging to the same class for each party shall occur separately in the following order:[13] (a) for general disqualification; (b) for implied bias; (c) for actual bias; and (d) for a peremptory challenge. The adverse party may except the challenge for insufficiency, and the court will rule as to whether insufficiency exists.[14] A challenge may occur for want of any of the qualifications listed earlier.[15]

A challenge for implied bias may be sustained for any of the following causes:[16] being related to either party;[17] standing in the relation of guardian and ward, attorney and client, landlord and tenant to the adverse party; being a partner in business, in the employment for wages, being surety or standing bail in the action of or for the adverse party; or having served as a juror on a previous trial in the same action, or in another action between the same parties for the same cause of action, or in a criminal action by the state against either party with substantially the same facts.

A challenge for actual bias will be upheld if the potential juror cannot try the issue impartially without prejudice to the substantial rights of the challenging party.[18] A juror, who admits to being prejudiced in the matter to be tried, must be excused.[19] Yet, a simple opinion or preconceived ideas about the case are not sufficient to sustain a challenge so long as the court believes that the juror is able to hear the case impartially.[20]

---

11. In prosecutions for capital offenses, both parties may challenge peremptorily 12 jurors each and for criminal offenses punishable by sentence to a penitentiary, 6 jurors each. Wash. Crim. R. 6.4(e)(1).
12. RCW 4.44.130.
13. RCW 4.44.220.
14. RCW 4.44.230 to .240.
15. RCW 4.44.160 and .170.
16. RCW 4.44.180. An objection to a juror was waived because a challenge of implied bias was not made. Basil v. Pope, 165 Wash. 212, 5 P.2d 329 (1931).
17. In a personal injury suit against the city, the spouse of a city employee should have been disqualified. Washington v. Seattle, 170 Wash. 371, 16 P.2d 597 (1932). As far as blood relatives are concerned, implied bias will be found if they are related by fourth degree or less.
18. RCW 4.44.170; RCW 4.44.190.
19. State v. Moser, 37 Wash.2d 911, 226 P.2d 867 (1951).
20. RCW 4.44.170 and .190; State v. White, 60 Wash.2d 551, 374 P.2d 867 (1962).

A peremptory challenge to a juror is one for which no reason need be given, but upon which the court shall dismiss that juror.[21] Each side alternately challenges potential jurors until all peremptory challenges are used or until using this process is waived by one or both sides.[22]

---

21. RCW 4.44.140.
22. RCW 4.44.210.

5C.2

Expert Witnesses[1]

Expert witnesses may testify as to matters about which the trier of fact (whether judge or jury) has general knowledge so long as the expert's opinion would aid in understanding the issues. They may even provide an opinion as to the ultimate fact(s) to be found by the trier of fact.[2] Frequently, MHPs are called to testify as expert witnesses on many issues.

(A) Qualifying as an Expert Witness

A witness will be *qualified* (allowed by the court to testify) as an *expert* if he or she has amassed scientific, technical, or other specialized knowledge by skill, experience, training, or education that will help the trier of fact to understand the evidence or to decide a fact in issue.[3] The trial court judge decides whether the person is qualified to testify as an expert witness, and such a ruling will not change on appeal except for manifest abuse of discretion.[4]

---

1. RCW 5.60.020.
2. Swartley v. Seattle School District No. 1, 70 Wash.2d 17, 422 P.2d 477 (1966). For instance, an expert witness may give an opinion as to whether the plaintiff is disabled and whether the disability prevents the person from gaining employment. Seattle-Tacoma Shipbuilding Co. v. Department of Labor and Industries, 26 Wash.2d 233, 173 P.2d 786 (1946).
3. Wash. R. Evid., 702. Practical experience may qualify a witness as an expert. A physician without psychiatry certification who had worked for four years in a mental hospital performing mental status examinations, forming treatment plans, and treating patients pharmotherapeutically, was qualified as an expert. State v. Smith, 88 Wash.2d 639, 564 P.2d 1154 (1977).
4. Vangement v. McCalmon, 68 Wash.2d 618, 414 P.2d 617 (1966); Mason v. Bon Marche Corp., 64 Wash.2d 177, 390 P.2d 997 (1964).

(B) Form and Content of Testimony

After the expert has been qualified, direct examination proceeds, and the expert provides opinions or draws inferences from the facts of the case. These are facts known before or discovered during the hearing. So long as these facts are of a type relied upon by similar experts in the particular field in forming opinions, the expert may depend on them.[5] The practical effect of this rule enables the mental health expert to depend on the patient's history, evaluation, and treatment; the reports of others about the patient's behavior; or social science data relevant to the case. Such testimony will not be prevented because of the rules of evidence.[6]

The expert is cross examined and may be required to reveal the underlying facts or data on which the opinions or inferences were based.[7] Opposing counsel may attempt to impeach the expert's credibility by questioning the expert about research findings or treatises that the expert admits are authoritative and inconsistent with the testimony. In addition, an expert may be subjected to cross-examination techniques used against nonexpert witnesses, such as proof of prior inconsistent statements[8] or of introducing facts that display the expert's bias in the outcome of the hearing. On redirect examination, counsel will ask questions of the expert that will clarify any conflicts in the testimony.

(C) Experts Protected

If a lawyer retains the services of an expert to consult about aspects of a particular case, such a consultation can be protected from discovery or trial.[9] In addition, the lawyer that employed the expert is liable for the fees of the expert absent an express agreement to the contrary.[10]

---

5. Wash. R. Evid., 703.
6. For example, the hearsay rule. Kennedy v. Monroe, 15 Wash.App. 39, 547 P.2d 899 (1976); Department of Fisheries v. Gillette, 27 Wash.App. 815, 621 P.2d 764 (1980).
7. Wash. R. Evid., 705.
8. Young v. Group Health, 85 Wash.2d 332, 534 P.2d 1349 (1975).
9. Crenna v. Ford Motor Co., 12 Wash.App. 824, 532 P.2d 290 (1975).
10. Copp v. Breskin, 56 Wash.App. 229 (1989).

An expert witness is also immune from lawsuit based on the acts and communications that occurred as a result of preparing for testimony and providing testimony even if compensated by one party[11] rather than appointed by the court.[12]

---

11. Bruce v. Bryne-Stevens & Associates Engineers, Inc., 113 Wash.2d 123, 776 P.2d 666 (1989).
12. Bader v. State, 43 Wash.App. 223, 716 P.2d 925 (1986).

5C.3

Polygraph Examinations and Polygraph Evidence

The state of Washington does not regulate or certify polygraphs, license polygraph operators, or provide standards for training polygraph operators. Results of polygraph examinations are not admissible at trial absent an agreement from both parties,[1] nor may evidence be entered at trial indicating that a party refused to submit to a polygraph examination.[2] If both parties stipulate that the polygraph results are admissible, and if procedural safeguards in conducting the examination and admitting the results as evidence are met, the court will enforce the stipulation and admit the results of the polygraph examination.[3] MHPs may incorporate polygraph results into their evaluations for courtroom testimony under these circumstances.[4]

(A) Submission to Polygraph Examination as Condition of Employment

It is unlawful for any public or private agency in the state of Washington to require any employee or prospective employee to take any polygraph or similar test as a condition of employment

---

1. State v. Grisby, 97 Wash.2d 493, 647 P.2d 6 (1982), *cert. denied*, 459 U.S. 1211 (1982); State v. Young, 89 Wash.2d 613, 574 P.2d 1171, *cert. denied*, 439 U.S. 870 (1978).
2. Industrial Indem. Co. v. Kallevig, 114 Wash.2d 907, 792 P.2d 520 (1990).
3. State v. Renfro, 96 Wash.2d 902, 639 P.2d 737, *cert. denied*, 459 U.S. 842 (1982).
4. *See* chapter 5D.25, Services for Sex Offenders; in using polygraph results, MHPs must adhere to specific standards; WAC 246-930-310(7) and (8).

or continued employment. Such a test may be used only for persons making initial application to law enforcement agencies, for persons who may be engaging in the manufacturing or distribution of controlled substances as defined in Chapter 69.50 RCW, or for persons directly involved in national security.[5]

Any person compelling another to submit to such an examination may be guilty of committing a misdemeanor (a criminal offense).[6] In a civil action alleging violation of this law, the court may award to the prevailing employee or prospective employee a penalty for $500 in addition to any award of actual damages and reasonable attorneys' fees and costs.[7]

---

5. RCW 49.44.120.
6. RCW 49.44.130.
7. RCW 49.44.135.

Competency to Testify

Every person of sound mind and discretion may be a witness in any action or proceeding.[1] A witness in a civil and criminal trial must have the mental capacity to testify accurately and reliably. Whenever reasonable doubt exists as to the competency of the witness, opposing counsel or the court should raise the issue. MHPs may assess and testify as to the competency of a witness to testify.

(A) Legal Test of Competency to Testify

The following persons shall not be competent to testify at the time of the legal proceeding:[2] if of unsound mind when they are to testify, or if they appear incapable of conveying their impressions about the facts or of relating them truly during their testimony.

(B) Determination of Witness Competency

Whether a witness is competent to testify is the trial judge's decision. It will not be overturned on appeal, except for a manifest

---

1. RCW 5.60.020.
2. RCW 5.56.050.

abuse of such discretion.[3] Counsel may produce evidence to show mental infirmity, or an expert witness may be called to testify as to the witness' competency.[4]

For persons of unsound mind, the burden of proof remains with the party attempting to prove a witness' incompetency. If a person has been adjudicated to be mentally ill, a presumption of incompetency to testify arises, but it is rebuttable.[5] Prior drug and alcohol use will not necessarily affect the finding of a witness' competency.[6]

Only children, no matter what their age,[7] who are incapable of perceiving or truthfully relating the facts of the case are considered to be incompetent.[8] The judge will decide if a child is

---

3. Competency is a precondition to admitting testimony of a witness about statements and recollections. State v. Ridley, 61 Wash.2d 457, 378 P.2d 700 (1963); State v. Ryan, 103 Wash.2d 165, 691 P.2d 197 (1984). However, someone who is incompetent to testify does not prevent the use of excited utterances made by the person. State v. Bouchard, 31 Wash.App 381, 639 P.2d 761 (1982).

4. Once the judge determines that the witness is competent, the jury must determine the extent to which the witness has the required capacities to observe, recollect, and communicate truthfully. If, on cross examination, an attempt is made to show that the witness had little recollection of the events because of an emotional condition, an expert witness may testify about the effect of the emotional condition on the testimony of the witness. State v. Froehlich, 96 Wash.2d 301, 635 P.2d 127 (1981). A defendant is not entitled to a state-appointed expert to examine the competency of a witness before a competency hearing, unless the alleged mental condition of the witness might prevent her from understanding the nature of the oath to tell the truth or give a correct account of what she had heard or seen: State v. Mines, 35 Wash.App. 932, 671 P.2d 273 (1983). An attack on the credibility of a witness in a case involving a crime against a child, however slight, may justify corroborating expert witness evidence, especially if the defendant denies the acts charged and the child asserts their commission. State v. Petrich, 101 Wash.2d 566, 683 P.2d 173 (1984).

5. Although a 38-year-old witness with a mental age of four years was severely retarded, the court did not abuse its discretion in allowing the testimony because the witness understood the obligation to tell the truth and was able to report basic facts about the incident. State v. Smith, 97 Wash.2d 801, 650 P.2d 201 (1982).

6. The court did not abuse its discretion by refusing to order a psychiatric examination to decide whether prior drug use affected the witness' competency. State v. Wood, 57 Wash.App. 792, 790 P.2d 220, review denied, 115 Wash.2d 1015, 797 P.2d 514 (1990). It was left to the jury to decide whether a witness was too drunk to remember events on the night of the crime. State v. Robinson, 35 Wash.App. 932, 671 P.2d 273 (1983).

7. State v. Ridley, 62 Wash.2d 457, 378 P.2d 700 (1963).

8. State v. Ryan, 103 Wash.2d 165, 691 P.2d 197 (1984). To decide whether a young child is competent as a witness, the child must understand the obligation to speak the truth as a witness and have possessed sufficient mental capacity at the time of the occurrence to receive an accurate impression, to retain an independent recollection, to express the memory in his or her words, and to understand simple questions. State v. Johnson, 28 Wash.App 459, 624 P.2d 213, affirmed, 96 Wash.2d 929, 639 P.2d 1332 (1981); State v. Smith, 30 Wash.App 251, 633 P.2d 137, affirmed, 97 Wash.2d 801, 650 P.2d 201 (1981).

competent to testify by observing whether the child's demeanor and manner of the answers are sufficient to permit the court to infer that, at the time of the occurrence about which the child is testifying, the child had the mental capacity to receive an accurate impression of those occurrences.[9]

---

9. The child's testimony that she knew who her school teachers were and what her performance had been in school justified the judge's deciding that she had sufficient memory to permit her to retain independent recollection of occurrences leading to the events described in the criminal prosecution. State v. Sardina, 42 Wash.App. 533, 713 P.2d 122 (1986). Inconsistencies in the testimony of a six-year-old child were left to the jury to assess her credibility. State v. Woodward, 32 Wash.App. 204, 646 P.2d 135 (1982).

5C.5

Psychological Autopsy

The motivations and mental state of a person before death are frequently issues in subsequent litigation. For instance, whether a gift was made by the person "in contemplation of death" can cause significant tax consequences.[1] Similarly, a finding that a person committed suicide rather than died accidentally may settle whether insurance benefits will be paid.[2] Expert witness opinions about such issues are referred to as coming from a "psychological autopsy." Opinions formed by an mental health expert about a dead person whom the expert never interviewed in person, but rather formed an opinion about from other peoples' reports or clinical records, may not be viewed as very compelling evidence if allowed at all. In cases involving testamentary capacity (see chapter 5B.7), such experts who provided testimony based upon a review of the clinical records and hypothetical questions posed during trial were found to have presented "the weakest and most unsatisfactory evidence."[3]

---

1. *See* Shaffer, The Psychological Autopsy in Judicial Opinions Under Section 2035, 3 *Loy.L.A.Rev.*, 1 (1970).
2. *See* Curphey, The psychological autopsy: The role of the forensic pathologist in the multi-disciplinary approach to death, 39 *Bull. Suicidology* (1968).
3. In re Estate of Reilly, 78 Wash.2d 623 (1970); In re Estate of Bottger, 14 Wash.2d 676, 129 P.2d 518 (1942); In re Miller's Estate, 10 Wash.2d 258, 116 P.2d 526 (1941).

Criminal Matters

5D.1

Screening of Police Officers

The legislature has created a Criminal Justice Training Commission to provide programs and standards for the training of county, city, state, and port criminal justice personnel within the state of Washington.[1] Other states have mandated that MHPs play a role in assessing the mental fitness of personnel as one of the minimum qualifications of recruitment or appointment for criminal justice positions. Washington's commission has established no such qualifications. Presumably, the screening of emotional instability, or alcoholism, or drug addiction occurs among aspiring criminal justice personnel, although it is unregulated.

---

1. RCW 43.101.020-020.

5D.2

Competency to Waive the Rights to Silence, Counsel, and a Jury

Persons taken into custody by police officers for a criminal offense may waive the rights to silence and to counsel that are guaranteed by the constitutions of the United States and of the state of Washington.[1] Criminal defendants may waive these rights and the rights to a jury trial during their prosecution. MHPs may be asked to examine criminal defendants and testify about whether they are competent to waive these rights during the investigation and arrest or at the trial.

(A) Right to Silence

Once an individual who is taken into custody by a police officer indicates in any manner, either before or during questioning, that he or she wishes to remain silent, all questioning must cease.[2] The suspect may waive the "Miranda rights"[3] and provide any information requested by the police, including a confession. However, to establish the waiver of a Miranda right, the prosecution must demonstrate by a preponderance of the evidence that the waiver was a voluntary, knowing, and intelligent relinquish-

---

1. U.S. Constitution, fifth and sixth amendments; Constitution of the state of Washington, Art.1 [4,06] 22.
2. State v. Wheeler, 43 Wash.App. 191, 716 P.2d 902 (1986) citing Miranda v. Arizona, 384 U.S. 436 (1966).
3. Before questioning, the police officers must state to the suspect that she or he has the right to remain silent, the right to counsel (as well as the appointment of counsel if the person is indigent), and that any statements made, may be used at trial. These rights are referred to as the Miranda rights. *See* Miranda v. Arizona, 384 U.S. 436 (1966).

ment.[4] When a statement by an accused is to be offered into evidence at a criminal trial, the judge will consider the following factors in determining the validity of waiving a previously asserted right to remain silent:[5] was the right to cut off questioning scrupulously honored; did the police engage in further words or actions amounting to interrogation before obtaining a valid waiver; did the police engage in tactics that tended to coerce the suspect to change his mind; and was the subsequent waiver given knowingly and voluntarily.

MHPs may be called upon to testify about whether the defendant possessed sufficient "sensibility and cognition" at the time to be aware that the right existed.[6] If a defendant is found to lack the capacity to stand trial, this does not necessarily indicate that the defendant lacked the capacity to waive his right to be silent at the time of the admission;[7] nor does a defendant's mental retardation[8] or mental illness[9] preclude the court finding that a valid waiver occurred. The court will hear testimony about the entire situation surrounding the statement or admission.

In one case, the following combination of factors led the court to find that statements had been made involuntarily:[10] the defendant made a statement while incompetent to stand trial and his mental illness had resulted in his being hospitalized; he experienced adverse reactions to the medications that he was taking; he attempted to plea bargain while waiving his rights without assistance of his attorney; and he was not provided with a narrative summary of facts about the crime (the leading questions of the officer had obtained "Yes" or "No" statements).

(B) Right to Counsel

A defendant is entitled to be represented by a lawyer in any criminal prosecution in which a judgment of guilty could result in imprisonment. This right attaches as soon as possible after the defendant is taken into custody. The lawyer not only represents the defendant at all the legal proceedings, but also acts as an advocate during further direct questioning by the police; when the right to counsel is invoked, questioning of the defendant that

---

4. State v. Kaiser, 34 Wash.App. 559, 663 P.2d 839 (1983).
5. State v. Wheeler, 43 Wash.App. 191, 716 P.2d 902 (1986).
6. State v. McDonald, 89 Wash.2d 256, 571 P.2d 930 (1977).
7. Id.
8. State v. Ortiz, 104 Wash.2d 479, 706 P.2d 1069 (1985).
9. State v. Ratow, 4 Wash.App. 321, 481 P.2d 20 (1971); State v. Anderson, 94 Wash.2d 176, 616 P.2d 612 (1980).
10. State v. Sergeant, 27 Wash.App. 947, 621 P.2d 209 (1980).

occurs without the presence of defense counsel will likely be found to have violated the right.[11]

To decide whether the defendant is competent to waive the right to counsel, the court must find that the person attempting to waive the right did so while understanding[12] the nature of the charges, the statutory offense included within them, the range of allowable punishments, possible defenses to the circumstances in mitigation, and all other facts essential to a broad understanding of the entire matter. The latter include facts about the background, experience, and conduct of the defendant as well as the awareness of the dangers and disadvantages of being tried without counsel.[13] If the defendant is incompetent to stand trial (see chapter 5D.5, Competency to Stand Trial), the court would not find that a waiver of the right to counsel was made knowingly and intelligently.[14]

11. *Id.*
12. RCW 10.77.020.
13. State v. Hahn, 106 Wash.2d 805, 726 P.2d 25 (1986).
14. State v. Sergeant, 27 Wash.App. 947, 621 P.2d 209 (1980).

5D.3

Precharging and Pretrial Evaluations

In some states, the prosecutor in a criminal case may request a mental health evaluation before determining whether to charge a person or to divert the person to the mental health or other social services system. The Washington legislature has established recommended prosecuting standards for charging and plea dispositions.[1] A prosecuting attorney has the discretion not to prosecute, although technically sufficient evidence to prosecute exists.[2] Presumably, a prosecutor may depend upon a mental health evaluation in determining whether to charge a person with a crime.

---

1. Sentencing Reform Act of 1981; RCW 9.94A.430 to .450.
2. RCW 9.94A.440.

5D.4

Bail Determinations

At the preliminary appearance for a criminal offense, the court may release the accused on personal recognizance or may impose the least restrictive set of conditions, including bail.[1] Detention of the accused pending trial may affect materially the ability to help in the preparation of a defense. The court must balance the defendant's rights to be treated as innocent until proven guilty and to a fair, impartial trial with the competing concerns of assuring the appearance of the accused at trial and preventing a new violent crime from being committed or witnesses being intimidated.[2] MHPs may contribute to a pretrial release determination by evaluating the accused and providing to the court an opinion about the person's mental health and dangerousness in an affidavit or under examination.

(A) Determining What Type of Release Is Appropriate

Unless grounds for continued detention exist, an accused must be released from detention within 24 hours after a preliminary appearance.[3] The court will impose conditions upon the accused before release, if the court finds that[4] personal recognizance will not reasonably assure the appearance of the accused in court; a

---

1. Criminal Court Rule 3.2(a). Bail is used to assure that the accused will appear at later hearings.
2. *Id.*; State v. Trickel, 16 Wash.App. 18, 553 P.2d 139 (1976).
3. Criminal Court Rule 3.2(d)(3).
4. Criminal Court Rule 3.2(a).

likely danger exists that the accused will commit a violent crime; or the accused may intimidate witnesses. In deciding the conditions of release, the court may consider any relevant information about the accused, not limited to the following:[5]

1. length and character of residence in the community;
2. employment status, history, and financial condition;
3. family ties and relationships;
4. reputation, character, and mental condition;
5. history of response to legal process;
6. criminal record;[6]
7. willingness of responsible members of the community to vouch for the reliability of the accused and assist the accused in complying with conditions of release;
8. nature of the charge;
9. any other factors indicating the ties of the accused to the community;
10. past record of threats to victims or witnesses or interference with witnesses in the administration of justice;
11. present threats or intimidation directed to witnesses;
12. record of committing offenses while on pretrial release, probation, or parole; and
13. record of use of or threatened use of deadly weapons or firearms, especially to victims or witnesses.

The court may impose the least restrictive of the following conditions, combination of conditions, or any other condition that is necessary to prevent the accused from committing a violent crime, intimidating witnesses, or interfering with the administration of justice:[7]

1. place the accused in custody and supervision of a designated person or organization;
2. impose restrictions on travel, association, or place of abode;
3. require the execution of an unsecured bond in a specified amount;
4. require the execution of a bond in a specified amount along with cash or other security not to exceed 10% of the bond amount;

---

5. Criminal Court Rule 3.2(b).
6. State v. James, 70 Wash.2d 624 (1967).
7. Criminal Court Rule 3.2(a).

5. require the execution of a bond along with sufficient solvent sureties backing the bond; or

6. require the accused to return to custody during specified hours.

Upon a showing that a substantial danger of the above exists, the court may impose one or more of the following restrictive conditions to prohibit the accused from[8]

1. approaching or communicating in any manner with particular persons or classes of persons;

2. going to certain geographical areas or premises;

3. possessing any dangerous weapons or firearms, engaging in certain high risk activities, or consuming any intoxicating liquors and drugs not prescribed;

4. disappearing by having to report regularly to and remain under the supervision of an officer of the court or other person or agency;

5. committing any violations of criminal law; or

6. violating the conditions of release by posting a secured or unsecured bond, conditioned on compliance with all conditions of release.[9]

The conditions of release may be modified at any time, under the inherent discretionary power of the court to control its own proceedings.[10] However, if conditions are modified during the trial, the court must do so without the jury being able to construe the court's action as a comment about the evidence at trial.[11] Due process of law also requires an opportunity for the accused to be heard before the conditions are adjusted.[12] The conditions of release, including a bail obligation, are discharged when the accused is found not guilty or found guilty, sentenced, and committed to the custody of law enforcement personnel.[13]

---

8. Criminal Court Rule 3.2(c).
9. This is to be imposed only if no other condition(s) would assure the safety of the community or the appearance of the accused in court.
10. State v. Trickel, 16 Wash.App. 18, 553 P.2d 139 (1976).
11. *Id.*
12. State v. Holland, 7 Wash.App. 676, 501 P.2d 1243 (1972).
13. State v. Ransom, 34 Wash.App. 819, 664 P.2d 521 (1983).

5D.5

Competency to Stand Trial

No incompetent person may be tried, convicted, or sentenced for the commission of a crime.[1] The defendant must understand the nature of the proceedings against him and be able to help in the defense. This fundamental right, originating in the common law, (case law) is guaranteed under the U.S. Constitution.[2] Whenever a reasonable doubt exists as to the defendant's competency, at least two qualified mental health experts, one of whom must be approved by the prosecuting attorney, must examine and report upon the mental condition of the defendant.[3]

(A) Legal Determination of Competency

(A)(1) Test of Competency

In addition to finding that a person is suffering from a mental illness or defect, the court must decide whether the accused lacks the capacity to understand the nature of the proceedings and to assist legal counsel rationally in the defense.[4]

The courts are cautious about possible defendant malingering. Even someone who has sustained a permanent cognitive deficit still may be found to understand his position and be able to

---

1. RCW 10.77.050.
2. Drope v Missouri, 420 U.S. 162 (1975); State v. O'Neal, 23 Wash.App. 899, 600 P.2d 570 (1979).
3. RCW 10.77.060(1); State v. Israel, 19 Wash.App. 773, 577 P.2d 631 (1978); State v. Wicklund, 96 Wash.2d 798, 638 P.2d 1241 (1982).
4. RCW 10.77.010(6); State v. Wicklund, 96 Wash.2d 798, 638 P.2d 1241 (1982).

assist counsel.[5] In addition, a defendant can be "insane" at the time of the offense yet competent to stand trial and vice versa (see chapter 5D.9).[6] For example, a person may be suffering from schizophrenia yet still be competent to stand trial.[7] In another example, retrograde amnesia, caused by a closed head injury from an automobile accident in which the defendant was charged for negligent homicide, was insufficient to render the defendant unable to comprehend his position or to assist counsel.[8] In other cases of memory loss,[9] a failure of memory will not necessarily result in a finding of incompetency. This is particularly true if the defendant can reconstruct the offense through other means.[10]

If the mental illness is treatable, a defendant may be found competent even though the person would be incompetent if taken off medications. Because the medication enables the defendant to understand the proceedings and assist in the defense, he or she will be found competent.[11]

(A)(2) Raising the Competency Issue

A concern about the defendant's competency may be raised at any time during the action and before judgment. The issue of whether a defendant is competent to stand trial is raised usually by the defense attorney after difficulties in communication have occurred. Additional concerns tend to arise after instances of irrational behavior on the part of the defendant, because of his or her demeanor, or because of the opinion of an MHP about the defendant's competence.[12] The prosecutor also has a duty, and the court has the inherent power to ensure that an incompetent defendant is examined.[13]

The decision about whether to commit the defendant for examination is left to the discretion of the court.[14] When the court has a reasonable doubt regarding the defendant's competency, it then has a duty to order a competency examination.[15] If the

---

5. State v. Ortiz, 104 Wash.2d 479, 706 P.2d 1069 (1985). The defendant was mildly retarded and had difficulty remembering past events.
6. State v. Jones., 84 Wash.2d 823, 529 P.2d 1040 (1974).
7. State v. Hahn, 106 Wash.2d 885, 726 P.2d 25 (1986).
8. State v. Swanson, 28 Wash.App.759, 626 P.2d 527 (1981).
9. Id.; for example in cases in which the defendant was either intoxicated, drugged, in a state of panic, or suffered from psychopathic delinquency.
10. Id.; Robinson v. Rhay, 4 Wash.App. 1, 479 P.2d 109 (1971).
11. RCW 10.77.090(5); U.S. v. Hayes, 509 F.2d 811 (5th Cir. 1979) cert. denied, 444 U.S. 847. A defendant could refuse to take medications (see chapter 6.2, Right to Refuse Treatment).
12. State v. O'Neal, 23 Wash.App.899, 600 P.2d 570 (1979).
13. RCW 10.77.060; State ex rel. MacKintosh v. Superior Court, 45 Wash. 248, 88 P. 207 (1907); State v. Tate, 74 Wash.2d 261, 444 P.2d 150 (1968); State v. Israel, 19 Wash.App. 773, 577 P.2d 631 (1978).
14. State v. Wicklund, 96 Wash.2d 798, 638 P.2d 1241 (1982).
15. State v. O'Neal, 23 Wash.App. 899, 600 P.2d 570 (1979).

defense elects to determine competency by a manner other than that specified by the statutes, this action forms a waiver of the specific statutory procedure.[16]

(A)(3) Competency Evaluation

If the court learns that reasonable grounds for an examination exist, it must appoint or request the secretary of DSHS to designate at least two experts. One of the experts shall be approved by the prosecuting attorney, and both will examine and report about the mental condition of the defendant.[17] Presumably, any licensed or certified MHP, who has developed an expertise at evaluating competency, could perform the examination.

The court may commit the defendant to a suitable facility to be examined, but for no longer than 15 days.[18] The defendant has the right to be assessed by an expert of his or her choice, and if indigent, the court must appoint the expert upon the defendant's request.[19] This retained or appointed expert may be present at the examination performed by the two other experts. Also, the expert is allowed reasonable access to the defendant and is provided full access to all information obtained during the other evaluations.[20] The experts file a report concerning their evaluations that must include the following information:[21]

1. a description of the nature of the examination;
2. a diagnosis of the mental condition of the defendant;
3. an opinion as to competence, if the defendant suffers from a mental disease or defect;
4. an opinion as to the defendant's sanity at the time of the act if the defendant has shown an intention to rely on the defense of insanity (see chapter 5D.9, Criminal Responsibility);
5. when directed by the court, an opinion as to the capacity of the defendant to have a particular state of mind that is an element of the offense charged (see chapter 5D.7, Mens Rea);
6. an opinion about whether the defendant is a substantial danger to other persons or presents a substantial likelihood of committing felonious acts that would jeopardize the public safety (see chapter 5D.4, Bail Determinations).

---

16. *Id.*; State v. Brooks, 16 Wash.App. 535, 557 P.2d 362 (1976). During the trial, the defendant refused to appear, and defense counsel requested that he appoint two experts; the prosecution did not object, and the court approved the request. The experts found the defendant competent.
17. RCW 10.77.060(1).
18. *Id.*
19. RCW 10.77.060(2).
20. *Id.*; RCW 10.77.070.
21. *Id.*

(B) Confidentiality and Privileged Communications

Anything said or done by the defendants during an evaluation as to their sanity at the time of their criminal acts is relevant to their mental conditions and is admissible.[22] Because the same experts tend to evaluate competency and sanity during one examination, all the information obtained would be admissible, and they could be called as witnesses.[23]

(C) Disposition of Those Incompetent to Stand Trial

If at anytime, a defendant is found to be incompetent, the court must order the proceedings to be stayed.[24] The court may commit a defendant charged with a felony for evaluation and treatment until competency is regained, but in any event, for no longer than 90 days.[25]

After the first 90-day period lapses, if the court finds by a preponderance of the evidence that the defendant remains incompetent, the court may extend the order of commitment or alternate treatment for an additional 90 days.[26] The court must establish a date for a prompt hearing to decide on the defendant's competency before the end of the second 90-day period; at that point, any party may demand a jury trial.

If the defendant remains incompetent upon the expiration of the second 90-day period, the charges must be dismissed without prejudice, and either civil commitment proceedings must be begun or the court will release the defendant.[27] However, criminal charges must not be dismissed if the defendant is found to be a danger to others or presents a likelihood of committing other felonious acts, and a substantial probability exists that the defendant will regain competency within a reasonable period. In this event, one last six-month period may be used to return the defen-

---

22. State v. Huson, 73 Wash.2d 660, 440 P.2d 192 (1968), *cert. denied*, 393 U.S. 1096 (1969); State v. Bonds, 98 Wash.2d 1, 653 P.2d 1024 (1982).
23. RCW 10.77.100.
24. RCW 10.77.090(1).
25. *Id.* For other crimes, the court may stay or dismiss the proceedings. The defendant may be detained for sufficient time to allow the county MHP to commence proceedings under Chapter 71.05 RCW, if appropriate (*see* chapter 5E.4, Involuntary Civil Commitment of Mentally Ill Adults).
26. RCW 10.77.090(1).
27. RCW 10.77.090(3).

dant to a competent state.[28] If the defendant remains incompetent, the charges must be dismissed without prejudice, and either civil commitment proceedings must be begun or the court will release the defendant.

---

28. *Id.*

5D.6

Provocation

In some jurisdictions, the law recognizes a mitigating factor of *adequate provocation* as a partial defense to a charge involving a homicide or an assault. Generally, adequate provocation is construed to mean conduct or circumstances sufficient to deprive a reasonable person of self-control. Washington does not recognize the defense of provocation. However, it does recognize self-defense as a complete defense to a charge involving a homicide or an assault. The state has the burden to prove beyond a reasonable doubt the absence of self-defense once it is raised as a defense.[1]

MHPs may be called to testify at a trial in which the issue of self-defense is raised. For instance, if the state's chief witness is the victim of the alleged crime and the mental disability of the witness is apparent, the disability may affect his or her credibility. If this witness is suffering from a mental disorder and its existence is established, an expert witness may testify about the consequences of the disorder.[2]

In addition, the legitimacy of the defendant's self-defense may be evaluated in light of all the facts and circumstances known at the time of the conduct.[3] For examples of how providers would testify for a defendant who raised such a defense, see chapter 5D.10, Battered Women Syndrome.

---

1. State v. Despenza, 38 Wash.App. 645, 689 P.2d 87 (1984).
2. *Id*. State v. Froehlich, 96 Wash.2d 301, 635 P.2d 127 (1981).
3. State v. Allery, 101 Wash.2d 591, 682 P.2d 312 (1984). Such testimony about comments or acts observed by witness before the killing or assault may help to establish the victim's state of mind as it related both to the issue of self-defense and to the defendant's premeditation. State v. Cameron, 100 Wash.2d 520, 674 P.2d 650 (1983).

5D.7

Mens Rea

The criminal code requires that each offense be performed with a "guilty mind," called *mens rea*. For particular offenses, a specific mental state is a necessary element to be proven by the prosecution at trial. Unless the element is proven to the fact-finder(s) beyond a reasonable doubt, the defendant will not be convicted of the offense. MHPs may testify about whether a defendant's mental disorder prevents the formation of a particular mental state at the time of the crime. This evidence may negate the prosecution's proof about a particular mental state or mitigate the grade of the offense by showing that only a less culpable mental state was possible.[1]

(A) Culpable Mental States

Most criminal offenses require either intentional or knowing conduct. Four hierarchical types of culpable mental states are delineated by the Code:[2]

1. *intentionally* or *with the intent to* means that a person acts with the objective or purpose of achieving a result that constitutes a crime;

2. *knowingly* or *with knowledge* means that either a person is aware of a fact, facts, circumstances, or a result described by a statute defining an offense, or the person has information that would

---

1. State v. Edmon, 28 Wash. App. 98, 621 P.2d 1310 (1981). This case specifies the foundational requirements needed before an expert may give an opinion about the defendant's ability to form a mental state.
2. RCW 9A.08.010.

lead a reasonable person in the same situation to believe that the specified facts exist (the facts are described by a statute defining an offense);

3. *recklessly* means that a person knows of and disregards a substantial risk that a wrongful act may occur and that the disregard of such a substantial risk is a gross deviation from conduct that a reasonable person would exercise in the same situation;

4. *criminally negligent* or *with criminal negligence* means that a person fails to be aware of a substantial risk that a wrongful act may occur, and the failure to be aware of such substantial risk forms a gross deviation from the standard of care that a reasonable person would exercise in the same situation.

The law applied in the particular case will define what mental state must be proved.

In addition to these mental states, first-degree murder requires that intentional conduct occurred and that the conduct was premeditated.[3] Premeditation is the element that distinguishes first- from second-degree murder. It requires the mental process of thinking beforehand, with deliberation, reflection, weighing, or reasoning for a period of time, however short.[4]

---

3. RCW 9A.32.030(1)(a).
4. State v. Brooks, 97 Wash.2d 873, 651 P.2d 217 (1982). In this case, the court held that excessive consumption of alcohol is insufficient to negate the element of specific intent in a prosecution for first-degree murder, but that evidence is not precluded as bearing on the element of premeditation. Expert testimony may be relevant for determining whether the defendant was capable of premeditated conduct.

5D.8

Diminished Capacity

Washington recognizes the defense of *diminished capacity*. The effect of intoxication from substances (alcohol or drugs) or the presence of a mental condition is admissible evidence to prove the lack of a particular mental state.[1] If the defendant's capacity was diminished at the time of the crime, such evidence could lead to a finding of no guilt or of a reduction of the crime to a lesser offense. MHPs may qualify as experts and provide evidence as to a defendant's inability to form a particular mental state or specific intent.[2]

(A) Foundational Requirements

In a recent decision, the Court of Appeals clearly delineated the foundational requirements that must be satisfied before an expert may give an opinion about a defendant's diminished capacity:[3]

---

1. The defense may be raised whether or not insanity is pled. State v. Welsh, 8 Wash.App. 719, 508 P.2d 1041 (1973); State v. Ferrick, 81 Wash.2d 942, 506 P.2d 860 (1973). *See* chapter 5D.7, Mens Rea for a discussion of the various mental states that must be proven.
2. State v. Edmon, 28 Wash.App. 98, 621 P.2d 1310 (1981). Specific intent includes premeditation (*see* RCW 9A.08.010(1)(a) and State v. Carter, 5 Wash.App. 802, 490 P.2d 1346 (1971)) or knowledge (*see* RCW 9A.08.010(1)(b)).
3. Mental disorder of diminishing capacity was addressed in State v. Edmon, 28 Wash.App. 98, 621 P.2d 1310 (1981). As to intoxication, *see* State v. Zamora, 6 Wash.App. 130, 491 P.2d 1342 (1971); State v. Thompson, 17 Wash.App. 639, 564 P.2d 820 (1977); State v. King, 24 Wash.App. 495, 601 P.2d 982 (1979); State v. Simmons, 30 Wash.App. 432, 635 P.2d 745 (1981).

1. the defendant lacks the ability to form specific intent because of a mental disorder not amounting to insanity;
2. the expert is qualified to testify on the subject;
3. the expert personally examines and diagnoses the defendant and can testify to an opinion with reasonable certainty;
4. the expert's testimony is based on substantial supporting evidence in the record relating to the defendant's condition and cannot consist of uncertain estimates or of speculation;[4]
5. the cause of the inability to form a specific intent must be due to intoxication or to a mental disorder, not to emotions such as jealously, fear, anger, and hatred;
6. the intoxication or mental disorder must be causally connected to a lack of specific intent, not just to reduced perception, overreaction, or other irrelevant mental state;
7. the inability to form a specific intent must have occurred at the time of the offense;
8. the intoxication or mental disorder must substantially reduce the probability that the defendant formed the alleged intent; and
9. the expert opinion must contain an explanation of how the mental disorder or intoxication cause the lack of intent rather than a simple conclusion.

If the defendant's offer of proof satisfies these foundational requirements, the court must admit the expert's testimony as to the defendant's lack of capacity to form a specific intent.

The underlying purpose of promoting equal justice also has caused Washington courts to rule that a defendant is entitled to the services of an expert. This will occur if the subject matter on which the expert will testify constitutes a significant factor in the defense.[5] Therefore, an expert will be provided to indigent defendants so that testimony of diminished capacity can be conveyed.[6]

---

4. *Id.* The determination of whether substantial evidence exists is a question of law for the court to decide. In the case of intoxication, lay witnesses must be able to testify about nature and extent of the substance consumption and the time period involved during the consumption.
5. State v. Poulsen, 45 Wash.App. 706, 726 P.2d 1036 (1986).
6. *Id.*

(B) Effect of Diminished Capacity

Once evidence has been allowed at trial, a diminished capacity jury instruction must be given by the court at the end of the trial if a two-pronged test has been met:[7]

1. substantial evidence of such a condition was admitted into evidence during the trial; and

2. such evidence connected the defendant's alleged condition with the inability to possess the required level of specific intent or mental state required for the crime charged.

If this test is met, failure to give a diminished capacity instruction, if requested, will be viewed by a higher court as a prejudicial error.[8]

After hearing the instruction and reviewing the evidence, if a reasonable doubt is raised in the minds of the jury about whether the defendant possessed the required mental state while committing the act, the jury may find the defendant not guilty or guilty of a lesser offense.[9]

---

7. State v. Griffin, 100 Wash.2d 417, 670 P.2d 265 (1983). An example of such an instruction was cited in a case involving intoxication that allegedly led to diminished capacity: "No act committed by a person while in a state of voluntary intoxication is less criminal by reason of that condition, but whenever the actual existence of any particular mental state is a necessary element to constitute a particular kind of degree of crime, the fact of intoxication may be taken into consideration in determining such mental state." See State v. Mathews, 38 Wash.App. 180, 685 P.2d 605 (1984) and State v. Simmons, 30 Wash.App. 432, 635 P.2d 745 (1981) citing WPIC 18.10, 11 Wash. Prac. 122 (1977).

8. Id.

9. State v. Welsh, 8 Wash.App. 719, 508 P.2d 1041 (1973).

5D.9

Criminal Responsibility

MHPs may serve as evaluators of criminal defendants who plead not guilty because of insanity. They would provide evidence as to the defendant's mental state to the court. Such a verdict may be warranted if the perceptual and cognitive functioning of the defendant, at the time of the crime, caused a loss of contact with reality so complete that the person would not be influenced by the criminal law.[1]

(A) Legal Determination of Insanity[2]

As an affirmative defense, the defendant must establish by a preponderance of the evidence that, at the time of the commission of the offense, because of mental disease or defect, the mind of the actor was affected to such an extent that[3]

1. the defendant was unable to perceive the nature and quality of the act for which he or she is charged; or
2. the defendant was unable to tell right from wrong concerning the particular act.

An example of the first type of legal insanity is a person so psychotic that delusions have caused the person to view his

---

1. State v. White, 60 Wash.2d 551, 374 P.2d 942 (1962).
2. *Id.* Washington has followed the M'Naghten rule since a statute was enacted in 1907, although the legislature of 1909 attempted to abolish insanity as a defense. This later legislation was held unconstitutional as the court found that the minimum requirements of *mens rea* required such a defense. State v. Strasburg, 60 Wash. 106, 110 P. 1020 (1910).
3. RCW 9A.12.010.

mother-in-law as a "Scarlet Whore Beast" who wanted him to kill her.[4] This defendant was unable to know the nature and quality of his act because he viewed his mother-in-law as an evil spirit rather than as a person.

An example of the second type of legal insanity is a person so psychotic that her command hallucinations have caused her to believe that God has decreed that she should kill her infant child.[5] In this case, the command was specific and perceived as a righteous act preventing the defendant from knowing that the act was wrong.

Mental disease or defect must cause the perceptual or cognitive dysfunction of legal insanity. Voluntary alcohol and drug intoxication that results in a perceptual or cognitive dysfunction is not sufficient to warrant an insanity instruction;[6] nor is chronic addiction, by itself, sufficient.[7] If, however, alcohol or drug intoxication combines with a preexisting, underlying psychotic disorder, the resulting perceptual or cognitive symptoms may cause legal insanity.[8] It appears though that the severity of the underlying psychotic disorder must be such that, by itself, it would be responsible for the legal insanity; otherwise, the insanity will be viewed as voluntarily caused by alcohol and drugs.[9] Alcohol and drug use may mitigate the sentence (see chapter 5D.15, Sentencing).

(B) Statutory Framework and Burden of Proof

The defense can be raised by the defendant. When the insanity defense is raised, the trier of fact must decide whether[10]

1. the state has proven beyond a reasonable doubt that the defendant committed the felonious act;

2. the defendant has shown by a preponderance of the evidence that insanity existed at the time of the act charged;

---

4. State v. Cameron, 100 Wash.2d 520, 674 P.2d 650 (1983).
5. State v. Crenshaw, 98 Wash.2d 789, 659 P.2d 488 (1983) citing People v. Schmidt, 216 N.Y. 324, 110 N.E. 945 (1915).
6. RCW 10.77.010(7); State v. Wicks, 98 Wash.2d 620, 657 P.2d 781 (1983); State v. Bower, 73 Wash. 2d 634, 440 P.2d 167 (1968).
7. Seattle v. Hill, 72 Wash.2d 786, 435 P.2d 692 (1967), *cert. denied*, 393 U.S. 872 (1968).
8. State v. Wicks, 98 Wash.2d 620, 657 P.2d 781 (1983).
9. *Id.*
10. Hickey v. Morris, 722 Wash.2d 543 (1983) citing RCW 10.77.030(2), .040, and .110.

3. the state has shown by a preponderance of the evidence that the defendant is a substantial danger to other persons unless kept under further control;

4. the state has shown by a preponderance of the evidence that the defendant presents a substantial likelihood of committing felonious acts and of jeopardizing public safety or security unless kept under further control; and

5. the state has shown by a preponderance of the evidence that the best interests of the defendant and others require that the defendant be detained in a state mental hospital instead of a less restrictive treatment.

If a reasonable doubt exists as to the defendant's legal insanity at the time of the crime, the court or any party may file a motion for experts to examine and report on the mental condition of the defendant.[11]

(C) Mental Examination

Once a motion for an examination is made, the court must either appoint or request that the DSHS appoint two experts, one of whom must be approved by the prosecuting attorney.[12] This would include any licensed or certified professional who could be qualified as an expert. The expert must have acquired sufficient experience for evaluating and treating people suffering from mental illness.[13]

In addition, the defendant may retain experts who would witness the examination and gain full access to all information obtained by the court-appointed experts.[14] Reasonable access is permitted for the experts to conduct an examination.[15] If the defendant is indigent, upon request, the court must assist in obtaining an expert, which includes paying for the services.[16]

---

11. RCW 10.77.060(1).
12. RCW 10.77.060(1).
13. Qualification as a clinical psychologist or psychiatrist is unnecessary. Practical experience in performing forensic evaluations can be sufficient to qualify a witness as an expert. Whether a witness possesses the skill and knowledge necessary to qualify as an expert is at the discretion of the court. State v. Smith, 88 Wash.2d 639, 564 P.2d 1154 (1977) citing State v. J-R Distribs., Inc., 82 Wash.2d 584, 512 P.2d 1049 (1973), *cert. denied*, 418 U.S. 949 (1974) and State v. Jacobsen, 78 Wash.2d 491, 477 P.2d 1 (1970); *see* chapter 5C.2, Expert Witnesses.
14. RCW 10.77.060(2).
15. RCW 10.77.070.
16. RCW 10.77.060(2); Criminal Rules of Procedure 3.2(f).

All experts have a right to file a report; the report must include the following:[17]

1. a description of the nature of the examination;
2. a diagnosis of the mental condition of the defendant;
3. a finding about whether the defendant suffers from mental disease or defect, and an opinion as to his or her competency;
4. an opinion as to the defendant's sanity at the time of the act if the defendant has indicated an intention to rely on the defense of insanity;
5. when directed by the court, an opinion as to the capacity of the defendant to have a particular state of mind that is an element of the offense with which charged; and
6. an opinion about whether the defendant is a substantial danger to other persons or presents a substantial likelihood of committing felonious acts jeopardizing public safety, unless kept under greater control.

The examination can be conducted on an outpatient basis. However, the court may order the defendant committed to a suitable facility for a sufficient amount of time to complete the examination, not to exceed 15 days.[18] It is possible that the defendant may continue to be hospitalized for a longer period of time if, during the examination, the defendant appears incompetent to stand trial.[19]

(D) Confidentiality and Privileged Communications

Statements made by a defendant to the court's experts or to the defense's expert are not confidential or privileged if the defendant has raised the insanity defense.[20] As a result, the prosecution may see all the information raised in the defense expert's examination. This is believed to prevent an abuse of process by the defendant because[21] the defense expert generally examines the defendant much earlier than the other experts, and access to the defendant's recollections is clearer with less opportunity for the defendant's

---

17. RCW 10.77.060(3).
18. RCW 10.77.060(1).
19. RCW 10.77.090; see chapter 5D.5, Competency to Stand Trial.
20. State v. Bonds, 98 Wash.2d 1, 653 P.2d 1024 (1982).
21. State v. Bonds, 98 Wash.2d 1, 653 P.2d 1024 (1982); State v. Johnson, 69 Wash.2d 264, 418 P.2d 238 (1966); State v. Huson, 73 Wash.2d 660, 440 P.2d 192 (1968), cert. denied, 393 U.S. 1096 (1969).

mental condition to change; the defendant, having undergone one examination, may attempt to tailor later responses to strengthen the defense at subsequent examinations; and the defendant is likely to provide a more accurate impression of the mental condition to the expert retained by defense counsel.

(E) Disposition of Defendants Found Not Guilty by Reason of Insanity

(E)(1) Acquitted of a Felony

The court must order hospitalization, or a less restrictive alternate treatment, if the defendant is acquitted because of being legally insane but remains a substantial danger to other persons or presents a substantial likelihood of committing felonious acts.[22] The defendant may not contest being detained because of claiming that he or she did not commit the acts with which charged.[23]

If the defendant is neither a danger to others nor likely to commit further felonious acts, the court may direct a conditional release for a defendant who requires monitoring.[24] If monitoring is not required, the court can direct a final discharge.[25]

(E)(2) Confinement or Conditional Release

Confinement to the hospital or a period of conditional release may extend to the maximum term of imprisonment allowed for the crime at the time of the acquittal.[26] Each person hospitalized or conditionally released must be examined by one or more experts at least every six months to decide whether an existing mental condition warrants granting a discharge.[27]

If a petition for final discharge is filed by application of the secretary of the DSHS or if a petition for final discharge or conditional release is filed by the petitioner independently, no subsequent petition filed by the petitioner can be considered by the court until one year has lapsed since the last determination.[28] The petitioner must prove fitness by the preponderance of the evidence with the court approving the discharge, even if the hospital decides that the petitioner is fit.[29]

---

22. RCW 10.77.110.
23. RCW 10.77.080.
24. *Id.*
25. *Id.*
26. In re Kolocotronis, 99 Wash.2d 147, 660 P.2d 731 (1983).
27. RCW 10.77.140.
28. RCW 10.77.200; State v. Kolocotronis, 34 Wash.App. 613, 663 P.2d 1360 (1983).
29. *Id.*

Experts will evaluate the defendant's readiness to be conditionally released and the conditions that would protect the public.[30] After considering the reports of the experts, the secretary will forward recommendations to the court.

Any reasonable conditions can be imposed upon the person acquitted of insanity. If the conditions are violated, any professional responsible for monitoring that person, the secretary, the prosecuting attorney, or the court may move to modify the terms of the conditional release.[31] The person may be taken into custody until the modification hearing is held if the defendant is likely to commit a felony that would endanger the safety or security of others.[32]

Both the prosecuting attorney and the defendant have a right to request an immediate mental examination. If the conditionally released person is indigent, the court or secretary, upon request, must help in obtaining an expert to conduct the examination.[33]

(E)(3) Acquitted of a Misdemeanor

A defendant acquitted by reason of insanity for a crime that is a misdemeanor must be released from custody. However, he or she may be held for a reasonable period to allow a county-designated MHP to evaluate the need for an involuntary civil commitment.[34] The state has the burden of proving, by a preponderance of the evidence, that the acquitted defendant should not be discharged.[35]

Often, the testimony of the experts who examined the defendant will provide evidence about whether the acquitted defendant is dangerous to others or likely to commit another felony that would jeopardize public safety or security.[36] The court also will consider the violent nature of the crime itself in determining whether the defendant is still dangerous.[37] The burden is not met if the defendant represents a danger only to a particular item of property.[38]

---

30. RCW 10.77.150.
31. RCW 10.77.190.
32. *Id.* State v. Thompson, 28 Wash.App. 728, 626 P.2d 51 (1981). A court may consider previous evidence presented at prior revocation hearings in determining whether to revoke the conditional release.
33. *Id.*
34. RCW 10.77.110; *see* chapter 5E.4, Involuntary Civil Commitment of Mentally Ill Adults.
35. In re Herman, 30 Wash.App. 321, 634 P.2d 310 (1981).
36. State v. Smith, 88 Wash.2d 639, 564 P.2d 1154 (1977).
37. *Id.*, *citing* Thompson v. Snell, 46 Wash. 327, 89 P. 931 (1907).
38. In re Herman, 30 Wash.App. 321, 634 P.2d 310 (1981). The defendant in this case was likely to direct his attacks against a particular statue in a Bremerton cemetery.

5D.10

Battered Woman's and Child's Syndrome

Battered woman's syndrome is sufficiently accepted in the scientific community and is considered to be outside of a lay person's competence, therefore, expert witness testimony is allowed to describe this syndrome at a criminal trial.[1] Testimony about battered child syndrome also is allowed.[2] Such evidence, provided by an MHP, can be offered to aid the jury in understanding[3]

1. the mentality and behavior of battered women generally;

2. the reasonableness of a defendant's apprehension of imminent death or bodily injury at the time of the crime; and

3. why a battered woman remains in a relationship that is both psychologically and physically dangerous.

It is evidence that can buttress the claim of self-defense.[4] It may assist the jurors in placing themselves in the position of the defendant when deciding the legitimacy of her act in light of all circumstances at the time.[5]

---

1. State v. Allery, 101 Wash.2d 591, 682 P.2d 312 (1984).
2. State v. James, 64 Wash.App. 134, 822 P.2d 1238 (1992).
3. State v. Warnow, 88 Wash.2d. 221, 559 P.2d 548 (1977), requires that the fact finder(s) evaluate the defendant's actions in light of her subjective impressions and of all circumstances known to her at the time of the incident.
4. Washington recognizes self-defense as a complete defense to a charge involving a homicide or an assault. The state has the burden to prove beyond a reasonable doubt the absence of self-defense once it is raised as a defense. State v. Despenza, 38 Wash.App. 645, 689 P.2d 87 (1984).
5. Even if such evidence does not lead to a jury concluding that the defendant acted in self-defense, the jury may find that the defendant lacked the requisite intent for murder (see chapter 5D.7, Mens Rea). Such evidence could also convince a judge to sentence the offender to an exceptional sentence, reducing the length of confinement required by the presumptive sentencing standards. State v. Pascal, 108 Wash.2d 125 (1987).

(A) Procedural Import of Battered Woman's and Child's Syndrome

Although expert witness testimony may be presented about these three issues, the court will not view the testimony as being offered as evidence of a pertinent trait of character.[6] As a result, the prosecution may not present evidence of prior acts of defendant misconduct in rebuttal because character is not an element of a self-defense claim.[7]

---

6. Under the rules of evidence, expert witness testimony about a pertinent trait of character is not permitted. State v. Woodard, 26 Wash.App. 735, 617 P.2d 1039 (1980).
7. Normally, under the evidence rules (ER 405(a)), if an accused offers evidence of a pertinent trait of character, it may be rebutted by cross examination of character witnesses (never expert witnesses) or by proof of a contrary reputation in the community. State v. Kelly, 102 Wash.2d 188, 685 P.2d 565 (1984).

5D.11

Rape Trauma
Syndrome

Rape trauma syndrome describes the behavioral, somatic, and psychological sequelae of an attempted or successful rape. In some states, the law allows a party to introduce expert testimony that an alleged victim is suffering from rape trauma syndrome. This may assist in a prosecution when the defendant acknowledges that sexual intercourse has occurred but claims that it was consensual. The presence of rape trauma syndrome may disprove consent. Also, the syndrome has been asserted as a defense for an assault or murder. The rape victim argues that guilt for the crime against the rape offender cannot be found because the syndrome creates an inability to form the necessary intent to commit the crime. In Washington, expert testimony based on new scientific theories is admissible only if the scientific principle from which deductions are made is sufficiently established to have gained general acceptance in the scientific community.[1]

The Washington Supreme Court has held that rape trauma syndrome is not sufficiently accepted in the scientific community. Therefore, an expert witness cannot testify that the existence of the syndrome proves that a rape occurred or that the victim did not consent to the sexual acts.[2] Along with methodological flaws in research studies about the syndrome, the court cited extensive contradictory scientific literature that suggested that no "typical" response to rape occurs; a wide-ranging variety of symptoms is

---

1. State v. Canaday, 90 Wash.2d 808, 585 P.2d 1185 (1978) *citing* Frye v. U.S., 293 F. 1013 (D.C. Cir. 1923). This standard has been applied frequently to determine the admissibility of scientific evidence. *See* State v. Allery, 101 Wash.2d 591, 682 P.2d 312 (1984) (expert witness testimony about battered woman syndrome is held admissible).
2. State v. Black, 109 Wash.2d 336, 745 P.2d 12 (1987).

possible and would provide a questionable means of identifying victims of rape.[3] Evidence of emotional or psychological trauma suffered by the alleged victim may be offered by lay testimony because permitting an expert to testify may unfairly prejudice the jury about the defendant by creating an aura of scientific reliability.[4]

---

3. *Id.*
4. *Id.; but see* Frazier & Borgida, *Juror Common Understanding and the Admissibility of Rape Trauma Syndrome Evidence in Court,* 12 Law Hum. Behav. 101 (1988). This empirical research article suggests that a strong consensus among experts about the current scientific database on rape trauma exists and that nonexperts remain poorly informed about rape-related issues.

5D.12

Hypnosis of Witnesses

A person who experiences stress or trauma while witnessing a legally important event may be unable to recount the event in sufficient detail. In some jurisdictions, hypnosis is used to alleviate stress or other conditions to enhance recall. Hypnotically induced or influenced information, used to form a basis for a search warrant or as evidence at a trial by a police officer or an attorney, is not permitted in many jurisdictions. MHPs with expertise in hypnosis may be able to obtain greater detail concerning a suspect or the details of a crime.

(A) Hypnotically Induced Information in a Police Investigation

No case law exists within Washington limiting the use of hypnotically induced statements. For instance, hypnosis might gain greater detail from a witness whose statements would form the basis for obtaining a search warrant. However, in view of the decisions concerning hypnotically induced courtroom testimony (see below), such statements are likely to be rejected by a magistrate. At the very least, the police presumably would have to base the warrant on other information that supports the statements obtained from a person under hypnosis.

(B) Hypnotically Induced Courtroom Testimony

The Washington Supreme Court found that the reliability of hypnotically induced testimony has been questioned by the experts in the field as a means to enhance recall. Such a technique may lead to[1] suggestibility and greater compliance by the subject; a subjective conviction in the truth of the memory after hypnosis that eliminates the fear of perjury as a factor to ensure reliable testimony; an impediment to effective cross examination as the witness cannot distinguish between facts known before the hypnosis, facts confabulated during hypnosis, and facts learned after hypnosis; adverse effects to jury observations as the witness, influenced by the hypnosis, will maintain an absolute subjective conviction about a particular set of events in spite of the objective reality. As a result, posthypnotic testimony will not be admitted and only the prior recall of the witness, properly preserved and documented, will be allowed into evidence.[2]

In two subsequent cases, the court excluded all posthypnotic testimony. It treated the point of hypnosis as a time barrier after which no admissible identifications of an offender could be made, although in both cases, the witnesses had given detailed descriptions of the offender before hypnosis.[3]

To overcome the legal presumption against the testimony of a witness who has been previously hypnotized, the party offering the prehypnotic statement must provide some independent verification of the witness's prehypnotic memory. For instance, a record could preserve the recollections regarding the event in question before hypnosis.[4] Any party who intends to offer such a record of a witness who later undergoes hypnosis must make a timely disclosure of such information to the court and to opposing counsel.

---

1. State v. Martin, 101 Wash.2d 713, 684 P.2d 651 (1984).
2. *Id.*
3. State v. Laureans, 101 Wash.2d 745, 682 P.2d 889 (1984); State v. Coe, 109 Wash.2d 832, 750 P.2d 208 (1988).
4. State v. Martin, 101 Wash.2d 713, 684 P.2d 651 (1984).

5D.13

Eyewitness Identification

Jurors tend to rely on the testimony of an eyewitness (who may be a party to the action, a victim, or a bystander). In many trials, such testimony is critical to a trial's outcome. Yet, jurors are often unaware of several factors that may influence the accuracy of the testimony.[1] MHPs can contribute experimental and clinical expertise to aid the jury or the court in evaluating the reliability of eyewitness testimony.

(A) Admissibility of Expert Testimony on Eyewitness Identification

Expert witness testimony regarding eyewitness identification lies within the discretion of the trial court.[2] However, the Court of Appeals has ruled that expert testimony should be allowed when[3]

1. the identification of the defendant is the principal issue at trial;

2. the defendant presents an alibi defense; and

---

1. Loftus, E. F. (1979). *Eyewitness Testimony.* Cambridge, MA: Harvard University Press.
2. State v. Guloy, 104 Wash.2d 412, 705 P.2d 1182 (1985), *cert. denied,* 106 S.Ct. 1208 (1986); State v. Jordan, 39 Wash.App. 530, 694 P.2d 47 (1985); State v. Cook, 31 Wash.App. 165, 639 P.2d 863 (1982); State v. Barry, 25 Wash.App. 751, 611 P.2d 1262 (1980); State v. Brown, 17 Wash.App. 587, 564 P.2d 342 (1972).
3. State v. Hanson, 46 Wash.App. 656, 731 P.2d 1140 (1987), *review denied,* 108 Wash.2d 1003 (1987); State v. Moon, 45 Wash.App. 692, 726 P.2d 1263 (1986).

3. there is little or no other evidence linking the defendant to the crime.

If the above three factors are present, trial courts should exercise their discretion liberally.

Expert testimony can address the particular factors of the case that affect the reliability of the identification. This is particularly critical if the eyewitness identification is uncorroborated.[4] The following are factors that have been raised in the scientific literature:[5] (a) what questions are asked and how they are phrased when the police interview the eyewitness; (b) people of other races are identified unreliably; (c) in the case of violent crimes, perceptions are clouded by the additional stress; (d) perceptions are influenced more readily when viewing conditions are poor; (e) substance use reduces the likelihood of accurate perceptions; and (f) memories about perceptions are contaminated by police practices, such as showing a composite or picture of an alleged offender before a lineup identification procedure.

---

4. *Id.*
5. *Id.*

5D.14

Competency to Be Sentenced

No incompetent person can be sentenced for a conviction of a crime so long as mental incapacity continues, and the defendant is unable to understand the proceedings or assist in the defense.[1] This rule, its application, and its implications for MHPs are discussed in detail in chapter 5D.5.

---

1. RCW 10.77.050.

5D.15

Sentencing

The Sentencing Reform Act of 1981 provided sentencing guidelines that greatly limit the discretion of a judge in deciding the sentence of an offender.[1] The period of confinement, community supervision, or community service work, and/or a fine of a specific amount of money is based on the offender score.[2] Points are accrued for the type and number of past convictions and the nature of the present conviction.[3] For instance, several past violent felony convictions combined with a present conviction for another violent felony would produce an offender score at the high end of the presumptive sentencing range for figuring out the sentence.[4]

Departures from the guidelines are possible if the sentencing court finds that an exceptional sentence, outside the standard range, should be imposed because of mitigating or aggravating circumstances.[5] The presumptive sentencing range and a few other factors are established in a presentence investigation conducted by the Department of Corrections; other reports may be submitted separately and may raise any information relevant in

---

1. Other purposes of the Act may justify an exceptional sentence and include ensuring that the punishment is proportionate to the seriousness of the offense and the offender's criminal history; protecting the public from further crime; providing an opportunity for self-improvement (i.e., vocationally and educationally); and expending the state's resources frugally. See RCW 9.94A.010. The balance of these interests led the legislature to create the particular presumptive sentence ranges. In some cases, such reasons may be used by the court to justify an extraordinary sentence: State v. Pascal, 108 Wash.2d 125, 736 P.2d 1065 (1987).
2. RCW 9.94A.030(10).
3. RCW 9.94A.360.
4. RCW 9.94A.310 to .320.
5. RCW 9.94A.390.

deciding the sentence.[6] MHPs may become involved with the process at this point. The offender's mental health or alcohol/ drug evaluations may influence what little discretion a judge has in deciding the penalty, the type of sentence (probation vs. incarceration), term of imprisonment, length of community service, and amount of fine.

(A) Procedures Before Sentencing

Within three days after a plea, finding, or verdict of guilt for a felony, the court may order a presentence investigation to be conducted by the Department of Corrections. It must contain the criminal history and such information about the defendant's characteristics, financial condition, and the circumstances affecting the defendant's behavior as may be relevant in imposing sentence.[7] Either party may produce new evidence to refute any part of the presentence report.[8] In addition, any interested person also may submit a separate report.[9] Finally, the trial court can order whatever investigation it deems necessary to find sufficient information about the offender's past life and personal characteristics.[10]

Mental health and alcohol or drug evaluations by experts, particularly for first-time offenses, can lead the court to declare an exceptional sentence. Such a sentence must be supported by written findings that show that the sentence imposed is neither too excessive nor too lenient when compared with the presumptive guidelines. Unless a higher court finds that no reasonable person would have imposed the sentence, the exceptional sen-

---

6. Wash. Crim. R. 7.1(b) and (d).
7. Wash. Crim. R. 7.1(b).
8. Both parties will have seven days to examine the presentence report. A three-day notice is required if either is going to produce evidence to controvert the presentence report at an evidentiary hearing held before sentencing. Wash. Crim. R. 7.1(a)(3) and (c). Unless the state presents adverse evidence about the presentence report, no public funds need be spent to provide expert evidence for the defense at this stage of the trial. State v. Melos, 42 Wash.App. 638, 713 P.2d 138 (1986).
9. Wash. Crim. R. 7.1(d).
10. State v. Russell, 31 Wash.App. 646, 644 P.2d 704 (1982). The court may not use the information unless admitted to or acknowledged by the plea agreement or at the time of sentencing. If any source is referred to in the presentence reports, unless objected to by a party, the information provided by the source will be deemed to be acknowledged. If material facts are disputed, an evidentiary hearing must be held to prove the real facts by a preponderance of the evidence. RCW 9.94A.370; State v. Wood, 42 Wash.App. 78, 709 P.2d 1209 (1985).

tence will stand, and no abuse of judicial discretion will be found.[12]

---

11. State v. Pascal, 108 Wash.2d 125, 736 P.2d 1065 (1987). Defendant was charged with second degree murder and manslaughter. The jury found that she lacked the requisite intent to murder the victim and was convicted of manslaughter. The presumptive sentencing range of 31 to 41 months of incarceration was disregarded by the court. Instead, she was sentenced to 30 days of confinement, 30 days of partial confinement, 240 hours of community service, and an additional year of community supervision (*see* chapter 5D.16, Probation) because of the following mitigating circumstances: The victim had battered her repeatedly and was a willing participant in the incident; the crime occurred under duress insufficient to constitute a complete defense; and the offender responded as if she suffered from battered woman syndrome (*see* chapter 5D.10). In another case, an offender convicted of indecent liberties was sentenced by the court to an exceptional sentence twice the length of the presumptive confinement range of 15 to 20 months. One of the aggravating factors that the judge cited was Western State Hospital's previous diagnosis of sexual deviancy and a finding that he was unamenable to treatment. The higher court ruled that such an exceptional sentence could be justified if the written record indicated that the longer confinement was necessary to protect society or to permit treatment of the offender. State v. Wood, 42 Wash.App. 78, 709 P.2d 1209 (1985).

5D.16

Probation

The granting of probation is at the discretion of the court.[1] No constitutional guarantee exists for receiving a deferred sentence, with probationary conditions being established.[2] Nor are the sentencing recommendations binding upon the court.[3] After conviction by a plea or a verdict of guilty for any crime, the court, upon application or on its own motion, may grant or deny probation. In the presence of the defendant, the court may decide the conditions of probation. To do so, it considers evidence about the defendant, the prior criminal record, the family surroundings and environment, and the circumstances of the crime.[4] Such evidence may include affidavits or testimony about the mental health of the defendant. Recommendations about probationary conditions may involve mental health or alcohol and drug evaluations and treatment.[5]

(A) Probationary Conditions

In granting probation, the court may suspend the execution of the sentence. The defendant must comply with the conditions for such a time as designated by the court, which is not to exceed the maximum term of the sentence or two years, whichever is longer.[6]

---

1. State v. Joy, 34 Wash.App. 309, 661 P.2d 994 (1983).
2. State v. Damon, 16 Wash.App. 298, 666 P.2d 390 (1983).
3. State v. Skinner, 3 Wash.App. 367, 475 P.2d 129 (1970).
4. RCW 9.95.200.
5. RCW 9.95.210.
6. State v. Damon, 16 Wash.App. 298, 666 P.2d 390 (1983).

Requiring that the defendant be evaluated, apply for appropriate treatment based on the evaluation results, and make satisfactory progress in treatment as determined by the treatment program, are common conditions of probation.[7] The only statutory limitations on the court's discretion are that the defendant may not be imprisoned in the county jail for a period exceeding one year, and the defendant may not be fined any sum exceeding the statutory limit for the offense committed.[8] Attendance at a residential treatment facility may be imposed as a term of probation without being considered imprisonment.[9]

(B) Modification or Revocation of Probation

At any time, the court may modify or revoke its order to suspend the execution of the sentence. Absent exigent circumstances,[10] a probationer must be given notice of a hearing to modify the probationary conditions and to the right of assistance from counsel.[11] The presence of the probationer at a revocation of probation is mandatory.[12]

Revocation of probation occurs at the discretion of the trial judge. It will be overturned on appeal only in cases in which no reasonable person would take the view adopted with regard to the proof about the probation violations.[13] A probationer's lack of intent to violate a condition of probation does not prevent the probation from being revoked. This is particularly true if the

---

7. State v. Osborn, 87 Wash.2d 161, 550 P.2d 513 (1976); State v. Ralph, 41 Wash.App. 770, 706 P.2d 641 (1985).
8. *Id.*
9. State v. Walker, 27 Wash.App. 544, 619 P.2d 699 (1980).
10. These arise if an *ex parte* hearing (a hearing without the probationer present) is necessary to preserve jurisdiction over the probationer.
11. State v. Campbell, 95 Wash.2d 954, 632 P.2d 517 (1981). The probationer threatened to kill his mother and the state sought a probation revocation. Defense counsel requested a stay of proceedings because the probationer was not competent to understand the nature of the hearing. He was committed for determination of incompetency, which prevented his being tried, convicted, or sentenced while incompetent (*see* chapter 5D.5). This tolled the term of probation. The probation period was extended to cover the number of days tolled. In another case, a period of probation was tolled for a probationer who remained outside the jurisdiction, contrary to the terms of probation. State v. Haugen, 22 Wash.App. 785, 591 P.2d 1218 (1979).
12. *Id.*
13. State v. Joy, 34 Wash.App. 369, 661 P.2d 994 (1983). The probationer failed to enter and to complete successfully an alcohol treatment program.

violation suggests that rehabilitation is impossible under the circumstances.[14]

(C) Dismissal of Information or Indictment after Probation

When the reformation of the probation warrants, the court may end probation and discharge the person.[15] Every probationer who has fulfilled the conditions of probation may request the court to dismiss the information or indictment against the probationer and release the probationer from all disabilities resulting from the conviction.[16]

---

14. State v. Bennett, 35 Wash.App. 298, 666 P.2d 390 (1983). The probationer entered the 90-day evaluation period at Western State Hospital but was found unamenable to treatment which left him unable to satisfy the condition of completing treatment in a sex offender program.
15. RCW 9.95.230.
16. RCW 9.95.240. However, in any subsequent prosecution for any other offense, this prior conviction may be pled and proven and shall have the same effect as if probation had not been granted or if the information or indictment had not been dismissed.

5D.17

Dangerous Offenders

In some states, the criminal sentencing law has provisions for increasing the term of imprisonment for "dangerous offenders." The legal decision of whether an offender is dangerous may depend on psychological characteristics that could be assessed by an MPH.

In Washington, the Sentencing Reform Act of 1984 has established sentencing guidelines that extend the range of confinement if a violent offense or a history of violent offenses has occurred.[1] In addition, a sentence may be imposed outside the standard range of the sentencing guidelines if certain aggravating circumstances are part of the offense.[2] Such aggravating circumstances include the following factors: (a) the offender was deliberately cruel to the victim; (b) the offender knew or should have known that the victim was particularly vulnerable or incapable of resistance because of extreme youth, advanced age, disability, or ill health; and (c) the current offense involved multiple victims or multiple incidents per victim (e.g., the offender sexually abused the same child multiple times during a prolonged period).[3] Mental health evaluations may delineate these aggravating factors.[4]

---

1. RCW 9.94A.310 to .320; RCW 9.94A.360.
2. RCW 9.94A.390(2).
3. *Id.*
4. State v. Wood, 42 Wash.App. 78, 709 P.2d 1209 (1985). In this case, a diagnosis of sexual deviancy and a finding that the offender's condition could not be meaningfully treated, because he was unamenable to treatment, were the aggravating circumstances that led the judge to impose a lengthier sentence outside the standard range.

5D.18

Habitual Offenders

The Sentencing Reform Act of 1984 modified many statutes within the Code. The habitual criminal section became inapplicable.[1] Other states that use this type of discretionary criminal sentencing law do so to increase the terms of imprisonment for offenders with a history of criminal convictions. Also in some states, a determination about whether a person is likely to commit additional offenses in the future is an issue about which MHPs provide testimony. In Washington, the sentencing guidelines increase the terms of imprisonment for certain types of criminal history on a systematic basis.[2]

---

1. RCW 9.92.090.
2. RCW 9.94A.360.

5D.19

Competency to Serve a Sentence

The law in several states provides that a criminal defendant must be competent while serving a sentence. In Washington, if a prisoner becomes incompetent during the sentence, confinement may continue only in a mental health facility located wholly within a correctional institution.[1]

---

1. RCW 10.77.220.

5D.20

Mental Mealth Services in Jails and Prisons

Screening, referral, and care of mentally ill and retarded prisoners or of prisoners addicted to alcohol and drugs are services that must be provided as part of the total health care program. Services must be furnished to incarcerated persons whether they are in local detention or in state correctional facilities.[1] Health care standards with written operating procedures approved by the responsible physician and governing unit of each facility must delineate how these services are to be dispensed.[2]

If the initial screening of a prisoner fails to identify a need for mental health or alcohol and drug treatment services, the guards of the facilities are responsible for reporting a prisoner's symptoms to health care staff for appropriate evaluation and treatment.[3] MHPs may provide services as employees of the facilities or act in a consulting capacity.

(A) Informed Consent

All mental health services must be consented to by the prisoners except as necessary to prevent the spread of communicable disease or to relieve imminent danger to self or to others.[4] The prisoner must be provided a clear statement about the diagnosis

---

1. WAC 289-20-205(1)(l). Health care includes preventive, diagnostic, and rehabilitation services provided by licensed health care professionals and/or facilities. RCW 70.48.020.
2. *Id.*
3. WAC 289-20-260(2)(a).
4. WAC 289-20-260(1).

and treatment process.[5] If the prisoner refuses treatment, the procedures required by Chapter 71.05 RCW must be followed to determine whether involuntary treatment is required.[6] Physical restraint must be directed by a physician when necessary for medical reasons; an acutely disturbed or violent prisoner may be controlled with restraints, but physician review and direction of the health care staff must be promptly obtained.[7]

(B) Limitations on Treatment Options

Without due process, electroconvulsive therapy (ECT)[8] and antipsychotic medications[9] may not be conducted or administered to a prisoner who does not consent to such treatment. These treatments require a judicial hearing at which the state must prove by clear and convincing evidence that the treatment is both necessary and effective to further a compelling state interest. Interests include

1. preservation of life;
2. protection of third parties interests;
3. prevention of suicide; and
4. maintenance of the ethical integrity of the medical profession.

A prisoner must be given reasonable notice and time to prepare for the hearing, be represented by counsel, and be present at the hearing.[10] Included in the requirement of a judicial hearing are the rights to present evidence, to cross examine witnesses, to be proceeded against under the rules of evidence, to remain silent, and to view and to copy all petitions and reports in the court file.[11] The court must set forth findings about the state's interest in the treatment, the necessity and effectiveness of the treatment, and the desires of the patient, or a substituted judgment by the court.[12] If the court grants the order for involuntary ECT or medication, it may place time limits and conditions upon the administration of these.[13]

---

5. *Id.*
6. *Id.*
7. WAC 289-20-260(2)(e).
8. In re Schuoler, 106 Wash.2d 500, 723 P.2d 1103 (1986).
9. Harper v. Washington, 110 Wash.2d 873, 759 P.2d 358 (1988), *overruled*, 494 U.S. 210 (1989). *See* chapter 6.2, Right to Refuse Treatment, for a detailed discussion about the treatment with antipsychotic medications of inmates within correctional institutions.
10. *Id.*
11. *Id.*
12. *Id.*
13. *Id.*

(C) Credit for Hospital Time

The equal protection clause of the state constitution requires that credit be given for time involuntarily spent in mental health facilities whether the detention occurs before or after the defendant begins serving a sentence.[14] Persons sent to prison and then transferred to a state hospital must be evaluated for early release determinations using the same standards applied to those persons confined in state correctional facilities.[15]

(D) Responsibility for Cost of Health Care

The governing unit, the county, city, or state department fiscally responsible for operating the facility incarcerating the prisoner, must bear the cost of providing health care services.[16] Local facilities can obtain reimbursement for health care services only if the person is eligible under the DSHS's public assistance medical program. The local facility inmate will not lose "confined status" by being hospitalized without a guard. The governing unit operating the facility from which the prisoner came will be responsible for paying for the services.[17]

(E) Records

All health care records must be maintained separately from other jail records to protect the confidentiality of the prisoner.[18] The records can be released to other persons and agencies only with the consent of the prisoner. However, MHPs can disclose to jail authorities information necessary for the protection of the welfare of the prisoner, other prisoners' management in the jail, or the maintenance of jail security and order.[19]

---

14. In re Knapp, 102 Wash.2d 466, 687 P.2d 1145 (1984).
15. RCW 72.68.031.
16. RCW 70.43.130.
17. Harrison Memorial Hospital v. Kitsap County, 103 Wash.2d 887, 700 P.2d 732 (1985).
18. WAC 289-20-150(2)(a).
19. WAC 289-20-150 (2)(b) and (3).

5D.21

Transfer from Penal to Mental Health Facilities

If the welfare of an inmate requires, the person will be moved for observation, diagnosis, or treatment of mental illness. The transfer would be initiated after the secretary of corrections received a detailed medical evaluation and recommendations.[1] Then, the secretary of corrections, with the consent of the secretary of the DSHS, will authorize the transfer.[2] Such a transfer could be to a facility for the care of the mentally ill run by a state correction system.[3] MHPs will be involved with the evaluation and treatment of the inmate.

(A) Regular Transfer

Any inmate involuntarily transferred to a mental health facility is entitled to a judicial hearing. At the hearing, the following due process safeguards exist:[4] the right to counsel, the right to call and cross examine witnesses, and the right to obtain testimony from an expert witness chosen by the inmate. In addition, if treatment at the mental health facility involves intrusive measures of ECT or antipsychotic medications, a separate due process hearing is required to decide the necessity of such treatment (see chapter 5D.20, Mental Health Services in Jails and Prisons).[5]

---

1. WAC 137-91-060.
2. RCW 72.68.031.
3. RCW 72.68.035
4. Harmon v. McNutt, 91 Wash.2d 126, 587 P.2d 537 (1978).
5. Harper v. State of Washington, 110 Wash.2d 873, 759 P.2d 358 (1988), *overruled*, 494 U.S. 210 (1989).

During the treatment, the sentence of the transferred inmate will continue to run as if confined in a correctional facility until the involuntary treatment is no longer necessary or the maximum term of the sentence is reached.[6] If the maximum term of the sentence is reached and the inmate still requires involuntary treatment at a state mental health facility, a civil involuntary commitment due process hearing may be held to decide the necessity of continued treatment.[7] Substantially similar opportunities for parole or an early release determination must be followed for the transferred inmate.[8]

(B) Emergency Transfer

In case of an emergency,[9] an inmate confined to a state correctional facility may be transferred and treated at a mental health facility.[10] However, a judicial hearing with all the due-process safeguards must follow promptly.[11]

(C) Notice of Transfer and Confidentiality

A notice of the transfer must be sent to the relatives, attorney, or guardian, if any, of the inmate.[12] Medical records must be maintained separately from other correctional records to protect inmate confidentiality. None of the records may be released to other persons or agencies without the written authorization of the prisoners.[13] Exceptions would involve the necessity of protecting the welfare of the inmate or other prisoners, or maintaining jail security and order.[14] At the time of a transfer, information regarding the serious health problem must be communicated to any transferring officer or receiving correctional institution.[15]

---

6. RCW 72.68.031.
7. Chapter 71.05 RCW.
8. *Id.*
9. Emergency is undefined in the statutes or case law. Presumably, an emergency involves a mental disorder that presents a danger to self or others and that, without immediate treatment in a mental health facility, may result in substantial physical harm or serious illness.
10. RCW 72.68.032.
11. *Id.*
12. RCW 72.68.037.
13. WAC 289-20-150(2).
14. WAC 289-20-150(3).
15. WAC 289-20-150(4).

5D.22

Parole Determination

Parole is a conditional release from imprisonment that entitles the parolee to serve the remainder of the term outside the confinement of a prison.[1] It differs from probation in that the convicted person must first serve a period in a prison. MHPs may be asked to provide information that may influence decisions regarding parole.

(A) Eligibility for Parole and Parole Criteria

The Indeterminate Sentence Review Board[2] transferred all of its powers, duties, and functions regarding persons convicted of crimes committed before July 1, 1984, to the Superior Courts of Washington.[3] The Board prepared recommendations on each of these prisoners about the suitability for parole and appropriate parole conditions.[4] The sentencing judge or the successor judge will have sole authority to decide the date of parole release for persons convicted of crimes after July 1, 1984.[5]

The Superior Court must not release a prisoner on parole unless rehabilitation has been completed, the prisoner is fit for

---

1. RCW 9.95.110.
2. RCW 9.95.001. Once called the Board of Prison Terms and Paroles, it ceased to function on June 30, 1992.
3. RCW 9.95.0011.
4. *Id*.
5. *Id*. The judge's authority is limited to a great extent by the presumptive sentence ranges established by the Sentencing Reform Act of 1981, Chapter 9.94 RCW (*see* chapter 5D.15, Sentencing).

release, and at least two-thirds of his sentence has been served in prison.[6] Parole of life-term prisoners cannot be considered until after they have served at least 20 consecutive years, less earned good time.[7] The secretary of corrections prepares plans and recommendations for conditions of supervision under which each prisoner eligible for parole may be released from custody; at the discretion of the court, such plans may be approved, rejected, or revised, and special conditions of supervision may be assigned for the parole officer to carry out.[8]

In determining whether a prisoner is fit for release and the conditions of parole sufficient, the Superior Courts may hear additional evidence about the fitness of the prisoner or the appropriate treatment possibilities on the basis of independent evaluation results.

(B) Violation of Parole Conditions

Violation of parole conditions, including failing to comply with treatment conditions, may lead to the immediate arrest, suspension of parole, and reconfinement of the prisoner without a warrant.[9] The prisoner is entitled to a hearing on the charges of the violation within 30 days of arrest near the site of the alleged violation(s) of parole.[10] Within 15 days of arrest and detention, the prisoner will be served a copy of the factual allegations about the violation(s) of parole.[11]

The prisoner has a right to be represented by a lawyer even if an appointed lawyer must be provided by the state because the prisoner is indigent.[12] The revocation hearing will be conducted under the same due process rights established for other criminal proceedings. However, a violation of parole need only be proven by a preponderance of the evidence.[13]

If the parolee is accused of breaking a law and is acquitted at a criminal trial with the toughest burden of proof in effect (i.e., beyond a reasonable doubt) that acquittal does not bar the state

---

6. RCW 9.95.100 to 110.
7. RCW 9.95.115. Time credit reductions for good behavior are recommended by the superintendent of the prison for prisoners whose conduct and work have been meritorious. RCW 9.95.070.
8. RCW 72.04A.070.
9. RCW 72.04A.090.
10. RCW 9.95.120.
11. RCW 9.95.121.
12. RCW 9.95.122.
13. RCW 9.95.123 to .125. Such due process rights entitle the parolee to present witnesses, to receive notice of the violation, to cross examine adverse witnesses, and to receive a transcript of the hearing. Morrisey v. Brewer, 408 U.S. 471 (1972); Petition of Haverty, 98 Wash.2d 621, 618 P.2d 1011 (1980).

from conducting a parole revocation hearing on the basis of the same incident.[14] When the evidence is considered with the lower burden that is used for the revocation hearing, the parole may be revoked.

---

14. State v. Dupard, 93 Wash.2d 268, 609 P.2d 961 (1980).

5D.23

Competency to Be Executed

A few states require that a prisoner who is sentenced to death must be competent at the time of execution. The practical purpose of this type of law is to prevent the execution of a person who is unable to pursue postconviction appeals because of a mental disease or defect. Washington requires a mandatory review of a death sentence by its Supreme Court.[1] Although Washington's incompetency law does not specifically apply to prisoners appealing their conviction, presumably the mandatory nature of the review would require the prisoner to possess the capacity to understand the nature of the proceedings and to assist in the defense.

---

1. RCW 10.95.100.

5D.24

Pornography

The state law that prohibited any involvement in the preparation, distribution, or sale of obscene materials was repealed by the legislature in 1982.[1] The remaining statutes restrict the distribution and exhibition of erotic materials to adults,[2] and the visibility of sexually explicit materials from a public thoroughfare.[3] Laws preventing the sexual exploitation of any person under the age of 18 years prohibit minors from being involved in any sexually explicit conduct for commercial gain.[4]

Although the state law restricting the preparation, distribution, or sale of obscene materials is repealed, municipal laws may restrict the viewing of lewd acts in a public place.[5] Yet, state statutes or municipal ordinances must not violate the First Amendment rights of the U.S. Constitution that protect freedom of expression. Often, a defense to violating such statutes or ordinances is that they are too broad and cause a chilling effect on the privileges of the First Amendment. To avoid impinging upon the First Amendment, the fact finders in the case must decide whether the average person, applying contemporary community standards, would find that the work taken as a whole appeals only to the prurient interest or is patently offensive and lacks

---

1. RCW 9.68.010.
2. RCW 9.68.015 to .120.
3. RCW 9.68.130.
4. Chapter 9.68A RCW. Sexually explicit conduct in return for a fee includes the sexual exploitation or abuse of children who would be photographed, or made part of a live performance, or patronized as a juvenile prostitute. RCW 9.68A.001 to .100. State v. Danforth, 56 Wash.App. 133, 782 P.2d 1091 (1989), held that an adult engaging in consensual activity (not prostitution) with 16- and 17-year-old children does not violate this statute.
5. Seattle v. Jarrett, 33 Wash.App. 525, 655 P.2d 1209 (1982).

serious literary, artistic, political, or scientific value.[6] Although not necessary to defining how any average person applies contemporary community standards, an MHP may testify about contemporary community standards.[7]

---

6. State v. Regan, 97 Wash.2d 47, 640 P.2d 725 (1982) *citing* Miller v. California, 413 U.S. 15 (1973), Hamling v. U.S., 418 U.S. 87 (1974), Smith v. U.S., 431 U.S. 291 (1977), Pinkers v. U.S., 436 U.S. 293 (1978).
7. State v. J. R. Distributors, Inc., 82 Wash.2d 584, 512 P.2d 1049 (1973). A psychiatrist's empirical study about people's attitudes toward pornography was admitted into evidence.

5D.25

Services for Sex Offenders

MHPs may become involved in evaluating an alleged offender, testifying in court, or providing treatment. Sex offender evaluation and treatment providers are regulated under the provisions of Chapter 18.155 RCW. The legislature found that

1. such providers play a vital role in protecting the public from sex offenders who remain in the community following conviction;

2. the qualifications, practice techniques, and effectiveness of sex offender evaluation and treatment providers varied widely; and

3. the courts' ability to decide the appropriateness of granting sentencing alternatives and of monitoring the offender to ensure continued protection of the community was undermined by the lack of regulation of health care providers working with sex offenders.

(A) Certification

The regulations defining the certification process[1] for sex offender evaluation and treatment providers contain several categories of certification depending on the applicant's ability to meet all of the educational, training, and experience requirements. Applicants

---

1. WAC 246-930 *et seq.*. The certification process applies to any evaluation and treatment provider who provides services to adult offenders under the Sex Offender Sentencing Alternative, RCW 9.94A.120(7), or to juvenile sex offenders under RCW 12.40.160.

with affiliate or provisional certification under the regulation may provide services under the direct supervision of a fully certified provider.[2]

(A)(1) Underlying Credential

To obtain certification as a sex offender evaluation and treatment provider, the individual must already possess an underlying credential as a health care professional. The regulations allow for certification of individuals whose health credentials are issued by a state other than that of Washington.[3] The regulations also tie continued certification to maintenance of the underlying credential in good standing; if the underlying credential is allowed to lapse or is revoked, the sex offender treatment provider certification will be immediately revoked.[4]

Full certification is contingent on meeting certain education,[5] professional experience,[6] and training requirements.[7] Affiliate certification can be obtained by an individual possessing a bachelor's degree and a total of 2,000 hours of evaluation and/or treatment experience obtained during the preceding seven years.[8]

(B) Standards of Professional Conduct

In addition to being subject to the provisions of the Uniform Disciplinary Act,[9] sex offender treatment providers are subject to other codes of professional conduct unique to the certification.[10] For example, certified sex offender treatment providers are required to report to the Department of Health any unprofessional conduct by any other certified sex offender treatment provider.[11] The standards for professional conduct and client relationships

---

2. WAC 246-930-075.
3. WAC 246-930-020(2).
4. WAC 246-930-020(3).
5. WAC 246-930-030.
6. WAC 246-930-040.
7. WAC 246-930-200.
8. WAC 236-930-060(1) and (2).
9. Chapter 18.130 RCW.
10. WAC 246-930-010 *et seq.*
11. WAC 246-930-300. In addition, many other individuals are charged with the responsibility of reporting the same information, including (a) the president, chief executive officer, or designated official of any professional association or society whose members are certified providers; (b) prosecuting attorneys and deputy prosecuting attorneys; (c) community corrections officers employed by the Department of Corrections; (d) juvenile probation or parole counselors and designated officials of any public or private agency that employs certified sex offender treatment providers; and (e) the president, chief executive officer, or designated official of any credentialing agency for the health professionals.

cover such topics as competence in practice,[12] confidentiality,[13] conflicts of interest,[14] fee setting and client interactions,[15] termination and alteration of therapist–client relationships,[16] and the use of plethysmography and polygraphy.[17] These standards are presented in considerable detail, and professionals should carefully examine individual provisions for possible conflicts with standards of conduct under other health profession credentials.

The regulations also contain detailed standards for the form and content of assessment and evaluation reports[18] and standards for treatment.[19] The standards for treatment of adult and juvenile sex offenders provide specific standards for planning and intervention, treatment methods, monitoring of treatment and sentence requirements, contacts with victims and vulnerable children, documentation of treatment, and completion of court-ordered treatment. Finally, there are standards for communicating with other professionals, including corrections and probation officers, other supervising law enforcement agencies, and the Department of Social and Health Services.[20] Taken as a whole, these standards closely define the activities and responsibilities of certified sex offender treatment providers, and any failure to abide by them subjects the provider to loss of certification.

---

12. WAC 246-930-310(2).
13. WAC 246-930-310(3).
14. WAC 246-930-310(4).
15. WAC 246-930-310(5).
16. WAC 246-930-310(6).
17. WAC 246-930-310(7) and (8).
18. WAC 246-930-320.
19. WAC 246-930-330.
20. WAC 246-930-340.

5D.26

Services for Victims of Crimes

Crime victims, survivors, and witnesses are eligible for benefits and services.[1] MHPs may become involved with this class of clients because of the evaluation and treatment of the emotional effects resulting from criminal acts.

(A) Compensation

If a criminal act has resulted in bodily injury or death, the benefits and services available to injured workers under Chapter 51 RCW are extended to the innocent victims of such acts.[2] The act must be punishable as either a felony or a misdemeanor.[3] However, an acquittal in the prosecution of the act or in the absence of any prosecution does not preclude recovering compensation.[4] Compensation would be denied to a victim who consented to, provoked, or invited the criminal act. It also would be denied to a person confined or living in any institution operated by the Department of Social and Health Services or the Department of Corrections.[5] However, an effort to prevent a criminal act or to

---

1. Chapter 7.68 RCW, Victims of Crimes: Compensation Assistance Act; Chapter 7.69 RCW; Chapter 7.69A RCW.
2. RCW 7.68.010.
3. RCW 7.68.020(2).
4. Id.; Department of Labor & Industries v. Sargeent, 27 Wash.App. 1, 615 P.2d 519 (1980). Absence of state jurisdiction, because the act occurred on the Yakima Reservation, does not prevent victims' heirs from recovering.
5. RCW 7.68.070(3); Stafford v. Department of Labor & Industries, 33 Wash. App. 231, 653 P.2d 1350(1982).

apprehend a person suspected of engaging in a criminal act that results in bodily injury may be compensated.[6]

The criminal act must be reported to the police department or sheriff's office within 72 hours of its occurrence or within 72 hours of the time during which a report could have been made in order for benefits under this chapter to be secured.[7] It appears not to matter who reports the criminal act.

An application for benefits must be received by the Department of Labor and Industries within one year of the date on which the criminal act was reported to the authorities or the date on which the rights of dependents or beneficiaries accrued.[8] The person making the application remains eligible for the benefits only if reasonable cooperation is given to law enforcement authorities.[9]

(A)(1) Types of Compensation

In the case of the death of an innocent victim, payments may be made for burial expenses and for small, lump-sum survivor payments to the spouse and children of the victim.[10] If the victim is left with a permanent total disability, variable monthly payments will be made to the victim depending on the victim's employment status[11] and number of children at the time of the crime.[12] Permanent partial disability benefits can be obtained[13] as well as temporary total disability proceeds.[14] In the case of partial disability or temporary total disability, vocational rehabilitation benefits can be provided (see chapter 5B.3, Vocational Disability Determinations). Counseling services are specified for victims of sexual assault and may include counseling for members of the victim's family other than a perpetrator of the assault.[15]

Although innocent victims may be compensated for their injuries, monetary ceilings limit the benefits to no more than $20,000 depending on the extent of the disability. [16] Reimburse-

---

6. RCW 7.68.020(3); Hansen v. Department of Labor & Industries, 27 Wash.App. 223, 615 P.2d 1302 (1980), found that a victim who could have ignored derogatory remarks was not innocent because he confronted the attacker by crossing the street and backing the attacker against the wall.
7. RCW 7.68.060(b).
8. RCW 7.68.060(a).
9. RCW 7.68.070(11).
10. RCW 7.68.070(4).
11. RCW 7.68.070(5); RCW 51.32.060.
12. Id.; RCW 51.08.018.
13. RCW 7.68.070(6); RCW 51.32.080.
14. RCW 7.68.070(7); RCW 51.32.090.
15. RCW 7.68.070(12). Fees for such counseling shall be determined by the DSHS in accordance with RCW 51.04.030.
16. RCW 7.68.085. Examination costs incurred by a hospital or other emergency medical facility when performed for gathering evidence for prosecution are paid for by the state. RCW 7.68.170.

ment for medical services is capped at $150,000.[17] Furthermore, the benefits to be paid by the Department of Labor and Industries must first be reduced by the amount of any other public or private insurance available to the innocent victim or family.[18] If a victim or a beneficiary files a civil lawsuit for damages against the person liable for the injury or death, the victim or beneficiary is entitled to full compensation and benefits under the Chapter only if the law suit is lost.[19] However, benefits will be paid out after the lawsuit is filed. The Department of Labor and Industries will be entitled to be reimbursed for benefits paid if the lawsuit is successful.[20]

(B) Confidentiality

Data in the claim files about the victim are deemed confidential and not open to public inspection.[21] However, information may be released if related to the performance of the official duties of public employees or to the examination and treatment needs of physicians retained by the victim or by the Department.[22] Information must be released by an institution and a health care provider if sought by the Department, and it pertains to a claim for benefits.[23]

(C) Services of County Victim Witness Programs

Comprehensive programs can be established by the county prosecuting attorney and approved by the Department of Labor and Industries.[24] The services are funded by penalty assessments levied against criminals in addition to fines or bail forfeitures.[25]

---

17. RCW 7.68.070(13); RCW 51.32.040, .055, .100, .110, .120, .130, .135, .140, .150, .160, .210.
18. RCW 7.68.130. In the case of life insurance proceeds, the first $40,000 shall not be considered in the reduction of Labor and Industries benefits. Social security benefits are not considered to be insurance. Standing v. Department of Labor & Industries, 92 Wash.2d 463, 598 P.2d 725 (1979).
19. RCW 7.68.050.
20. The Department can file a lien for benefits on the amount to be received from the assailant in a personal injury action. Department of Labor and Industries v. Dillon, 28 Wash.App. 853, 626 P.2d 1004 (1981).
21. RCW 7.68.140.
22. *Id*.
23. RCW 7.68.145.
24. RCW 7.68.035.
25. *Id*.

The program is responsible for informing the known victim or surviving dependents about the contents of this chapter and the application procedures, helping victims during the restitution and adjudication process, and preparing and presenting their claims to the department.[26]

(D) Rights of Victims, Survivors, and Witnesses

A reasonable effort must be made by law enforcement agencies, prosecutors, and judges to ensure the following rights for victims, survivors, and witnesses:[27]

1. to be informed of the final disposition of the case;
2. to be notified if their appearance during a court proceeding to which they have been subpoenaed will not occur as scheduled;
3. to receive protection from harm and threats of harm and to be provided with information as to the level of protection available;
4. to be informed about and assisted in receiving any witness fees;
5. to be provided a secure waiting area during court proceedings away from the defendant and family or friends of the defendant;
6. to have stolen property returned when no longer needed as evidence (most property can be photographed and returned to the owner within 10 days);
7. to be provided employer intercession services to minimize an employee's loss of pay and other benefits resulting from court appearance;
8. to access immediate medical assistance without being detained for questioning;[28]
9. to schedule the court appearances of victims and survivors as early as practical in the proceedings so that they can be physically present during the trial after testifying;

---

26. RCW 7.68.035(4).
27. RCW 7.69.010; RCW 7.69.030.
28. The law enforcement agency staff may accompany the person and question the person about the circumstances of the criminal act if it does not hinder the administration of medical assistance. RCW 7.69.030(8).

10. to be informed, if requested, as to the time and place of trial and of the sentencing hearing for felony convictions;

11. to receive, if requested, victim impact statements, and all presentence reports about the offender;

12. to present a statement personally or by representation at the sentencing hearing for felony convictions; and

13. to be provided restitution in all felony cases unless extraordinary circumstances exist that suggest restitution is inappropriate in the court's judgment.

If a victim is incapacitated or otherwise incompetent, such a person will have a representative designated by the prosecuting attorney without formal legal proceedings being necessary.[29] No cause of action can result in civil liability against a person for failing to ensure the rights of victims, survivors, or witnesses.[30] However, discipline complaints could be filed with the Washington State Bar Association or the Commission of Judicial Conduct depending on whether the person is a lawyer or a judge.

(E) Child Victims and Witnesses

Reasonable efforts must be made by law enforcement agencies, prosecutors, and judges to ensure that the children victims and witnesses of crimes are provided with additional rights:[31]

1. to have explained to them, in language easily understood all of the details in the case;

2. to be provided a secure waiting area during court process and to be accompanied by an advocate or support person during the court proceedings;

3. to remain anonymous to everyone except to people involved with the prosecution of the case or to the agency that provides the services;

4. to allow an advocate[32] to inform the prosecuting attorney about the ability of the child to cooperate with the prosecution and the potential effects of such cooperation;

5. to allow an advocate to provide information to the court about the child's ability to understand the nature of the proceedings;

---

29. RCW 7.69.040.
30. RCW 7.69.050.
31. RCW 7.69A.030.
32. RCW 7.69.040.

6. to provide appropriate referrals to social service agencies who could assist the child and the child's family with the emotional impact of the crime and the subsequent investigation and judicial proceedings in which the child is to be involved;

7. to allow an advocate to be present in court while the child testifies to provide emotional support to the child;

8. to provide to the court information as to the need of other supportive persons to be present while the child testifies; and

9. to allow assistance of other professional personnel during the interviewing of the child victim.

The failure to make a reasonable effort to assure that child victims and witnesses are afforded these rights shall not result in civil liability so long as the failure was not grossly negligent.[33] Discipline complaints could be filed with the Washington State Bar Association or the Commission of Judicial Conduct depending on whether the person is a lawyer or a judge.

---

33. RCW 7.69A.040.

Voluntary or Involuntary Receipt of State Services

5E.1

Medicaid

Medicaid is a federally supported program that permits the states to make direct payments to providers of health care services for individuals receiving cash payments under the programs of old-age assistance, aid to needy families with dependent children under 21 years of age or in foster care, subsidized adoption or care facilities for the mentally retarded, aid to the blind, and aid to the disabled.[1] In Washington, the program is called *medical assistance* and is administered by the DSHS to comply with the federal requirements of Medicaid reimbursement.[2] MHPs may be reimbursed for their services under this law.

(A) Coverage

Medical assistance excludes only routine foot care and dental services.[3] Many of the recipients of medical assistance are enrolled by the DSHS in one of the managed health care systems that provide health care services directly or by contract.[4]

Inpatient care for alcohol or drug treatment and mental health services is reimbursed through medical assistance.[5] However, only outpatient mental health services appear to be reimbursed through medical assistance.[6]

---

1. Title XIX of the Social Security Act, 42 U.S.C. § 1396 *et seq.*
2. RCW 74.09.500.
3. RCW 74.09.520.
4. RCW 74.09.522.
5. WAC 388-86-050.
6. WAC 388-86-067.

(B) Confidentiality

For MHPs, one aspect of medical assistance remains particularly chilling for the clients. The court has interpreted in very broad terms the requirement of review and audit of records for participant service providers for the medical assistance program.[7] Whenever the DSHS seeks to review or to audit the records of medical assistance recipients, it may gain access to the entire record.[8]

The confidentiality of alcohol and drug treatment records for health care providers who work within state-approved alcohol and drug treatment settings are regulated by both state and federal laws. The federal law supersedes state law in conflict unless the state law is more restrictive.[9]

---

7. 42 U.S.C. § 1396a(a)(27) and (30).
8. Social & Health Services v. Latta, 92 Wash.2d 812, 601 P.2d 520 (1979).
9. RCW 70.96A.150; WAC 275-19-074, -075; WAC 248-18-235; WAC 248-22-041; WAC 248-18-235; Public Health Service of the Department of Health and Human Services of the United States, pursuant to section 408 of the Drug Abuse Prevention, Treatment, and Rehabilitation Act (42 U.S.C. § 290dd-3), see 42 C.F.R. § 2.1 et seq. See chapter 4.2, Confidential Relations and Communications.

5E.2

Washington Health Care Access Act

In 1987, the legislature found that most of the population in the state did not have available insurance or other coverage of the costs of necessary, basic health care services.[1] This lack led to substantial expenditures for emergency and remedial health care. The legislature believed that the use of managed health care systems would reduce the growth of health care costs incurred by the people of the state generally, and by low-income pregnant women specifically, who are in a vulnerable position along with their children. Because of these findings, it enacted an experimental program to provide necessary, basic health care services to working persons and others who lacked coverage. MHPs may be reimbursed for services rendered to some of the persons covered by the program.

(A) Who Is Covered

The legislature specified that the following groups of people could apply for coverage: displaced forest products workers, those less than 65 years of age and not eligible for Medicare, and those without a gross family income above 200% of the federal poverty guideline.[2] The program limits strictly the number of individuals who can participate and the specific areas within the state of Washington.

---

1. RCW 70.47.010.
2. Id.

(B) What Services Are Provided

The program can contract with the managed health care system to provide basic health care services; the system includes health care providers, insurers, health care service contractors, health care maintenance organizations, or any combination of the above that provide, by contract, basic health care services.[3] Some parts of the managed health care system do provide mental health services. Whether mental health and alcohol or drug treatment is covered depends on the individual managed health care program.

(C) Program Limitations

A sunset law will terminate the program, absent compelling evidence as to detailed cost benefit savings.[4] In addition to this limitation, the basic health plan trust account cannot be overdrawn in any year by 95% of the anticipated spending for the purchase of services.[5]

---

3. RCW 70.47.020.
4. RCW 70.47.010.
5. RCW 70.47.030.

5E.3

Voluntary Civil Admission of Mentally Ill Adults

Both private and public inpatient facilities may admit voluntary patients, that is adult persons suffering from a mental disorder.[1] Washington has promulgated many statutes and rules to regulate inpatient treatment. One goal of the legislation was to curb the past abuses of inappropriate commitments of mentally disordered persons that have led to the violation of individual rights.[2] Also, regulations were imposed by the legislature to encourage the provision of services within the community on an outpatient basis.[3] However, the legislature has not foreclosed the alternative of providing voluntary evaluation and treatment services in inpatient facilities for persons with serious mental disorders. MHPs may become involved in this process by referring a client to inpatient treatment or by evaluating and treating a person while within inpatient treatment.

(A) Differences Between Voluntary and Involuntary Admission

Any person voluntarily admitted to an inpatient facility must be released immediately upon request.[4] Involuntarily admitted patients are released only after elaborate due process procedures are exhausted.

1. WAC 275-55-030, -040; see chapter 5A.19, Voluntary Admission and Civil Commitment of Minors.
2. RCW 71.05.010.
3. Id.
4. RCW 71.05.050.

(B) Voluntary Evaluation and Treatment

(B)(1) Consent and the Rights Due to a Voluntary Patient

Any adult entering an inpatient facility must voluntarily consent to admission in writing and be provided with a list of rights specified by regulations.[5] Voluntary patients must be advised, both orally and in writing, of all their rights,[6] including the right[7] to immediate release upon request, unless involuntary commitment proceedings are initiated; to receive written communications about their admission, evaluation, or treatment; to adequate care and individualized treatment; to wear their own clothes and to keep and use their personal possessions; to keep and spend a reasonable amount of money while hospitalized; to individual storage space for private use; to see visitors at reasonable times; to have reasonable access to a telephone booth to make and receive confidential calls; to have ready access to writing material and stamps to send and receive uncensored correspondence; to refuse shock treatment, surgery, or neuroleptic medications unless ordered by a court;[8] to avoid psychosurgery under any circumstance; to dispose of property and sign contracts unless adjudicated incompetent and not be presumed incompetent because of receiving evaluation and treatment; to object to detention and request release; the right of access to attorneys, courts, and other forms of legal redress; and to have all information remain confidential.

At any point during the treatment, the patient must be released immediately upon request unless the staff believes that, because of a mental disorder,[9] the person is at imminent risk of attempting serious injury to self or others or remains gravely disabled.[10] If such a concern arises at the time of the request, the staff may detain the person for no longer than one judicial day so that a designated county MHP may assess the need for involuntary treatment.[11]

---

5. WAC 275-55-040.
6. WAC 275-55-211.
7. WAC 275-55-241.
8. *See* chapter 6.2, Right to Refuse Treatment.
9. *Mental disorder* refers to any organic, mental, or emotional impairment that has substantial adverse effects on an individual's cognitive or volitional functions. RCW 71.05.020(1).
10. *Id. Gravely disabled* refers to a condition caused by a mental disorder or escalating loss of cognitive and volitional control that results in the person failing to provide for his own essential human needs of health or safety.
11. *Id.*

The status of a voluntary patient must be reviewed at least once every 180 days to decide whether further inpatient treatment is required.[12] If further treatment is not necessary, the person is to be released.

(C) Legal Effect of Voluntary Admission

No person shall be presumed incompetent or lose any civil rights as a consequence of being evaluated or treated voluntarily for a mental disorder.[13] A separate hearing must occur to declare someone incompetent and to appoint a guardian, if such a finding is made.[14]

(D) Confidentiality and Privilege

All information compiled, obtained, and maintained during the course of a voluntary hospitalization is regulated by the same statute that applies to involuntarily treated patients.[15] The statute and how it establishes protections for patient confidences is discussed thoroughly in chapter 5E.4.

---

12. RCW 71.05.050.
13. RCW 71.05.450; *see* In re Quesnell, 83 Wash.2d 224 (1973).
14. *See* chapter 5A.2, Guardianship for Adults.
15. RCW 71.05.390, .440, .610 to .690.

5E.4

Involuntary Civil Admission of Mentally Ill Adults

In 1973, the legislature dramatically changed the procedures of involuntary civil commitment to meet several objectives:[1]

1. to end inappropriate, indefinite commitment of mentally disordered persons and to eliminate legal disabilities that arise from such commitment;

2. to provide prompt evaluation and short-term treatment of persons with serious mental disorders;

3. to safeguard individual rights;

4. to provide continuity of care for persons with serious mental disorders;

5. to encourage the full use of existing agencies, professional personnel, and public funds to prevent duplication of services and unnecessary expenditures;

6. to encourage, whenever appropriate, that services be provided within the community; and

7. to protect public safety.

MHPs decide whether to summon a county designated MHP to evaluate the necessity of involuntarily treating their client or patient, testify in court about evidence that supports the necessity of involuntary treatment, and provide services within the facility or within an outpatient facility in the community for the committed person. All MHPs may use the involuntary treatment process if the condition of their patient or client meets certain prerequisites.

---

1. RCW 71.05.010.

(A) Terms and Definitions

Many legal definitions exist within this area of the law that do not necessarily fit the common-sense conception of the words. For the purpose of understanding the involuntary commitment laws, the following definitions are applied:

1. *mental disorder* refers to any organic, mental, or emotional impairment having substantial adverse effects on an individual's cognitive or volitional functions, classified by the current diagnostic and statistical manual of the American Psychiatric Association;[2]

2. *gravely disabled* refers to a condition in which a person, because of a mental disorder, (a) is in danger of serious physical harm resulting from a failure to provide for his or her essential human needs of health or safety, or (b) manifests severe deterioration in routine functioning evidenced by repeated and escalating loss of cognitive or volitional control over his or her actions and is not receiving such care as is essential for his or her health or safety;[3]

3. *likelihood of serious harm* refers to (a) a substantial risk that physical harm will be inflicted by an individual upon his or her own person, as evidenced by threats or attempts to commit suicide or inflict physical harm on one's self; (b) a substantial risk that physical harm will be inflicted by an individual upon another, as evidenced by behavior that has caused such harm or that places another person or persons in reasonable fear of sustaining such harm; or (c) a substantial risk that physical harm will be inflicted by an individual upon the property of

---

2. WAC 275-55-020(17). The developmentally disabled, senile, or those impaired by chronic alcoholism or drug abuse shall not be judicially committed by reason of that condition unless the condition causes a person to be gravely disabled or, as a result of a mental disorder, the condition has caused a danger to self or others. RCW 71.05.040.

3. RCW 71.05.020(1). The state must demonstrate through recent, tangible evidence that serious physical harm will occur to the person because his or her significant loss of cognitive or volitional control creates an inability to provide for the essential human needs of food, clothing, shelter, and medical treatment. Weight loss, poor hygiene, delusions and disorganized thinking, losses of cognitive or volitional control immediately before and during the hospital stay, and the probability that if released the person would likely decompensate rapidly were sufficient to find grave disability. In re LaBelle, 107 Wash.2d 196 (1986).

others, as evidenced by behavior that has caused loss or damage to the property of others;[4]

4. *designated county mental health professional (DCMHP)* refers to a person appointed by the county to investigate whether to file a petition for initial detention;[5]

5. *detention* occurs when a person is held in a facility involuntarily pursuant to applicable sections of Chapter 71.05 RCW, and the person not being permitted willful physical movement beyond the facility without express prior permission;[6]

6. *emergency detention* occurs when a person is taken into an evaluation or treatment facility without prior notice of the proceedings for detention, usually by a police officer, because reasonable cause exists to believe that the person is suffering from a mental disorder and presents an imminent likelihood of serious harm to others or to self or is in imminent danger because of being gravely disabled;[7]

7. *initial detention* refers to the first 72-hour period required by a petition for initial detention, emergency detention, or a supplementary petition for initial detention that shall be computed to start on the time and date on which the facility accepts the person to be detained, but excludes Saturdays, Sundays, and holidays;[8]

8. *less restrictive alternative to treatment* means that, in considering all petitions for involuntary treatment, the professional person in charge of the inpatient facility must consider whether better or equal treatment could be provided by outpatient or other forms of residential treatment within the patient's community;[9] and

---

4. RCW 71.05.020(3). Involuntary treatment of someone who has committed no crime, functions reasonably well, and poses no threat to self or others, in spite of some degree of mental illness, was found to violate fundamental liberty interests unless the person was found to be dangerous. In re Levias, 83 Wash.2d 253, 517 P.2d 588 (1973). The finding that the person is likely to commit serious harm is indicated by behavior that has caused harm or creates a reasonable apprehension of harm, although a showing of imminent danger is required only for emergency detention. In re Harris, 98 Wash.2d 276, 654 P.2d 109 (1982). A recent overt act must have caused the harm or created the reasonable apprehension of harm. A husband threatening to kill an ex-husband if the wife left their marriage, coupled with his repeatedly ordering their two young children to sit on a teeter-totter while he abruptly jumped off to cause them to fall, was sufficient substantial evidence of recent overt dangerous acts. In re Meistrell, 47 Wash. App. 100 (1987).
5. WAC 275-55-020(6).
6. WAC 275-55-020(19); RCW 71.05.150.
7. RCW 71.05.150(2),(3), and (4).
8. WAC 275-55-020(20) and (21).
9. WAC 275-55-301.

9. *conditional release* refers to a transfer of an involuntary patient from inpatient to outpatient treatment, pursuant to conditions specified by the facility while remaining under the order of commitment.[10]

(B) Involuntary Treatment May Not Be Used for Certain Persons

Persons who are disabled because of mental retardation, cerebral palsy, epilepsy, autism, or other neurological condition closely related to mental retardation that has originated before their 18th birthday and is expected to continue indefinitely also may be detained under the laws of this Chapter.[11] However, they shall not be detained for evaluation and treatment solely because of that condition. Such a condition also must cause a person to be gravely disabled or, because of a mental disorder, to be likely to commit serious harm to self or others.[12]

(C) Initiation of Involuntary Treatment

Most involuntary commitments originate when the DCMHPs, who after receiving information that the person refuses treatment and is mentally ill and gravely disabled or a danger to self or others,[13] will file a petition for initial detention.[14] The DCMHP must personally interview the person in question (unless the person refuses), evaluate the reliability and credibility of the informant(s) who provided the information about the person, and find that the person will not seek voluntary treatment.[15]

From the petition, a judge of the Superior Court will determine whether, because of a mental disorder, the person is gravely disabled or a danger to self or others, and whether the person has refused to accept appropriate evaluation and treatment voluntar-

---

10. WAC 275-55-020(28).
11. Developmentally Disabled Persons, RCW 71A.10.015.
12. RCW 71.05.040. This standard also applies to the senile, the chronic alcoholic or drug abuse impaired person. Sexual psychopaths may be committed to treatment at facilities run by the DSHS; *see* chapter 5D.25, Services for Sexual Offenders.
13. Any person alleging in good faith that a person should be involuntarily committed shall not be civilly or criminally liable. RCW 71.05.500.
14. RCW 71.05.150(1)(a).
15. *Id.*

ily.[16] If necessary, the judge will order the person to appear within 24 hours to a designated evaluation and treatment facility for an evaluation.[17] The person usually will be permitted to remain within the community before the time of the evaluation. The order also will contain a designated attorney appointed to represent the person.[18]

During the evaluation, unless the presence of others would present a safety risk or interfere with the evaluation, one or more relatives, friends, an attorney, a personal physician, or other professional advisors can remain present.[19] After the order has been served on the person or the person's guardian, the DCMHP must schedule a probable cause hearing to be held within 72 hours of the date and time of the outpatient evaluation or inpatient detention for evaluation.[20]

If the person fails to appear on or before the date specified in the order, the facility must immediately notify the DCMHP.[21] The DCMHP may notify the police to take the person into custody for initial detention in the evaluation and treatment facility designated within the order.[22]

(C)(1) Emergency Detention

If a DCMHP concludes that the person, as a result of a mental disorder, presents an imminent likelihood of serious danger to self or others or is in imminent danger because of being gravely disabled, the person may be detained in emergency custody for 72 hours.[23]

In addition, a police officer may immediately deliver a person for evaluation and treatment when reasonable cause exists to believe that the person is suffering from a mental disorder and presents an imminent likelihood of serious harm to self or others or is in imminent danger because of being gravely disabled.[24] A person delivered to a facility under such circumstances may be

---

16. RCW 71.05.150(1)(b).
17. *Id.* Procedural due process safeguards are violated unless, in nonemergency situations, a judge finds that a substantial likelihood of physical harm would occur to the person or others as a result of the mental disorder, and that the DCMHP has sufficiently investigated and documented this probability while showing that all less restrictive means to detention have been exhausted. In re Harris, 98 Wash.2d 276, 654 P.2d 109 (1982).
18. *Id.*
19. *Id.*
20. RCW 71.05.150(1)(c). The 72-hour initial detention for inpatient evaluation begins when the facility accepts the petition and the person, not when the person is actually admitted. Matter of Swanson, 115 Wash.2d 21, 793 P.2d 962 (1990).
21. RCW 71.05.150(1)(d).
22. *Id.*
23. RCW 71.05.150(2).
24. RCW 71.05.150(4).

held for only 12 hours. An MHP must examine the person within three hours, and the DCMHP must file a supplemental petition for detention within 12 hours, with service also being made on the designated attorney for the person.[25]

(D) Fourteen-Day Commitment

Unless the person is released or voluntarily seeks treatment within 72 hours, the process will continue. Before the probable cause hearing and during the initial detention for evaluation and treatment, the person and, if possible, a responsible member of the immediate family or guardian must be notified that[26]

1. a hearing shall be held within 72 hours after the initial detention to decide whether probable cause exists to extend the detention to 14 days because the mental disorder presents a likelihood of serious harm to self or others or whether the person is gravely disabled;

2. the person has a right to communicate immediately with an attorney and, if the person is indigent, an attorney will be appointed to represent the person before and at the probable cause hearing;[27]

3. the person has the right to remain silent,[28] but any statement made by the person may be used as evidence;

4. the person may present evidence and cross examine witnesses who testify against him; and

5. the person may refuse all but emergency life-saving treatment beginning 24 hours before the probable cause hearing.

(D)(1) Evaluation and Outcome

Within 24 hours of initial detention, the person must be examined and evaluated by a licensed physician[29] and an MHP who will provide expert testimony about the patient at the hearing.[30] At the end of the 72-hour period, the detained person must be re-

---

25. RCW 71.05.150(5).
26. RCW 71.05.200(1).
27. The attorney rather than the guardian or guardian *ad litem* (if either is serving) becomes the principal representative of the person during the evaluation and adjudication process. In re Quesnell, 83 Wash.2d 224 (1973).
28. No inference of mental illness may be drawn from the person's deciding not to testify at the hearing. Dunner v. McLaughlin, 100 Wash.2d 832 (1984).
29. Note that a board-certified psychiatrist need not be present at the evaluation.
30. Defined as a psychiatrist, licensed physician, licensed psychologist, psychiatric nurse, a person with a masters degree, or a certified social worker. WAC 275-55-020 (33).

leased unless ordered to be held further because of the outcome of the probable cause hearing or the person voluntary consents to additional treatment.[31] The detained person or the attorney may postpone the hearing for an additional 48 hours.[32]

If, after the evaluation, the physician and the MHP decide that the person would be served better by placement in an alcohol treatment facility, the person shall be referred to an approved alcohol treatment facility.[33] If the physical condition of the person requires hospitalization, the person shall be transferred for appropriate treatment, and notice shall be given to the court, the attorney for the person, and the DCMHP; the court shall order a continuance of the proceedings as may be necessary but not for longer than 14 days.[34]

(D)(2) Procedures of 14-Day Commitment Probable Cause Hearing

A person may be detained for an additional 14 days (or 90 days of a less restrictive alternative to involuntary intensive treatment) if the following conditions are met:

1. testimony shows that because of the person's mental illness, the person is gravely disabled, or a danger to self or others exists;

2. the person requires treatment and has not volunteered for treatment;

3. a petition for a longer period of treatment has been signed by two physicians (or one physician and an MHP) who have examined the person and have found that the above conditions exist, and that a less restrictive alternative to detention was inappropriate for specifically stated reasons, or that a less restrictive alternative to detention was supported by specifically stated facts with the facility designated to provide treatment having agreed to assume the responsibility; and

4. a copy of the petition is served on the detained person, the attorney, and guardian within 12 hours after the person has been detained for evaluation.[35]

---

31. RCW 71.05.210.
32. RCW 71.05.240.
33. RCW 71.05.210. *See* chapter 5E.5, Voluntary Admission and Involuntary Comitment of Alcoholics and Drug Addicts.
34. *Id.*
35. RCW 71.05.230.

If the court finds, by a preponderance of the evidence,[36] that the person suffers from a mental disorder that causes a grave disability or presents a likelihood of resulting in serious harm to self or others, and that no less restrictive alternative to detention would meet the best interests of the person or others, then the court may order a 14-day commitment to a certified facility.[37] If treatment by less restrictive means is found to be in the best interests of the person or others, the court may order an appropriate less restrictive course of treatment that will not exceed 90 days.[38]

Along with the due process rights mentioned earlier, the person may present evidence, cross examine witnesses, remain silent, and view and copy all petitions and reports filed in court.[39] At this hearing and noted in writing, the person shall be informed by the court that, if additional involuntary treatment is sought beyond the 14-day detention or the 90-day less restrictive course of treatment, the person would retain a right to another full hearing or jury trial.[40]

Release from the commitment must occur at the end of the initial period if, in the opinion of the professional in charge of the treatment facility or the designee, the person no longer forms a likelihood of serious harm to self or others, or is no longer gravely disabled. Release from commitment also will occur if the person accepts voluntary treatment.[41]

(E) Additional Confinement

At the end of the 14-day period, a person may be confined for further treatment if the following statutory elements are met:

1. the mental disorder continues to cause grave disability or a likelihood of serious harm to self or others;
2. after being taken into custody for evaluation and treatment, the person has threatened, attempted, or inflicted physical

---

36. Due process requires a different burden of proof for the various lengths of commitment. A preponderance of the evidence standard that applies to hearings regarding 14-day detention was deemed sufficient by the court when coupled with the other due process protections, such as the right to be represented by an attorney, etc. In re LaBelle, 107 Wash.2d 196, 728 P.2d 138 (1986).
37. *Id.*
38. *Id.*
39. RCW 71.05.250.
40. RCW 71.05.240. A jury verdict does not have to be unanimous in an involuntary commitment proceeding. Due process guaranties are satisfied when a verdict is reached by 10 members of a 12-member jury or 5 members of a 6-member jury. Dunner v. McLaughlin, 100 Wash.2d 832 (1984).
41. RCW 71.05.260(1).

harm on self or others or substantial damage to the property of others because of a mental disorder; or

3. the person is incompetent to stand trial for acts forming a felony (but the charges have been dismissed because of the incompetency)[42] and meets the conditions required for civil involuntary commitment.[43]

(E)(1) Procedures for the Additional Commitment Hearing

The professional in charge of the facility, or the designee, or the DCMHP must petition the Superior Court for an order requiring the person to undergo additional 90-day treatment within three days of the expiration of the 14-day detention.[44] The petition must summarize the facts that support the need for more confinement and must be supported by the affidavits of two physicians (or a physician and an MHP) that describe in detail the behavior of the person that supports the petition, and what, if any, less restrictive alternative treatment to confinement is available to the person.[45]

At the filing of the petition, the clerk must notify the DCMHP and set a time for the person to appear before the court on the next judicial day, unless such an appearance is waived by the person's attorney.[46] As soon as possible, it is the DCMHP's responsibility to provide a copy of the petition to the person detained, his or her attorney, the guardian or conservator, and the prosecuting attorney.[47] The purpose of the appearance is to advise the person of the right to be represented by an attorney and to have the matter tried before a jury; if requested, the court also must appoint a reasonably available physician or psychologist designated by the detained person to testify on his or her behalf.[48] Within five judicial days after the appearance described in the above paragraph, the court must conduct a hearing. At the hearing, the court will decide whether 90 days of additional treatment are necessary. The matter may be continued for good cause at the request

---

42. RCW 71.05.280(3). The charges have been dismissed pursuant to RCW 10.77.090(3). A petition for a 180-day commitment may be filed without the person serving an initial detention or a 14-day detention. In re Harris, 94 Wash.2d 430, 617 P.2d 739 (1980); In re Patterson, 90 Wash.2d 144, 579 P.2d 1335 (1978). Before a person who has been committed under this provision may be released because a petition for an additional period of detention was not filed, the prosecuting attorney in the county in which the alleged felony occurred must be given a 30-day written notice about the release; such a notice must be sent even if the person is permitted to leave the facility temporarily. RCW 71.05.325.
43. RCW 71.05.280.
44. RCW 71.05.300.
45. RCW 71.05.290(2).
46. RCW 71.05.300.
47. *Id.*
48. *Id.*

of the person or his or her attorney (the continuance may not exceed five judicial days).[49]

If a jury trial is requested, the trial shall commence within 10 judicial days.[50] In addition to all of the due process safeguards listed above, the prosecutor must prove by clear, cogent, and convincing evidence[51] that further involuntary treatment is required because the person suffers from a mental disorder that causes a grave disability or presents a likelihood of resulting in serious harm to self or others, and that no less restrictive alternative to detention would meet the best interests of the person or others.[52] If these statutory elements have been proven, the period of treatment may not exceed 90 additional days.[53]

If no order is received within 30 days after the filing of the petition (not including the time of the person's continuances), the person shall be released.[54] After 90 days, the person is to be released from involuntary commitment unless another petition is filed and heard in court.

The court may order the person returned for an additional period of treatment not to exceed 180 days if the statutory elements described above are proven.[55] The person must be released unless successive periods of 180 day commitments are each proven to be a necessity.[56]

At anytime during the commitment period, if the person no longer presents a likelihood of serious harm to others, the professional in charge of the facility may release the person after notifying the court that committed the person.[57] However, before a detained person who has been declared incompetent to stand trial for a felony may be released,[58] the prosecuting attorney from the county in which the alleged felony occurred must be given a 30-day written notice about the release. Within 20 days of receiving the notice, the prosecuting attorney may petition the court to

---

49. RCW 71.05.310.
50. *Id.*
51. *Id.* The standard jury instruction need not suggest that the burden of proof by clear, cogent, and convincing evidence is much closer to beyond a reasonable doubt than the standard of the preponderance of the evidence. Matter of McLaughlin, 100 Wash.2d 832, 676 P.2d 444 (1984).
52. RCW 71.05.320(1).
53. RCW 71.05.320(1). If the incompetent person was unable to stand trial for a felony charge but meets the statutory conditions for commitment, less restrictive treatment could extend to 180 days.
54. RCW 71.05.310.
55. RCW 71.05.320(2).
56. *Id.*
57. RCW 71.05.330(1).
58. These following procedures also would apply if the person incompetent to stand trial were to gain a conditional release. *See* the next section of this chapter for more details about conditional release requirements.

review the decision.[59] Within 10 days, the court must decide whether the person remains a substantial danger to others or is likely to commit other felonious acts.[60] Unless the court finds substantial evidence to deny the early release, the person must be released.[61]

(F) Less Restrictive Alternative Treatment or Conditional Release

The following grounds and procedures apply both to less restrictive treatments and to conditional releases.[62] The person may be released early, contingent upon the person continuing with outpatient treatment, and the outpatient program agrees to assume such a responsibility. A copy of the condition(s) required of the person will be sent to the program, the DCMHP of the program's county, and the court of original commitment.[63] In addition, if the county in which the person is to receive outpatient treatment is the same in which the alleged felony occurred, the prosecuting attorney may transfer the hearing to the court within that county.[64]

Conditions for continued release may be modified as required if in the best interest of the person, and notification has been sent to all parties.[65]

The person may fail to follow the conditions of the release or the person's functioning may deteriorate substantially. At that point, the DCMHP or the secretary of DSHS may order the person apprehended and detained for a period of up to five days until a hearing can be scheduled to decide whether the person requires further detention.[66] Written notice must be provided of all the grounds that will be relied upon at the hearing to revoke the conditional release.[67]

---

59. RCW 71.05.330(2).
60. *Id.*
61. *Id.*
62. RCW 71.05.340(5).
63. RCW 71.05.340(1).
64. *Id.*
65. RCW 71.05.340(2). Notice must be provided to the person so that the change in the conditions can be contested. In re Cross, 99 Wash.2d 373, 662 P.2d 828 (1983).
66. RCW 71.05.340(3). In re Cross, 99 Wash.2d 373, 662 P.2d 828 (1983) upheld that the only basis for revoking or modifying an order for treatment less restrictive than involuntary treatment is a finding that the person violated a condition of the release. The hearing can be scheduled without detaining the person. RCW 71.05.340(4).
67. *Id.*

The court shall decide whether the person followed the conditions, whether the person's functioning has deteriorated substantially, and if either occurred, whether the person should be returned for further detention or for further outpatient treatment with modified conditions.[68] This hearing may be waived if all parties involved in the process agree to the waiver, and the person continues in treatment.[69] In case of revocation, the subsequent treatment period may be no longer than the period established in the original court order.[70]

(G) Additional Rights of the Involuntarily Detained Person

Involuntarily treated persons must be advised of all their rights,[71] both orally and in writing, including rights[72] to adequate care and individualized treatment; to wear their own clothes and to keep and use personal possessions; to keep and spend a reasonable amount of money while hospitalized; to individual storage space for private use; to receive visitors at reasonable times; to have reasonable access to a telephone to make and receive confidential calls; to have ready access to writing materials and stamps to send and receive uncensored correspondence; to send written communications about admission, evaluation, or treatment during detention; to refuse electroconvulsant therapy, surgery, or antipsychotic medications unless ordered by the court;[73] to avoid psychosurgery under any circumstance; to dispose of property and sign contracts unless adjudicated incompetent and not be presumed incompetent as a consequence of receiving evaluation and treatment; to object to detention and request release; to access to an attorney and the judicial process; and to have all information remain confidential.

No person shall be presumed incompetent or lose any civil rights as a consequence of being evaluated or treated voluntarily or involuntarily for a mental disorder.[74] A separate hearing must occur to declare someone incompetent and to appoint a guardian, if such a finding is made.[75]

---

68. *Id.*
69. *Id.*
70. RCW 71.05.340(6).
71. WAC 275-55-211.
72. WAC 275-55-241.
73. *See* chapter 6.2, Right to Refuse Treatment. RCW 71.05.215 establishes specific rules that limit the right to refuse antipsychotic medicine.
74. RCW 71.05.450; *see* In re Quesnell, 83 Wash.2d 224 (1973).
75. *See* chapter 5A.2, Guardianship for Adults.

(H) Confidentiality and Privilege

The fact of admission and all information and records compiled during voluntary or involuntary treatment at either a public or private agency shall be confidential.[76] Information and records may be disclosed under the following circumstances:[77]

1. in communications among professionals who are meeting the requirements of Chapter 71.05 RCW but not to professionals who lack a connection with the evaluating or treating facility except to a professional with medical responsibility for the patient, the DCMHP, or those who are providing services under the Community Mental Health Services Act, Chapter 71.24 RCW;

2. when the communications regard the special needs of the patient, and circumstances arise in which communications about the needs are necessary;[78]

3. when the person receiving services, or the guardian of the person, designates persons to whom the information may be released;

4. to the extent necessary to further a person' claim for aid, insurance, or medical assistance to which the person may be entitled;

5. for program evaluation or research that follows the rules established by the secretary of the DSHS;

6. to the courts as is necessary under this Chapter;

7. to law enforcement officers, public health officers, or corrections personnel if the person is committed to the custody of the Department of Corrections but only about the fact, place, and date of involuntary admission and the date of discharge to the last known address;[79]

8. to the attorney of the person;

9. to the prosecuting attorney, as necessary, about the treatment, prognosis, medication, behavior problems, and other records relevant to the person being released on conditional release; and

---

76. RCW 71.05.390.
77. Id.
78. In particular, this applies to the developmentally disabled patient.
79. Greater dissemination of information is allowed for persons committed under RCW 71.05.280(3) and .320(2)(c); after the dismissal of a sex offense; or if the patient and counsel believe that the release of information is necessary and upon a showing of clear, cogent, and convincing evidence.

10. to appropriate law enforcement agencies and to the reasonably identifiable victim about an actual threat of physical violence.

Any disclosure, the reason for the disclosure, and to whom the information was disclosed shall be documented within the patient's record.[80]

An additional limitation on a patient's right to confidentiality occurs if the patient refuses antipsychotic medications, and the court is called upon to decide whether such medications are necessary. Then, both the physician–patient privilege or the psychologist–client privilege is deemed waived.[81] As to all other hearings that arise under the laws regulating involuntary treatment,[82] the court may decide that a waiver of privilege is necessary to protect either the detained person or the public and order testimony from the professionals.[83] The waiver is limited to records or testimony that may prove that the person requires involuntary treatment; upon motion of the person or on its own motion, the court shall decide whether a record or testimony is within the scope of the waiver.[84]

(H)(1) Person Committed Following Dismissal of Sex or Violent Offense[85]—Notification of Conditional Discharge, Leave, Transfer, or Escape

At the earliest possible date and no later than 10 days before a conditional release, final discharge, leave, or transfer to a less restrictive facility than a state mental hospital, the superintendent shall send written notice about the intended occurrence to[86] the chief of police of the city and the sheriff of the county in which the person will reside, the victims or the witnesses of the sex or violent crime who have requested that such a notice be given in writing, or any other person specified in writing by the prosecuting attorney. The identity of the persons receiving such notices will not be disclosed to the committed person.[87]

If a person is committed following dismissal of a sex or violent offense escapes, the superintendent shall inform, by the most expedient means possible, the chief of police of the city and the sheriff of the county in which the person resided; if previously requested, the superintendent will also inform the witness(es),

---

80. *Id.*
81. RCW 71.05.215 and RCW 71.05.250.
82. In re LaBelle, 107 Wash.2d 196, 728 P.2d 138 (1986).
83. *Id.*
84. *Id.*
85. A sex or violent offense is defined by RCW 9.94A.030.
86. RCW 71.05.420.
87. *Id.*

the victim(s), and the victim's spouse, parents, siblings, and children, if the crime was a homicide.[88]

If the person is recaptured, the superintendent must renotify, within two days, all those who received the earlier notification.[89] The superintendent shall also notify the guardian or parent of any escapee who is under the age of 16 years.[90]

(H)(2) Limitations on Confidentiality to Increase the Continuum of Care

A number of new statutes relating to confidentiality became effective July 1, 1995 or when regional support networks[91] were established to increase the continuum of care. Treatment records of the person may be released without informed consent in the following circumstances:[92]

1. for program monitoring or evaluation;

2. when necessary for billing or collection purposes;

3. for purposes of research as permitted in Chapter 42.48 RCW;

4. under lawful order of a court;

5. to those responsible for deciding whether the person should be transferred to a less restrictive or more appropriate treatment modality or facility;

6. within the treatment facility, to those trainees or volunteers at the facility when necessary to the performance of their duties;

7. whenever necessary to coordinate the treatment of mental illness, developmental disability, alcoholism or drug abuse of a patient;

8. to a licensed physician who has determined that the life or health of the person is in danger, and that treatment without the information contained in the records could be injurious to the person's health;

9. to programs that admit the person, but the records shall be limited to a summary of previous somatic treatments, a discharge summary that may include a statement of the person's problem, the treatment goals, the type of treatment provided to date, and recommendations for future treatment; and

---

88. *Id.*
89. *Id.*
90. *Id.*
91. The legislature intended that the procedures and services authorized under Chapter 71.05 RCW be integrated with those of Chapter 71.24 RCW to maximize the continuum of care to the mentally ill. Under this latter chapter, the county authorities are to enter into operating agreements to provide a complete range of residential programs and services for adults and children who are chronically, acutely, or severely mentally ill.
92. RCW 71.05.630(2).

10. to staff members of the protection and advocacy agency or nonprofit corporation protecting and advocating the rights of a person with mental illness or developmental disabilities.

Following discharge, the detained person shall have a right to a complete record of somatic treatments prescribed and a copy of the discharge summary.[93] Each time in which written information is released from a treatment record, the patient shall have access to the release data, and a notation with the following information must be entered into the record:[94] the name to whom the information was released, the type of information released, the purpose of the release, and the date of the release.

(H)(3) Penalties for Violating Confidentiality

If the confidentiality of a person is violated, the statutes provide an action for unauthorized release of confidential information. Any person may bring a personal injury action against an individual who has willfully released confidential information for the greater of the following amounts:[95] $1,000 or three times the amount of actual damages sustained.

---

93. RCW 71.05.640(2).
94. RCW 71.05.650.
95. RCW 71.05.440.

5E.5

Voluntary Admission and Involuntary Commitment of Alcoholics and Drug Addicts

In 1972, the Uniform Alcoholism and Intoxication Treatment Act, Chapter 70.96A RCW, decriminalized alcoholism.[1] Rather than jailing untreated alcoholics and addicts, a continuum of care was established so that victims of these diseases could receive services from[2]

1. free-standing detoxification centers;[3]
2. inpatient treatment centers;
3. recovery houses for those requiring additional support after inpatient care;
4. long-term treatment centers and shelters for the more severely debilitated, chronic addicts;
5. a secure treatment center for alcoholics committed involuntarily; and
6. outpatient treatment for those not requiring residential services or those wishing aftercare support.

In 1987, the Alcohol and Drug Addiction Treatment and Support Act (ADATSA), Chapter 74.50 RCW, established the process of providing treatment to those alcoholics and addicts who were using their welfare grants to purchase more alcohol and drugs;

---

1. Aripa v. Department of Social and Health Services, 91 Wash.2d 135 (1978) noted that the legislature attempted to prohibit the use of penal facilities for treatment of people afflicted with alcoholism.
2. Division of Alcohol and Substance Abuse (May, 1990), Report on Detoxification and Involuntary Treatment for Alcoholics and Other Drug Dependent Persons in Washington State.
3. Jailing increases the risk of death due to withdrawal and medical complications.

during the outpatient phase of ADATSA, clients could receive a monitored living stipend to assist them while they reentered the work force.[4] Finally, in 1989, Chapter 70.96A RCW was amended extensively[5] to provide the same continuum of care to the drug addict population; to enable law enforcement and alcohol/drug program staff to take persons incapacitated by drugs other than alcohol and to detain them in protective custody until no longer incapacitated for a maximum of 72 hours; and to commit involuntarily an alcoholic who is gravely disabled by alcohol and some other drug. MHPs may evaluate and treat dual disordered clients of alcohol and drug treatment programs. They also may refer their clients to such programs.

(A) Terms and Definitions

The following definitions are used by the statutes or administrative code and apply to voluntary admission and involuntary commitment of alcoholics:

1. *alcoholic* is a person who suffers from the disease of alcoholism;[6]

2. *alcoholism* is a disease characterized by a dependency on alcoholic beverages, loss of control over the amount and circumstances of use, symptoms of tolerance, physiological or psychological withdrawal if use is reduced or discontinued, and impairment of health or disruption of social or economic functioning;[7]

3. *chemical dependency* refers to alcoholism or drug addiction, or to a dependence on alcohol and on one or more other psychoactive chemicals;[8]

4. *designated chemical dependency specialist (DCDS)* is a person designated by the county alcoholism and other drug addiction program coordinator to perform the commitment duties;[9]

5. *drug addict* is a person who suffers from the disease of drug addiction;[10]

6. *drug addiction* refers to a disease characterized by a dependency on psychoactive chemicals, loss of control over the

---

4. *Id.*
5. *Id.*
6. RCW 71.96A.020.
7. *Id.*
8. *Id.*
9. *Id.*
10. *Id.*

amount and circumstances of use, symptoms of tolerance, physiological or psychological withdrawal if use is reduced or discontinued, and impairment of health or disruption of social or economic functioning;[11]

7. *gravely disabled by alcohol or other drugs* means that a person, because of the use of alcohol or other drugs, (a) is in danger of serious physical harm resulting from a failure to provide for his or her essential human needs of health or safety; or (b) manifests severe deterioration in routine functioning evidenced by a repeated and escalating loss of cognition or volitional control over his or her actions and is not receiving the care essential for his or her health or safety;[12]

8. *incapacitated by alcohol or other psychoactive chemicals* refers to persons whose judgment is so impaired by the use of alcohol or other psychoactive chemicals that they are incapable of realizing and making a rational decision with regard to their need for treatment and constitutes a danger to self, others, or property;[13] and

9. *treatment* refers to the broad range of emergency, detoxification, residential, and outpatient services and care, including diagnostic evaluation; chemical dependency education and counseling; medical, psychiatric, psychological, and social service care; and vocational rehabilitation and career counseling that may be extended to alcoholics and other drug addicts and their families.[14]

(B) Standards for Guiding Efficacious Treatment

The legislature directed the secretary of the DSHS to establish rules that would ensure that an alcoholic or drug addict would be[15] treated voluntarily rather than involuntarily; treated by an outpatient facility unless found to require residential treatment; treated without discrimination because of withdrawal from treatment on a prior occasion against medical advice or relapsed after earlier treatment; treated as directed by a current individualized treatment plan; and provided with a continuum of coordinated

---

11. *Id.*
12. *Id.*
13. *Id.*
14. *Id.*
15. RCW 70.96A.100.

treatment services so that further treatment would be available upon completion of any particular form of treatment.

(C) Voluntary Treatment of Alcoholics or Drug Addicts

Any person 14 years of age or older may voluntarily consent to receive treatment from any of the various programs provided by the continuum of care in the state of Washington.[16] If the person is refused treatment by a program, the administrator of the program must refer the person to another program, if possible.[17] If a person leaves an approved public treatment program on or against the advice of the program's administrator, reasonable provisions for transportation to another program or to the person's home must be made.[18]

Intoxicated persons may admit themselves for treatment. If the persons are intoxicated in public and they consent to the help proffered by the authorities, they may be assisted to their home or to an approved treatment program or other health facility.[19]

(D) Involuntary Treatment

(D)(1) Emergency Detention

A person who appears incapacitated or gravely disabled by alcohol or drugs, who is in a public place, or who has threatened or inflicted harm on self or another shall be brought to a treatment program by the police or staff designated by the county for a period of time not exceeding eight hours.[20] If no treatment facility is available, then the person must be taken to an emergency medical facility.[21] Such action by the authorities is not considered to be a crime, and no record shall be made of the person being arrested or charged with a crime.[22]

---

16. RCW 70.96A.095. The parent(s) or legal guardian of a patient younger than 18 years of age is not liable for the payment of care for the patient unless he or she also has consented to the care provided by the program.
17. RCW 70.96A.110.
18. *Id.* If the person has no home, he or she must be assisted in obtaining shelter.
19. RCW 70.96A.120(1).
20. RCW 70.96A.120(2).
21. *Id.*
22. *Id.* This standard applies when the intoxicated person has been apprehended for a crime, unless the crime is not related to the intoxication or the person was operating a motor vehicle.

After examination by a qualified person, the person may be admitted as a patient or, if necessary, referred to another facility for emergency medical treatment.[23] The referring program must arrange for transportation.[24]

A person who is found to be incapacitated or gravely disabled by alcohol or drugs, at or after the admission to a program, may not be detained for more than 72 hours unless an involuntary commitment petition is filed, or the person consents to remain in the program.[25]

(D)(2) Petition for Involuntary Commitment

In the state of Washington, only adults who are incapacitated by alcoholism and minors who are incapacitated by alcoholism and/or other drug addiction may be committed involuntarily.[26] When the DCDS receives information that such incapacitation exists, and an investigation shows the allegations to be reliable, the DCDS may file a petition with either the Superior or the District Court.[27] If the DCDS believes that the needs of the person would be served better within the mental health system, commitment may be pursued through either Chapter 71.05 RCW or 71.34 RCW.[28]

If treatment is available and appropriate, the petition must allege one or more of the following conditions:[29] in the case of an adult, alcoholism and/or addiction, or detoxification or treatment for alcoholism during the previous 12 months; in the case of a minor, alcoholism and/or drug addiction, prior detoxification or treatment; and in the the case of an adult or minor, threats, attempts, or infliction of physical harm on another person or the likelihood of inflicting harm unless committed. A refusal to enter treatment does not constitute sufficient evidence about lack of judgment concerning the need for treatment.[30]

Unless the person whose commitment is sought has refused to be examined medically, the petition is to be accompanied by the findings of a licensed physician that supports the allegations of the petition. The medical examination of the person must occur within five days before submission of the petition.[31] If the person

---

23. RCW 70.96A.120(3).
24. *Id.*
25. RCW 70.96A.120(4). The 72-hour period does not include week end days or holidays.
26. RCW 70.96A.140(1).
27. *Id.*
28. *Id.* These are the chapters that regulate involuntary commitment of adults and minors. *See* chapter 5E.4, Involuntary Civil Admission of Mentally Ill Adults.
29. *Id.*
30. *Id.*
31. *Id.*

has refused to be examined, and sufficient evidence exists at the hearing to affirm that the allegations in the petition are true, the court may order the person's commitment for five days to obtain more medical evidence.[32]

(D)(3) Involuntary Treatment Hearing

If the person is being detained at a treatment program, a hearing must be held within 72 hours, otherwise the hearing will occur two to seven days after the petition has been filed.[33] The date of the hearing may be extended upon a showing of good cause by a motion from the person whose commitment is sought or with the person's permission.[34] The DCDS shall serve a copy of the petition, the notice of the hearing, and the medical report on any person the court believes should be notified.[35]

At the hearing, all relevant testimony may be heard with information otherwise deemed privileged becoming accessible if the court finds that a waiver is necessary to protect either the detained person or the public.[36] The waiver is limited to records or testimony about the evaluation of the detained person.[37] Testimony may be by telephone.[38] However, any opinions about whether the person is an alcoholic or, in the case of a minor, an alcohol/drug addict, must be deleted from the record unless the person is available for cross examination.[39]

The person must be present during the hearing unless the court decides that such presence would be harmful to the person. If this is the case, a guardian *ad litem* will be appointed to represent the person's interests during the hearing.[40] The court shall order the commitment if it finds that the grounds have been established by clear, cogent, and convincing proof, and an appropriate treatment program is available.[41]

(D)(4) Additional Commitment

A person shall be committed only for 60 days unless discharged sooner.[42] At the end of the 60-day period, the person must be discharged unless another petition for recommitment is filed to

---

32. RCW 70.96A.140(3).
33. RCW 70.96A.140(2). Weekend days and holidays do not count.
34. *Id.*
35. *Id.*
36. RCW 70.96A.140(3).
37. *Id.*
38. *Id.*
39. *Id.*
40. *Id.*
41. RCW 70.96A.140(4).
42. RCW 70.96A.140(5).

detain the person for an additional 90 days.[43] Upon the filing, the court must hear the case within seven days of the filing and proceed as described earlier.[44]

(E) Less Restrictive Treatment and Conditional Releases

When in the opinion of the person in charge of the facility, the committed person can be served more appropriately by less restrictive treatment before the end of the commitment period, less restrictive treatment may be added as a condition for earlier release so long as the time in a less restrictive treatment does not exceed the period of commitment.[45]

The program that is to provide the less restrictive treatment must agree to accept such a responsibility in writing.[46] It may also modify the conditions for continued release.[47] If the person fails to follow the conditions of the release or a substantial deterioration of the patient's functioning has occurred, the DCDS shall notify the court of original commitment so that a hearing can occur within seven days to decide whether the person should be returned to the more restrictive treatment.[48]

The court will determine whether the person adhered to the conditions of the release, a substantial deterioration of the patient's functioning has occurred, and the conditions of the release should be modified or the person be returned to more restrictive treatment.[49] The hearing may be waived if all parties agree to such a waiver, and the person may be returned to involuntary treatment or be continued on a conditional release with the same or modified conditions.[50]

---

43. *Id.*
44. RCW 70.96A.140(6).
45. RCW 70.96A.140(12).
46. *Id.*
47. *Id.*
48. *Id.*
49. *Id.*
50. *Id.*

(F) All Facilities: Voluntary and Involuntary Clients' Rights

All approved treatment facilities, either public or private, shall take reasonable efforts to[51]

1. promote the client's dignity and self-respect without discriminating because of race, color, creed, national origin, religion, gender, sexual preference, age, or disability;

2. protect the client's privacy from being invaded;[52]

3. treat all clinical and personal information confidentially;

4. permit client review of own treatment records in the presence of the administrator or a designee during such times in which a treatment session would not be interrupted;

5. not deny communication with significant others in emergencies;

6. not subject clients to physical abuse, corporal punishment by facility staff or be denied food, clothing, or other necessities;

7. receive a copy of the facility's client grievance procedures;

8. instruct ADATSA recipients that they may report back to a community service office in the case of disciplinary discharge from treatment, and that they may request a hearing to challenge any departmental action that affects eligibility for ADATSA treatment or shelter assistance; and

9. receive a copy of these rights at admission and in the case of a disciplinary discharge.

(G) Additional Rights of the Involuntarily Committed

The court shall inform the involuntarily committed that, at every stage of the proceedings, they have a right to legal counsel or to appointed counsel if they are unable to obtain counsel.[53] If the court believes that they require counsel, the court will appoint counsel regardless of their wishes.[54] These patients also have the right to be examined by a physician of their own choosing.[55]

---

51. WAC 275-19-075.
52. Reasonable searches may be made for contraband being possessed and used on the premises.
53. RCW 70.96A.140(9).
54. Id.
55. Id.

(H) All Facilities: Confidentiality and Record Keeping Requirements

Registration and treatment records shall remain confidential except for the following limitations:[56]

1. according to the prior written consent of the person for whom such a record is maintained;

2. if authorized by an appropriate court order;

3. to comply with state laws mandating the reporting of suspected child abuse or neglect; and

4. when a person commits a crime on program premises or against program personnel or threatens to do so.

Outpatient and residential treatment facilities shall conduct intake interviews with each client that will collect the following information:[57]

1. a history about the volume, frequency, type, duration (date of first and last use) of each drug use, and involvement with alcohol;

2. a history about previous alcohol and drug treatment;

3. a medical history;

4. a description of the client's most recent living situation, genetic predispositions to chemical dependence, employment history, educational history, significant life events (e.g. moves, losses, and sexual or physical abuse or neglect); and

5. a history of the client's legal history.

On the basis of these data, a written assessment statement must include[58]

1. a diagnosis of the type of substances used and the degree of progression in the disease, if a diagnosis of alcoholism or other addiction is determined, and the signs and symptoms that prove the diagnosis;

2. a prognosis statement that will address the patient's motivation, the ability to maintain abstinence, the level of social support from family, friends, and employer, the physical and mental health status (a summation of the patient's assessment will be included), and the strengths and weaknesses as perceived by staff and the patient himself; and

---

56. RCW 70.96A.150.
57. WAC 275-19-165.
58. *Id.*

3. the treatment recommendations, including the modality and length of the treatment.

(H)(1) HIV/AIDS Intervention

An HIV/AIDS brief, risk intervention must occur with each client during which the patient's risk for HIV acquisition and transmission is assessed, and behaviors that increase the risk are detailed; when indicated, the patient must be referred for HIV/AIDS-related services that would include HIV antibody testing and counseling.[59] The patient must be informed of the results of the assessment and of the right to be referred to an approved treatment program offering services consistent with the results.[60] The evaluation and assessment must be completed within 21 days of admission or by the third visit to an outpatient facility, and within five days for an inpatient facility.[61]

(H)(2) Treatment Plan Detail

An individual treatment plan must include the specific issues to be addressed, the objectives to be accomplished by the treatment, the time and methods to be used in achieving the objectives, and the anticipated length of treatment.[62] Minimum treatment requirements are specified:[63]

1. at least one face-to-face group or individual session must occur during each month for outpatient treatment and every week for residential treatment;

2. all group counseling must be limited to not more than 12 patients to a group;

3. no more than 20% of treatment time shall consist of film or video presentations;

4. whenever possible, the facility must involve the patient's family and friends in the treatment (such involvement must be documented within the treatment record);

5. the facility must encourage all patients and their families to participate in self-help groups (e.g., Alcoholics Anonymous, Alanon, Alateen, etc.); and

6. every 90 days, if chemotherapy is being provided, a medication evaluation must be made unless the medication is prescribed by the patient's private physician.

---

59. WAC 275-19-030(31), (33), and (34); WAC 275-19-165(3).
60. WAC 275-19-165.
61. *Id.*
62. *Id.*
63. *Id.*

Documented treatment reviews that assess the adequacy of the plan must occur once every week for inpatient treatment, once every 20 hours of client service for intensive outpatient treatment, once every two weeks for recovery house or long-term residential treatment, and once each month for outpatient and extended care recovery house.[64]

(H)(3) Aftercare

Upon completion of the course of treatment, the facility must develop an aftercare plan to assist the patient in maintaining the treatment goals, identify agencies and services that can address unresolved problems listed on the treatment plan, and provide a copy of the plan to the patient upon discharge.[65] A discharge summary must be included within the record and must summarize the patient's progress toward each of the treatment goals.[66]

---

64. *Id.*
65. *Id.*
66. *Id.*

5E.6

Services for Developmentally Disabled Persons

The legislature recognizes the capacity of the developmentally disabled to be productive and to achieve a measure of independence and fulfillment.[1] The law states that the DSHS must provide, or arrange with other providers, services that include but are not limited to[2] architectural services, case management services, early childhood intervention,[3] employment services, family counseling, family support,[4] information and referral, health ser-

---

1. RCW 71A.10.015. Chapter 74.18 RCW is legislation that promotes the economic and social welfare of blind persons or visually handicapped persons from the distress of poverty through their complete integration into society. Some developmentally disabled people also are visually handicapped, and this chapter may apply to them and provide vocational rehabilitation services, grants of equipment and material, services for independent living, services for blind children and their families, and a business enterprise program.
2. RCW 71A.12.040.
3. *See* chapter 5A.20, Education for Handicapped and Highly Capable Children.
4. WAC 275-27-220. Such services are provided to allow the person to live in the most independent setting possible. They include but are not limited to emergency or planned respite care; attendant care; physical, occupational, communication, and behavior management therapies; the purchase, rental, loan, or refurbishment of specialized equipment; and environmental modification. A service is authorized for a period of time. If the requested service is not authorized, such action is deemed to be a denial of service and may be appealed. Family support services may include help with personal care (e.g., bathing, dressing, feeding, mobility, personal hygiene); and medical support (e.g., respirator, gastrostomy). Authorization is based on the risk that, without a particular service, the person's behavior may cause physical injury to self, others, and property; the number of primary care givers available to assist the person or the family; the availability of private, local, state, or federal resources; the likelihood of out-of-home placement; the person's or the family's relative need when compared with others in like circumstances.

vices and equipment, legal services, residential services and support,[5] respite care,[6] therapy services and equipment, and vocational services. MHPs can aid in the evaluation and treatment of the developmentally disabled.

(A) Terms and Definitions

Before discussing the statutes and administrative code that regulate provision of services, it is necessary to understand the legal meanings of terms that are within the law:[7]

1. *developmental disability* refers to mental retardation, cerebral palsy, epilepsy, autism, or other neurological conditions closely related to mental retardation or requiring treatment similar to that required for mental retardation.[8] The disability must arise before the patient attains the age of 18 years, form a substantial handicap, and continue or be expected to continue indefinitely (the disabling condition may not be diagnosed solely by an intelligence quotient score);

2. *eligible person* is one who has been found eligible for services by the DSHS; and

3. *habilitation services* are those provided by program personnel to help persons in acquiring and maintaining life skills and to raise their levels of physical, mental, social, and vocational functioning (such services include education, training for employment, and therapy).

(B) State Services

The DSHS is expected to develop and coordinate state services for persons with developmental disabilities; a continuum of services

---

5. Residential programs provide domiciliary care and other services, including state residential facilities (*see* Chapter 71A.20 RCW and WAC 275-27-300), group homes (*see* Chapter 71A.22 RCW and Chapter 275-36 WAC), skilled nursing home facilities, intermediate care facilities, congregate care facilities, boarding homes, children's foster homes, adult family homes, and group training homes. *See* WAC 275-27-020(9).
6. *Respite care* refers to temporary services provided to the developmentally disabled person and/or the person's family on either an emergency or planned basis without which the person would need a more dependent program (such a program would provide less opportunity for greater frequency and variety of community contacts or require greater hours of staff supervision/training/support). WAC 275-27-020.
7. RCW 71A.10.020.
8. Auditory or visual impairment may also require treatment similar to that required for mentally retarded individuals. WAC 275-27-030.

must be established to meet the needs of each person regardless of age, degree of handicap, or stage of the person's development.[9] However, such policy is limited specifically by the extent to which state, federal, or other funds are available for providing eligible persons with such services. Minimum standards for services are established.[10]

The DSHS may pay for nonresidential services that exceed the cost of caring at home. The services must be necessary to the care, treatment, maintenance, support, and training of developmentally persons and are established by an individual service plan approved by the DSHS.[11] For those persons placed in community residential programs, the DSHS will pay for services that are not covered by the estate of the person or by any other source from which the person is entitled to receive.[12]

9. RCW 71A.12.010.
10. RCW 71A.12.020.
11. RCW 71A.12.050.
12. RCW 71A.12.070.

Hospice Care

The legislature developed law regulating home health care and hospice care. The cost of medical care in general and hospital care in particular created the need to provide less expensive and more appropriate levels of care for the terminally ill patient. As a result, palliative, rather than curative, care and treatment have become more available.[1] Such care is planned and executed to cause a reduction of physical, psychosocial, and spiritual pain and to ease the person's illness.[2] Often, the quality of the patient's life is enhanced through such care. This permits the family and the patient to face the transition to the impending death openly and with greater compassion. MHPs may assist in this process by providing evaluation and treatment services.

(A) Hospice Care Center

These health care facilities are licensed and regulated through Chapter 70.41 RCW. They are operated to provide accommodations and palliative care during a continuous period for patients who are in the latter stages of an advanced disease that is expected to lead to death.[3] The hospice shall provide short-term care for the person as an inpatient, care for the person as an outpatient as indicated in the approved plan for treatment, and respite care in

---

1. RCW 70.126.001; WAC 248-21-001.
2. WAC 248-21-002(26).
3. WAC 248-21-002(18).

the most appropriate setting for a maximum of five days per three-month period of hospice care.[4]

An interdisciplinary care team composed of the patient, the family, and the professional providers plan and provide coordinated palliative care of the patient during, between, and after treatment in the facility with emphasis on symptom management that is specific to the needs of the individual patient.[5] Core team services shall include[6] care by a physician; monitoring of nursing services by a registered nurse; psychosocial services; spiritual counseling; bereavement care to be integrated into the individualized care plan; home care as indicated in the individualized care plan; facilitation of all prescribed diagnostic, treatment, or palliative services; and translation services to simplify communication when language barriers exist.

(A)(1) Record Keeping Requirements

An adequate clinical record must be maintained on each patient and be readily accessible to members of the interdisciplinary care team.[7] Each entry shall be legible, dated, and authenticated. Such a record must be retained for no less than 10 years after the ending of services.[8]

(B) Home Health Care

Home health care is accessed by prescription from a physician. With such a prescription, a private or public home health care agency that is certified by the DSHS could provide the following:[9] delivery of services from a registered nurse, licensed practical nurse, physical therapist, respiratory therapist, social worker, and home health aid on a part-time basis; supplies and equipment such as medication, rented durable medical apparatus, oxygen, catheters, needles; ambulance service; and any other services established by the physician as medically necessary for the patient's treatment, including bereavement care for family members.[10]

---

4. RCW 70.126.030.
5. WAC 248-21-025.
6. *Id.*
7. WAC 248-21-045.
8. *Id.*
9. RCW 70.126.20.
10. *Bereavement care* refers to consultation, support, counseling, and follow up with the client and the client's family before and after the death of the patient. WAC 248-21-002(6).

Limitations on
and Liability
for Practice

6.1

Informed Consent for Services

Before beginning treatment, all MHPs must furnish a written description about their services so that the patient could be expected to understand[1]

1. the nature and character of the proposed treatment;
2. the anticipated results of the proposed treatment;
3. the recognized possible alternate forms of treatment; and
4. the recognized serious possible risks, complications,[2] and anticipated benefits involved in the treatment and the recognized possible alternate forms of treatment, including nontreatment.

A signed consent form constitutes evidence that the patient provided consent for the administered treatment.[3] The failure of providers to obtain informed consent increases the likelihood of being held liable in a malpractice suit.[4] This procedure is called for specifically under the laws regulating psychologists[5] and

---

1. RCW 7.70.060. This standard of care applies to all persons licensed to provide health care or related services. RCW 7.70.020(1). A patient may elect, in writing, not to be informed of the necessary elements of the process before consent is obtained.
2. Providers have legally mandated duties to breach confidentiality under certain circumstances. Such potential complications to treatment should be disclosed. See chapter 4.2, Confidential Relations and Communications, for details.
3. RCW 7.70.060 specifies that the patient then assumes the burden of rebutting that consent by the preponderance of the evidence.
4. RCW 7.70.050. See chapter 6.5 for necessary elements of proof.
5. RCW.18.83.115.

counselors,[6] and noncompliance creates a risk of disciplinary action.

(A) Priority of Persons to Provide Consent for Incompetent Patients

A patient who lacks the capacity to make informed decisions about caring for self by reason of mental illness, developmental disability, senility, habitual drunkenness, excessive use of drugs, or other mental infirmity may be declared incompetent by a Superior Court after a guardianship proceeding.[7] A person under the age of majority also may lack the capacity to consent.[8] A minor 13 years of age or older can legally consent to mental health services.[9] Situations may arise in which the person lacks capacity, but guardianship has not been adjudicated. Informed consent to health care can be provided by a person authorized to act on the incapacitated patient's behalf. Such a person(s) must be a member(s) of a class in the following order of priority:[10]

1. an individual to whom the patient has given a durable power of attorney that encompasses the authority to make health care decisions;

2. the patient's spouse; or

3. children of the patient.

The provider must make a reasonable effort to locate and secure authorization from a person in the first or in one of the succeeding classes with authorization being acceptable from any person(s) in the class with priority.[11]

No person may provide informed consent to health care if a person from a class with higher priority has refused authorization or if two or more individuals in the same class object.[12] In such an event, a guardianship should be pursued.[13]

---

6. RCW 18.19.060. *Counselors* are those health care professionals who obtain certification as marriage and family therapists, mental health counselors, and social workers. RCW 18.19.020.
7. RCW 11.88.010; *see* chapter 5A.2.
8. *Id.* It is recommended that health care providers evaluate and document whether the minor patient has the capacity to make informed decisions about caring for self.
9. RCW 71.34.030.
10. RCW 7.70.065(1).
11. RCW 7.70.065(2).
12. *Id.*
13. RCW 11.88.010 et seq.

Before any person(s) may exercise authority to provide informed consent on behalf of the incapacitated patient, the person(s) must first decide, in good faith, whether the patient would have consented to the proposed health care.[14] If the patient would not have consented, then the decision to proceed can be made only if it is in the patient's best interests.[15]

(B) Community Mental Health Programs

Before providing treatment to patients in this public mental health setting, the patient or responsible other must consent to treatment by signing the initial treatment plan and whenever significant changes in the plan occur.[16] If any treatment with medications occurs, consent must be obtained before medications can be used,[17] except in case of emergency.

(C) Additional Requirements for Certain Providers

Counselors and psychologists must provide the following disclosure information to their clients before the beginning of treatment:[18]

1. the purposes and resources of the disciplinary process;[19]

2. the right of clients to refuse treatment;[20]

---

14. RCW 7.70.065
15. *Id.*
16. WAC 275-56-275. In the event that the patient refuses to sign, efforts to obtain the signature must be documented. *See* chapter 4.1 for details about the extensiveness of the treatment plan.
17. WAC 275-56-265. In the event that the patient refuses to sign, efforts to obtain the signature must be documented.
18. RCW 18.19.060, Counselors; RCW 18.83.115, Psychologists.
19. *Guidelines for Disclosure*, published by the Department of Licensing (August, 1987), recommend that, at a minimum, a written explanation must indicate that the law provides a complaint/discipline option and that the client may contact the Department of Licensing (at such an address and phone number) if any complaints remain unresolved between the provider and the client.
20. *Id.*, the right to request a change of therapy, a referral to another therapist, or an ending of therapy exists.

3. the responsibility of clients for choosing the provider and treatment modality that best suits their needs;[21]

4. the extent to which client confidences may be protected;[22]

5. the relevant education and training of the provider;[23]

6. the therapeutic orientation of the practice;

7. the proposed course of treatment where known;[24] and

8. any financial requirements.[25]

In addition, counselors must indicate that, even though they are certified by the Department of Licensing, such certification does not "necessarily imply the effectiveness of any treatment."[26] All of the disclosure information must be written and discussed with the client.[27]

Providers who are employed by a medical center, hospital, community mental health center, or organization that has developed its own disclosure statement are exempted from having to provide individual disclosure statements.[28]

---

21. *Id*. The client may raise questions about the therapist and the therapeutic approach and progress.

22. *See* chapter 4.2 for details.

23. *Guidelines for Disclosure*, published by the Department of Licensing (August, 1987): the provider acquired what degree, from where, with what specialty training if a specialty practice, and obtained what particular licensure or certification.

24. *Id.*, the type of assessment and treatment to be used, when the provider will become more specific about the treatment, how and when treatment might end.

25. *Id.*, the policies about fees and missed or canceled appointments.

26. RCW 18.19.060.

27. RCW 18.19.060, Counselors; RCW 18.83.115, Psychologists.

28. WAC 308-122-630(4).

6.2

Right to Refuse Treatment

Those who seek voluntary treatment through an informed consent process may refuse treatment and seek other services (see chapter 6.1, Informed Consent for Services). In the state of Washington, the right to refuse treatment for the involuntarily committed or for those who lack capacity is addressed by statute and case law. The law restricts the nature and scope of invasive services and details the judicial or administrative procedure to follow. MHPs may be involved with the evaluation and treatment of clients who refuse treatment.

(A) Regulation of Electroconvulsive Therapy (ECT), Antipsychotic Medications[1] and Nonemergency Surgery[2] in Civil Institutions

The involuntary treatment of people who are civilly committed with ECT and psychosurgery[3] and who are using antipsychotic

---

1. Defined as the class of drugs used primarily to treat thought disorders. RCW 71.05.020(18).
2. Psychosurgery can never be performed under any circumstances. RCW 71.05.370(9).
3. In re Schuoler, 106 Wash.2d 500, 723 P.2d 1103 (1986).

medications[4] is currently regulated by statute.[5] A court of competent jurisdiction must find, by clear, cogent, and convincing evidence, that a compelling state interest justifies overriding the patient's lack of consent to such medical procedures; the proposed treatment also must be necessary and effective with no alternate form of treatment available or likely to be effective.[6]

Specific findings of fact must be entered by the lower court concerning[7] the existence of one or more compelling state interests;[8] the necessity and effectiveness of the treatment; and the person's desires regarding the proposed treatment. If the patient lacks the capacity of making an informed decision about the proposed treatment, the court can make a substituted judgment for the patient as if the patient were competent to make such a determination himself.[9]

The patient is guaranteed the following due process rights:[10]

1. to be represented by an attorney;

2. to present evidence;

3. to cross examine witnesses;

4. to have the rules of evidence enforced;

5. to remain silent;

6. to view and to copy all petitions and reports in the court file; and

7. to be given reasonable notice and an opportunity to prepare for the hearing.

In cases involving ECT, the court must appoint a psychiatrist or psychologist to testify on behalf of the patient.[11]

Antipsychotic medications may be administered to a nonconsenting patient without a court order if[12]

---

4. The law was changed for these medications because the dicta, within a case involving an inmate of the Department of Correction, appeared to extend sweeping due process protections to involuntarily committed persons. Harper v. State of Washington, 110 Wash.2d 873, 759 P.2d 358 (1988), *overruled*, 494 U.S. 210 (1990).
5. RCW 71.05.370(7).
6. RCW 71.05.370(7)(a).
7. RCW 71.05.370(7)(b).
8. Four nonexclusive interests were delineated, In re Schuoler, 106 Wash.2d 500, 723 P.2d 1103 (1986), and reconfirmed by Harper v. State of Washington, 110 Wash. 2d 873, 759 P.2d 358 (1988), *overruled*, 494 U.S. 210 (1990): (a) preservation of life; (b) protection of third-party interest; (c) prevention of suicide; and (d) maintenance of the ethical integrity of the medical profession.
9. RCW 71.05.370(7)(b).
10. RCW 71.05.370(7)(c).
11. *Id.* For surgery and treatment with antipsychotic medications, the court may appoint such an expert.
12. RCW 71.05.370(7)(e).

1. the patient presents an imminent likelihood of serious harm to self or other;

2. medically acceptable alternatives to administration of medications are not available, have not been successful, or are not likely to be effective; or

3. the patient's condition constitutes an emergency requiring that the treatment be administered before a hearing can be held.

Such treatment must be followed with a petition filed on the next day for an order authorizing the administration of antipsychotic medications, the hearing shall be held within two judicial days, and the medications may be continued until the hearing is held.[13] An order for administration of antipsychotic medications remains effective for the duration of adjoining commitment periods.[14]

(B) Treatment with Antipsychotic Medications of Inmates Within Correctional Institutions

The Washington Supreme Court decision that greatly increased the due process protections of correctional inmates being involuntarily treated with ECT or antipsychotic medications has been overturned by the United State Supreme Court.[15] The Court found that the administrative review procedures of the institution sufficiently protected the liberty and due process interests of non-consenting inmates. It believed that such treatment relates sufficiently to the legitimate interests of the state in combating the danger posed by a violent, mentally ill inmate. If the inmate does not consent to such treatment, involuntary treatment with medications may occur only if he or she (a) suffers from a mental disorder, and (b) is gravely disabled or poses a likelihood of serious harm to self or others.[16]

A special committee composed of a psychiatrist, a psychologist, and an institutional representative, none of whom currently involved in the evaluation or treatment of the inmate, must hold a hearing. By a majority vote, they must find that the above condi-

---

13. *Id.*
14. RCW 71.05.370(7)(d). Such a judicial hearing about medication orders can occur at the hearing on petition filed pursuant to RCW 71.05.300 (90-day commitment).
15. State of Washington v. Harper, 110 Wash.2d 873, 759 P.2d 358 (1988), *overruled*, 494 U.S. 210 (1990).
16. *Id.*

tions exist before ordering such treatments. During the hearing process, the inmate has the following rights:[17]

1. to notice of the hearing;

2. to attend, present evidence, and cross examine witnesses;

3. to be represented by a neutral lay advisor versed in the issues of psychiatric treatment;

4. to appeal the decision to the superintendent of the institution;

5. to periodic review of the ordered involuntary medication; and

6. to state court review of the committee decision.

---

17. *Id.*

Regulation of Aversive and Avoidance Conditioning

No specific law exists within Washington that regulates aversive or avoidance conditioning. However, MHPs may violate a standard of care in conducting such treatments for certain patients under some circumstances. The more intrusive the treatment, the greater potential exists for exposure to civil liability.[1]

(A) Incompetent Clients

For those adjudicated to be incompetent,[2] such treatment requires court approval. A law within the guardianship regulations states that any procedure that is "intrusive on the person's body integrity, or physical freedom of movement" requires that the guardian petition the court for an order before treatment proceeds.[3]

(B) Involuntarily Treated Clients

Those patients who are involuntarily committed have a right to be "treated in a less restrictive alternate course of treatment."[4] This general limitation would appear to create a duty to attempt less invasive treatment options before using aversive and avoidance conditioning.

---

1. *See* chapter 6.6, Other Forms of Professional Liability.
2. *See* chapter 5A.2, Guardianship for Adults.
3. RCW 11.92.040.
4. RCW 71.05.370.

6.4

Quality Assurance for Hospital Care

Every hospital, public or private, must maintain a coordinated program for the identification and prevention of medical malpractice and include, at least, the following elements:[1]

1. a quality assurance committee[2] to oversee and coordinate the medical malpractice program and, based on the information collected, to review and revise hospital policies and procedures to improve the quality of medical care;

2. a medical staff privilege sanction procedure through which credentials, physical and mental capacity, and competence in delivering health care services are periodically reviewed as part of an evaluation of staff privileges;

3. the periodic review of credentials, physical and mental capacity, and competence in delivering health care services for all persons who are employed or associated with the hospital;

4. a procedure for the prompt resolution of grievances, by patients or their representatives, related to accidents, injuries, treatment, and other events that may result in claims of medical malpractice;

5. the maintenance and continuous collection of information concerning the hospital's experience with negative health care outcomes and incidents injurious to patients, patient grievances, professional liability premiums, settlements, awards,

---

1. RCW 70.41.200(1).
2. At least one member of the committee must be the a member of the governing board of the hospital but not otherwise affiliated with the hospital in an employment or contractual capacity.

costs incurred by the hospital for patient injury prevention, and safety improvement activities;

6. the maintenance of relevant information by physicians of data collected pursuant to 1 through 5 above;

7. education programs about public safety, injury prevention, staff responsibility to report professional misconduct, legal aspects of patient care, improved communications with patients, and causes of malpractice claims for staff personnel engaged in patient care activities; and

8. policies to ensure compliance with the reporting requirements of this section.

A gross negligence standard has been established to protect complainants or members of the quality assurance committee; a party who alleges injury must prove that the complainant or committee acted in bad faith or with reckless disregard.[3]

All information or documents prepared about health care providers in connection with quality assurance reviews are not subject to discovery nor may they be introduced into evidence in any civil action; no person attending the review may testify in civil actions about the content of such a proceeding.[4] However, such limitations do not preclude[5]

1. testimony of any person about facts that form the basis for the institution of such proceedings if the personal knowledge about the facts was acquired independently from the review;

2. testimony about information collected by the review committee in the case of restriction or revocation of a health care provider's clinical or staff privileges if sought or introduced by the health care provider;

3. disclosure that staff privileges were ended or restricted, including the specific restrictions imposed; or

4. discovery or introduction into evidence of the patient's medical records.

Any violation of any of the above shall not be considered negligence per se.[6]

---

3. RCW 70.41.200(2).
4. RCW 70.41.200(3).
5. *Id.*
6. RCW 70.41.200(6).

6.5

Malpractice Liability

A *malpractice suit* is a civil action brought by a patient or client against a professional service provider who, it is claimed, has failed to meet the standard of care that would be met by a reasonably prudent practitioner possessing the degree of skill, care, and learning that is possessed by other members of the same profession in the state of Washington. It must also be shown that the failure to meet that standard was the proximate cause of the injury complained of.[1]

(A) Malpractice Law

Washington law specifically provides for civil actions regarding injuries resulting from health care practice.[2] It defines a *health care provider* as

> A person licensed by this state to provide health care or related services, including, but not limited to, a certified acupuncturist, a physician, osteopathic physician, dentist, nurse, optometrist, podiatrist, chiropractor, physical therapist, psychologist, phar-

---

1. RCW 7.70.040. *See also* Watson v. Hockett, 107 Wash.2d 158, 727 P.2d 669 (1986); Even though involving a medical doctor practicing family medicine, it is the standard applied to all professional service providers in Washington whether providing health care or other professional service; it is virtually the same language used to state the standard of care for attorneys in Washington. *See* Hawkins v. King County, 24 Wash.App. 338, 602 P.2d 361. *See also* Washington Pattern Jury Instructions (WPI) 105.01 regarding claims of negligence involving any member of the healing arts.
2. RCW 7.70.010 *et seq.*

macist, optician, physician's assistant, nurse practitioner. . . paramedic. . . .[3]

The express language of the statute states that a psychologist and a psychiatrist (as a physician) may be sued for malpractice. Social workers, counselors, and those who must register under Washington law[4] as providing counseling to the public would fall under this statute, notwithstanding the word "licensed" used by this statute as opposed to the words "registered" or "certified" used in the law regulating these professions.[5]

All health care providers should be aware that a malpractice law suit is merely a particularized expression of four concepts fundamental to any negligence action:

1. the professional owed a duty;

2. the professional breached that duty;

3. a damage or injury occurred to the person whom the duty protected; and

4. a proximate causation existed between the breach and the injury.[6]

For example, a failure to protect a potential victim from an actual threat of physical harm made by a client could result in a malpractice claim against the provider by the victim (rather than against the client) because the provider breached the statutorily created duty to protect such potential victims.[7]

It may seem unusual to be sued for malpractice by someone who is not a client, but all four elements of a malpractice claim may be met by this situation: The duty is created by a statute (rather than by the therapeutic relationship with the client); the breach consists of the failure to report the actual threat of violent behavior to an identifiable victim; the damage consists of the injury done to the victim; and the proximate causation consists of the failure to take the steps described in the statute that would have allowed the victim to safeguard himself or herself.

---

3. RCW 7.70.020(1).
4. RCW 18.19.030. See chapters 1.4 to 1.8.
5. See RCW 18.130.020(9). It states that for purposes of the regulation of health professionals, the Uniform Disciplinary Act terms of licensed and registered are equivalent.
6. Harbeson v. Parke-Davis, 98 Wash.2d 460, 656 P.2d 483 (1983).
7. RCW 71.05.120(2) states: "This section does not relieve a person from. . .the duty to warn or to take reasonable precautions to provide protection from violent behavior where the patient has communicated an actual threat of physical violence against a reasonably identifiable victim or victims. The duty to warn or to take reasonable precautions to provide protection from violent behavior is discharged if reasonable efforts are made to communicate the threat to the victim or victims and to law enforcement personnel."

Under the language of the Washington statutes that bear directly on malpractice, however, the person bringing the claim as the plaintiff must prove one or more of the following propositions:

1. the injury resulted from the failure of a health care provider to follow the accepted standard of care;

2. the health care provider promised the patient or his representative that the injury suffered would not occur; or

3. the injury resulted from health care to which the patient or his representatives did not consent.[8]

Most malpractice suits would fall under Proposition 1 because this is a statutory restatement of the basic concept of malpractice. Many duties are created by statute, administrative code, or case law.

Proposition 2 would become relevant in a situation in which, for example, a physician reassured a patient or his representative that there would be no side effects from specific psychotropic medication, such as phenothiazenes. Although the use of such medication might not violate Proposition 1 because it may be within the standard of care of a prudent practitioner, should injurious side effects occur, it might run afoul of Proposition 2 because of the reassurance about side effects. Finally, Proposition 3 could be triggered by the practitioner's failure to obtain the informed consent from the patient or client before treatment. For psychologists and counselors, this proposition could be the basis of a claim for a failure to reveal information about treatment to a client as required by Washington law.[9]

For any health care provider, a claim under Proposition 3 can be established by showing that[10]

1. the health care provider failed to inform the patient or client of a material fact relating to treatment;

2. the patient or client consented to the treatment without being aware of the material fact;

3. a reasonably prudent patient or client would not have consented to the treatment if informed of such material fact; and

4. the treatment was the proximate cause of injury.

---

8. RCW 7.70.030.
9. *See* RCW 18.19.060 (e.g., informed consent requirements as required by "counselors") and 18.83.115 (e.g., informed consent requirements as required by psychologists). *See also* chapters 1.3, 1.4, 1.5, 1.8, and 6.1.
10. RCW 7.70.050; Washington Pattern Jury Instructions 105. *See also* chapter 6.1, this volume.

If the plaintiff can prove these elements, he or she will have a successful claim under Proposition 3 in the Washington statute and may recover for the injuries.

Malpractice actions can be brought under the Washington statutes against a hospital licensed by the state or any of the personnel of such hospital acting as agents of that hospital,[11] but only Proposition 1 and 2 will apply. Proposition 3, relating to informed consent, is expressly made inapplicable to such hospital by the statute.

(B) Expert Testimony In Malpractice Suits

In the absence of exceptional circumstances,[12] expert testimony is necessary to establish the proper standard of care given by a health care provider to meet the duty that is required.[13] This expert testimony may be provided by nonphysicians if they are found, by the court, to be qualified.[14] It is generally understood that it is up to the trial judge's discretion to accept a witness as an expert based on the witness's credentials presented to the judge at the trial (see chapter 5C.2).

The question is not whether the expert would have done things differently than the defendant health care provider, but whether the treatment used deviated unreasonably from the standard of care that would have been given by like professionals in the same or similar professional community. Usually, this means that the person bringing the claim must present an expert in the same discipline as the defendant so that the expert can testify that the defendant's actions failed to reach the level of care in that discipline in that community. A mistake in judgment, either an omission or an act of commission, will not violate the standard of care and breach the duty unless such a mistake was unreasonable to make.

---

11. RCW 4.24.290. *See* Pedroza v. Bryant, 101 Wash.2d 226, 677 P.2d 166 (1984).
12. Helling v. Carey, 83 Wash.2d 514, 519 P.2d 981 (1974). In this case, ophthalmologists were negligent as a matter of law in failing to administer a glaucoma test to a patient under the age of 40 years, in spite of uncontradicted testimony that it was the universal practice of ophthalmologists not to test patients younger than 40 years for glaucoma because of the low incidence of the condition in younger patients.
13. Douglas v. Bussabarger, 73 Wash.2d 476, 438 P.2d 829 (1968).
14. *Id.* Harris v. Groth, 99 Wash.2d 438, 663 P.2d 113 (1983).

(C) Proximate Cause

This is a legal term for the basic idea of cause and effect. The concept of proximate cause addresses the question of whether the acts of the health service provider were linked to the injury to the patient or client. Did the breach of the standard of care by the defendant bring about the injury to the plaintiff in such a manner that the two events could be said to be reasonably related? The plaintiff must introduce evidence that affords a reasonable basis for the conclusion that it is more likely than not that the conduct of the defendant was in fact a cause of the result.[15]

Two ideas that should be kept in mind when determining proximate cause are: (a) whether the injury resulting from the defendant's act was reasonably foreseeable; and (b) whether it was the primary reason for the injury. This is obviously a difficult proposition. It has caused lengthy debate in the law and is accepted as being particularly difficult to prove in the field of mental health.

(D) Avoiding Malpractice

The professional who wishes to avoid malpractice should begin by knowing the laws and regulations promulgated by the state and its licensing boards (see the relevant section in chapter 1). These guidelines, by their nature, constitute the standard of care in Washington because all members of the applicable discipline are required to follow them. Also, standards provided by national associations are helpful as they often establish the highest standard of care for the profession. However, as it has often been pointed out, the greatest prevention factor for malpractice suits is the development of a positive, cooperative relationship between therapist and patient.[16]

A second strategy involves seeking peer consultation whenever a doubt arises as to what would be a reasonable evaluation and treatment of the client, particularly if the client discloses material that may call for a disclosure because of the law, or if the

---

15. Prosser and Keeton on Torts (5th ed. 1984), [4,06] 41.
16. Pope et al., *Malpractice in Outpatient Psychotherapy*, 32 Am. J. Psychotherapy 593 (1978). Such a relationship is founded on the informed consent process that must be carried out within this state (*see* chapter 6.1) and forewarns clients about issues (*e.g.*, legal limitations on protecting client confidences, expectations about paying fees) that have caused hard feelings among clients in other jurisdictions and have led to malpractice actions against MHPs. Waitzkin, H., *Doctor–patient communication*, 252 *J.A.M.A.* 2441 (1984); Kovacs, A., *Bulletin*, Washington, D.C: Division 42, American Psychological Association (1985).

client's condition is worsening in spite of the clinician's care.[17] This contemporaneous action shows an attempt to establish what is the standard of care, taking into account the facts at hand; such an action may decrease the risk of being sued or, if sued, bolster the defendant's contention that he or she acted reasonably at the time.[18]

Finally, a last strategy involves documenting the rationale and procedures of evaluation and treatment. Brief documentation is sufficient, unless an extraordinary event occurs such as a threat of violence or the necessity of disclosing a confidence. At such a time, thorough documentation will establish that the MHP acted reasonably under the circumstances, particularly if combined with peer consultation.[19]

(E) Statute of Limitations

A *statute of limitations* is a law that limits the amount of time a plaintiff has to file a law suit. For a malpractice claim against a health care provider, it must be filed within three years of the act or omission alleged to have caused the injury, or one year from the time the injury was discovered or reasonably should have been discovered, whichever period expires later. However, in no event may such an action be commenced more than eight years from the act or omission. The knowledge of a guardian or of a custodial parent of a child under the age of 18 years shall be imputed to the person. The imputed knowledge will bar the claim of a ward or minor to the same extent in which an adult would be barred. The time limits described above will begin to run.[20]

However, a specific exception exists for actions based on the sexual abuse of a minor. In such cases, the suit must be filed within three years of the act or within three years of the time in which the victim discovered or reasonably should have discovered that the injury or condition was caused by the act, whichever expires later. This time limit is suspended for a child until the child reaches 18 years of age and the knowledge of a parent or guardian is not imputed to the minor.[21]

---

17. *Id.* Gutheil, T. G. & Appelbaum, P. S. (1982). *Clinical Handbook of Psychiatry and the Law.* New York: McGraw-Hill.
18. Benjamin, G.A.H. *Malpractice by Psychologists: A General Prevention Strategy.* Paper presented at the 93rd Annual Convention of the American Psychological Association, Los Angeles, CA (August 1985).
19. Pope et al., *Malpractice in Outpatient Psychotherapy,* 32 Am. J. Psychotherapy 593 (1978).
20. RCW 4.16.350
21. RCW 4.16.340.

Other Forms of Professional Liability

When clients sue a mental health service provider, the action generally takes the form of a suit for malpractice (see chapter 6.5). It is also possible that claims can arise that are more broadly based and are not arising from a wrong that was done to the client in the narrow context of the immediate diagnosis and treatment. It is even possible that a claim can have the character of being based on both sides of such a line and arise because of actions by the provider that were completely outside the treatment, but reflect directly on the quality of the professional service provided. An example of such a claim would be a suit based on the actions of a therapist who writes a book about a client without the client's permission.[1] While the professional service provided by the therapist might have been excellent, the decision to write a book about it could give rise to a law suit by the client that would be based on one of several theories of recovery only one of which might be the strict theory of malpractice. Other theories could be invasion of privacy or breach of confidentiality. MHPs should be aware of the other causes of action that may arise because of their misdirected behavior.

(A) Alternative Theories of Liability

One reason for which lawyers might seek alternative legal theories on which to base their clients' claims is the varying lengths of the statutes of limitation that attach to different theories. If a client waits too many years to sue on a malpractice theory, the claim

---

1. Doe v. Roe, 400 N.Y.S.2d 668 (1977).

might be barred by the time limit of the statute of limitations on malpractice actions (see chapter 6.5). But if the lawyer was able to find a different legal theory upon which to base the claim, there might be a longer period in which to bring the law suit.

Another reason for which a lawyer might seek alternate legal theories is to give a judge or jury choices on which to find in favor of the client. For example, if the jury did not believe that the provider malpracticed because he or she gave good professional service, but did believe that it was wrong to write a book about it, a recovery would be granted for the invasion of privacy if this theory was presented as an alternative cause of action to the malpractice claim.

This chapter discusses other types of claims that could be brought in addition to the strict malpractice law suit.

(A)(1) Defamation of Character

Defamation, in the legal sense, occurs when information that is communicated about the plaintiff to a third party causes harm to the reputation of the plaintiff. If the defamation is written, it is called *libel*. If it is oral, it is called *slander*. Truth is considered to be an absolute defense to an action in defamation. However, falsity does not make for absolute liability because the defendant might have the protection of a privilege to make such a communication.[2] There are forms of privilege that are virtually absolute, such as when an MHP has been appointed by the court to do an evaluation and report back to the court either by way of written report or courtroom testimony.[3] There are also privileges that are qualified or limited to a particular circumstance. An example would be when a former colleague, student, or employee gives your name as a reference, and you are contacted by the potential employer. Under such circumstances, you have a qualified privilege to express your honest opinion on the issue about which the inquiry is being made. You may not be sued by the person listing you as a reference because of their disappointment or disagreement with the accuracy of the opinion, provided that the inaccuracy, should there be one, is not motivated by malice and is, in fact, an honest mistake.

---

2. The privilege spoken of here is not the same as the privilege that one usually thinks of in a mental health setting, that is, the doctor–patient privilege, and that is based on a specific statute that grants the patient such special protection. The privilege in defamation cases arises from case law. Its purpose is to protect persons who communicates false information in certain instances.
3. Bader v. State, 43 Wash.App.233, 716 P.2d 925 (1986); Bruce v. Byrne-Stevens and Associates Engineers, Inc., 113 Wash.2d 123, 776 P.2d 666 (1989).

(A)(2) Crime-Related Actions

If a person commits an assault and battery, he or she can be charged by the state for such a crime. The person can also be sued by the victim of the assault and battery in a civil action to recover money damages for the injuries suffered. The difference between a criminal charge and a civil claim is that in the former, the wrong done by the defendant is to the peace and welfare of the body politic and it is the state, through its local prosecutor, who brings the charge. That is why in criminal cases the charge is worded as "The state of Washington v. John Doe, defendant." In a civil action, the wrong is called a *tort* and it is perpetrated on the victim/plaintiff directly. It is he or she who sues under the law of torts claiming an injury to themselves.

In the criminal action, if the defendant is found guilty, a penalty of imprisonment or fine is imposed. In the civil action (in a separate trial based on the same facts), if the defendant is found liable, a judgment for money damages is rendered. The money is awarded directly to the victim to compensate for actual out of pocket expenses such as doctor bills, lost income, future losses, and for general pain and suffering.

An example of a common duty that could result in a criminal penalty, if an MHP has failed to comply with the law, is the necessity of reporting any reasonable suspicion of child abuse (see chapter 5A.8).

(A)(3) Invasion of Privacy

This is an action that involves the public disclosure of private information. This type of suit usually presumes a broad disclosure of such information that goes beyond a single third party or small group. The publication of a book, as discussed earlier, might give rise to a claim based on invasion of privacy. However, such a claim against an MHP would also involve a breach of confidentiality, which in itself may be actionable under Washington law as described in chapters 6.5 and 4.2.

Two different theories of recovery might be involved as two separate counts in a single suit exist against the provider. This does not mean that a double recovery would be allowed. If one theory fails or cannot be proven for lack of specific evidence, the other theory may still be available because it may not require that particular evidence. Thus, if a provider discusses an identifiable patient in a consultation with a colleague, and the colleague writes a book about the patient, it is possible for the patient to sue the provider for breach of confidentiality, but not for invasion of privacy because the disclosure was so limited and was not, in fact, public. However, the patient could sue the colleague who wrote the book for invasion of privacy because the information was disclosed publicly; nevertheless, a claim for breach of confidentiality might not be successful against the colleague because no confidential relationship existed with the patient. The patient could name both as defendants in the same suit and proceed with alternate theories against them.

(A)(4) Supervision and Consultation

These are distinct activities that are often spoken of as one by people who are not familiar with the important difference between the two. Supervision presumes direct responsibility for the actions of the person supervised, therefore, the supervisor is answerable for the practices of the supervisee. Supervision is concrete and not abstract; it is real and not hypothetical. It has to do with the service provided to specific clients. This means that if the supervisee malpractices, the supervisor would most assuredly be named as a defendant in a law suit. This is particularly true if the fact of supervision is known to the client, who can then claim to have relied on the expertise of the supervisor as well as on that of the supervised service provider.

Consultation does not imply direct control over the person receiving the consultation. A provider may seek consultation on an approach or theory, but is not bound to accept the opinions or practices of the consultant. A consultation may reflect on hypothetical or abstract considerations; it is more in the nature of education as opposed to oversight. It may be within a teacher–student context or peer consultation group, but this does not suggest the monitoring of a practice as supervision does.

If called upon to supervise or consult, one should be careful to clarify the exact nature of the request because supervision makes one more vulnerable to law suits.

(A)(5) Insurance Fraud

Insurance fraud is a harsh phrase, but many health insurers are beginning to consider some billing practices by service providers as fraudulent, and they are filing law suits to recover payments.

There are some billing practices that everyone would agree are improper:[4]

1. Billing for sessions that did not occur and were never even scheduled.

2. Billing for sessions that were scheduled but did not occur because the client canceled with or without advance notice. This does not mean that the client should not be billed for

---

4. Kovacs, A. (1985). *Bulletin*. Washington, D.C.: American Psychological Association, Division 42.

missed appointments, if that is the office policy, but the insurer should not be billed, and the notice of the charge on the client's bill should be clearly indicated as a missed or canceled appointment.

3. Billing couples as two separate individuals when the treatment being provided is couples therapy or marriage counseling. This constitutes double billing, and it is inappropriate.[5]

4. Billing for services provided by an unlicensed provider. Even if services are properly supervised by the licensed provider, it is clearly misleading to the insurer to fail to indicate on the claim for reimbursement that the licensed provider plays a supervising role. The identity and credentials for the provider should also be clearly indicated on the form.

5. Failing to bill one's clients for their copayment and agreeing to accept the insurance reimbursement as full payment.[6]

Washington law makes it a crime to present a health care payor with a claim for health care payment knowing the claim to be false.[7] Although the Washington statute does not define specific practices that are unlawful, it states that a *deceptive claim* is one that contains a statement of fact or fails to reveal a material

---

5. It is equally inappropriate to designate marriage counseling, couples therapy, or family treatment as individual therapy even if the billing is for one hour to one identified patient. The question becomes more complex when one individual receives treatment for a diagnosable condition, but as part of the treatment, the partner, parent, or other family member attends the sessions. Such a situation may have to be determined on the basis of its own facts, but one should be sensitive to the view that some insurers are extremely skeptical of reimbursing for treatment when there is more than one person in the session. If there are doubts about the situation, the best approach is to speak to the service representative of the insurer. Certainly, the practitioner's treatment record should reflect the services that are provided to the identifiable client.

6. Providers are sometimes misled by their own instincts to help a client who cannot afford their usual rate. In such instances, they will sometimes agree to accept whatever the insurance company pays as their full fee. Such an agreement between the provider and the client constitutes collusion because both the provider and the client know that the insurance pays only a specified percentage of the usual rate of the provider. Even if well motivated, the provider should avoid this improper billing practice or any variation on this theme. The practice of raising the usual and customary rate for billing purposes and then accepting the insurance payment as full payment is wrong. The practice of lowering the rate for the client, but not for the insurance company, is also wrong. The practice of keeping the rate the same as that of the insurance provider, but failing to make reasonable efforts to collect the proper copayment from the client is specifically mentioned as improper by Department of Defense regulations governing CHAMPUS policies: The Department of Defense, Regulation 6010.8-R, Ch. IV, § F.

7. It is a Class C felony to present a claim for health care payment knowing the claim to be false. Upon conviction under this statute, the prosecutor will inform the provider's disciplinary board about the conviction: Chapter 48.80 RCW, Health Care False Claims Act.

fact leading the health care payor to believe that the represented or suggested state of affairs is other than what it actually is.

(A)(6) Excessive Detention

The Washington state law on involuntary treatment[8] (see chapter 5E.4) contains provisions that limit civil or criminal liability for providers acting under the directives of that law, provided that such acts were performed in good faith and without gross negligence.

Ordinary negligence is usually defined as a failure to exercise the degree of care that a reasonable person in the position of the actor would exercise under the same or similar circumstances (see chapter 6.5, Malpractice Liability). *Gross negligence* is usually defined as actions committed in wanton or in reckless disregard for the rights of others. These are clearly different standards, and it is only the former behavior that is protected when a provider is acting within the structure of the laws dealing with involuntary treatment of clients. If the provider is grossly negligent, he or she may be liable for such negligent acts.

The law on excessive detention[9] specifically states that a client who is detained for more than the number of days allowed in the statute by a provider who is acting knowingly, willfully, or through gross negligence shall be allowed to recover money damages against the provider. Furthermore, it is not necessary that the client suffer actual financial loss because of the excessive detention, but he or she may be compensated for general damages of pain and suffering because of the unlawful detention.

---

8. RCW 71.05.010 *et seq.*
9. RCW 71.05.510.

Criminal Liability

Washington has enacted only one criminal law that is directed at health care providers specifically. Any health care provider who "knowingly fails to make, or fails to cause to be made [a report to the Department of Social and Health Services] about the abuse, neglect, or exploitation of a child, elder, or adult developmentally disabled person" shall be guilty of a gross misdemeanor.[1] If found guilty beyond a reasonable doubt, the court could imprison the health care provider in a county jail for as long as one year or levy a fine of not more than $5,000 or both imprison and fine the offender.[2]

---

1. RCW 26.44.080.
2. RCW 9.92.020.

6.8

Liability of Credentialing Boards

The regulation of health professionals by the Uniform Disciplinary Act[1] includes psychiatrists, psychologists, and counselors.[2] It was the intent of the legislature to strengthen and to consolidate the regulation of the professions by providing a Uniform Disciplinary Act with standardized procedures.[3] The Act provides immunity to members of the disciplinary boards or an individual acting on their behalf from suit in any action, civil or criminal, if based on official acts performed during their duties.[4] This provision appears to create an absolute immunity to law suit rather than a qualified immunity. Before this law, if the official acts were performed in good faith, a qualified immunity applied to regulating physicians[5] and psychologists.[6] Presumably, the Uniform Disciplinary Act standard would be applied.

1. Chapter 18.130 RCW.
2. Chapter 18.19 RCW regulates marriage and family therapists, mental health counselors, and social workers, all referred to as counselors. RCW 18.130.040 specifically includes physicians, psychologists, and counselors.
3. RCW 18.130.010.
4. RCW 18.130.300.
5. RCW 4.24.240.
6. RCW 18.83.135.

Appendix

Table of Cases

References are to page numbers in this book.

State v. Wicks, 340
State v. Wood, 356, 357, 363
State v. Woodard, 346
State v. Woodward, 307
State v. Young, 49, 303
State v. Zamora, 335, 336
Strickland v. Deaconess Hosp., 270
Swartley v. Seattle School District No. 1, 299
Sykes v. Republic Coal Co., 254

T

Thompson v. Snell, 344
Tucker v. Tucker, 159
Tumelson v. Todhunter, 282

U

U.S. v. Bulman, .127
U.S. v. Hayes, 326
United Pacific Ins. Co. v. Buchanan, 275, 276

V

Vangement v. McCalmon, 300

W

Wallace v. University Hospitals of Cleveland 97, 100, 107
Washington State Nurses Association v. Board of Medical Examiners, 7
Washington v. Seattle, 297
Watson v. Hockett, 451
Welch v. Helvering, 94
Wilbur v. Department of Labor and Industries, 256
Wilson v. KeyTronic Corp., 272

Y

Young v. Group Health, 300

Table of Statutes

References are to page numbers in this book.

Revised Code of Washington

Table of Rules of Court

References are to page numbers in this book.

Table of Administrative Rules and Regulations

References are to page numbers in this book.

Washington Rules

Code of Federal Regulations

Index

References are to chapters.

PRISONS. *See* JAILS AND PRISONS
PRIVILEGED COMMUNICATIONS
    Generally, 4.3
PROBATION
    Generally, 5D.16
PRODUCT LIABILITY
    Generally, 5B.10
PROFESSIONAL CORPORATIONS
    Generally, 2.2
PROVOCATION
    As legal defense, 5D.6
PSYCHIATRIC NURSES
    Licensure, 1.2
PSYCHIATRISTS
    Licensure and regulation, 1.1
PSYCHOLOGICAL AUTOPSY
    Generally, 5C.5
PSYCHOLOGISTS
    Licensure and regulation, 1.3
    School, 1.6
    Unlicensed, 1.4
PUBLIC DISCLOSURE
    Generally, 4.5

Q

QUALITY ASSURANCE
    Hospital care, 6.4

R

RAPE TRAUMA SYNDROME
    Generally, 5D.11
RECORDS
    Access, 4.1
    Confidentiality, 4.2
    Extensiveness, 4.1
    Maintenance, 4.1
    Ownership, 4.1
    Public disclosure, 4.5
    Search, seizure, and subpoena, 4.4
REGISTRATION
    Family therapists, 1.5
    Marriage therapists, 1.5
REGULATION
    Aversive and avoidance
        conditioning, 6.3
    Hypnotists, 1.8
    Polygraph examiners, 1.9
    Psychiatric nurses, 1.2
    Psychiatrists, 1.1
    Psychologists, 1.3
    School psychologists, 1.6
    School social workers, 1.7

REIMBURSEMENT
    Insurance, 3.1
REPORTS
    Adult abuse, 5A.6
    Child abuse, 5A.8
RIGHTS
    Legal, competency to waive, 5D.2
    Parental, 5A.10
    To refuse treatment, 6.2

S

SCHOOL
    Special education, 5A.20
SCHOOL PSYCHOLOGISTS
    Certification and regulation, 1.6
SCHOOL SOCIAL WORKERS
    Certification and regulation, 1.7
SEARCH AND SEIZURE
    Generally, 4.4
SENTENCING
    Competency to be executed, 5D.23
    Competency to serve sentence,
        5D.19
    Dangerous offenders, 5D.17
    Generally, 5D.15
    Habitual offenders, 5D.18
    Probation, 5D.16
SEX OFFENDERS
    Mental health services for, 5D.25
SOCIAL WORKERS
    School, 1.7
SOLE PROPRIETORSHIPS
    Generally, 2.1
SUNSET LAWS
    Credentialing agencies, 1.10

T

TAX DEDUCTIONS
    Mental health services, 3.3
TERMINATION
    Parental rights, 5A.10
TRIAL LAW
    Adequate provocation defense, 5D.6
    Battered woman's and child's
        syndrome, 5D.10
    Competency to stand trial, 5D.5
    Competency to testify, 5C.4
    Competency to waive legal rights,
        5D.2
    Criminal responsibility
        determination, 5D.9
    Diminished capacity defense, 5D.8

Eyewitness identification, 5D.13
Hypnosis of witnesses, 5D.12
Mens rea, 5D.7
Psychological autopsy, 5C.5
Rape trauma syndrome, 5D.11

U

UNFAIR COMPETITION
Generally, 5B.11
UNLICENSED PSYCHOLOGISTS
Generally, 1.4

V

VOCATIONAL DISABILITY
Determinations, 5B.3

VOLUNTARY ADMISSION
Of alcohol and drug addicts, 5E.5
Of mentally ill adults, 5E.3
Of minors, 5A.19
VOTING
Competency, 5B.8

W

WILLS
Competency to sign, 5B.7

Z

ZONING
Community homes, 2.8

About the Authors

G. Andrew H. Benjamin, JD, PhD, is a clinical associate professor and director of the Parenting Evaluation Training Program in the Department of Psychiatry and Behavior Sciences at the University of Washington Medical Center. He also operates a half-time private practice that focuses on the evaluation and treatment of families in conflict, dual disordered patients, and legal professionals. In 1992, he was named Professional of the Year by the Washington State Bar Association's Family Law Section for creating the program mentioned above and for developing the Washington State Bar Association's Lawyers' Assistance Program to evaluate and treat distressed lawyers. Dr. Benjamin has contributed 18 articles to law, psychology, and psychiatry journals.

Laura Ann Rosenwald received a BA in history from Standford University and worked as a newspaper reporter for 11 years in Idaho, Washington (DC), Kentucky, and Washington state. She also worked in Taiwan as a teacher and textbook author. She received a JD degree in 1994 from the University of Washington School of Law, where she was editor-in-chief of the *Washington Law Review.* Currently, she is a law clerk for the Hon. Betty B. Fletcher, U.S. Court of Appeals for the Ninth Circuit. She has published several articles on issues of law and psychology.

Thomas D. Overcast, JD, PhD, is a graduate of the Law–Psychology Program at the University of Nebraska. Dr. Overcast worked for five years as a health care policy analyst and researcher, focusing on legal and regulatory issues affecting the provision of health care services. He is a member of the Nebraska and Washington bars and now practices law in Edmonds, WA, where he represents a variety of health care practitioners and groups in business, professional, and disciplinary matters. Dr. Overcast is an adjunct professor of psychology at Central Washington University, where he teaches courses on law and psychology. He is also a member of the editorial advisory board for the *Washington State Bar Journal.*

Stephen R. Feldman is a psychologist in private practice in Seattle, WA. His practice includes divorce mediation and consultation. He consults with psychologists regarding legal and ethical problems and advises attorneys about psychological issues in trial practice. He is on the clinical faculty of the University of

Washington School of Medicine and has served on the law faculties of Harvard and Georgetown universities and the University of Puget Sound.